Praise for

Healing with Stories

"George Burns has become the '*metaphor man.*' In this volume he showcases some of today's best therapists healing with metaphors. These rich *teaching stories* provide valuable tools for students as well as professionals. I consider this volume must reading for anyone wanting to improve their psychotherapy service."

Jon Carlson, PsyD, EdD, ABPP
Distinguished Professor, Governors State University

"*Healing with Stories* surveys the approaches of many leaders in field of therapeutic metaphors and gets into their heads to give readers a unique behind-the-scene understanding of how experts formulate metaphoric interventions."

Stephen Lankton, MSW, DAHB
Editor, *American Journal of Clinical Hypnosis*
Author of *Assembling Ericksonian Therapy* and *The Answer Within*

"I am an admirer of Burns' writing. His books are always well-written and useful. When he tackles a topic, as in this extremely practical casebook, no other book needs to be written about it. He covers the whole waterfront."

Bill O'Hanlon, MSc
Author of 27 books, including *Do One Thing Different*

"Aristotle said, 'The thing most important by far is the command of metaphor.' In *Healing with Stories,* George Burns has assembled a pantheon of 'old pros' whose classic methods add innovative scope and depth to the practice of contemporary psychotherapy."

Jeffrey K. Zeig, PhD
Director, The Milton Erickson Foundation

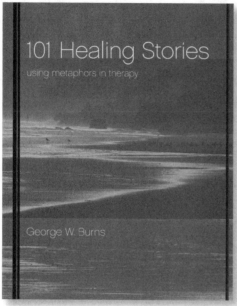
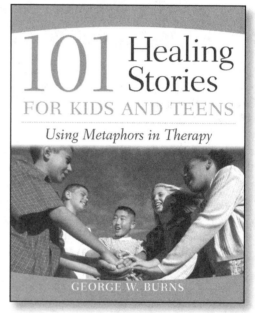
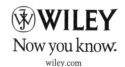

Healing with Stories

Healing with Stories

Your Casebook Collection
for Using Therapeutic Metaphors

Edited by

George W. Burns

BICENTENNIAL
1807
WILEY
2007
BICENTENNIAL

John Wiley & Sons, Inc.

Published by John Wiley & Sons, Inc., Hoboken, New Jersey.
Published simultaneously in Canada.

Wiley Bicentennial Logo: Richard J. Pacifico

Library of Congress Cataloging-in-Publication Data:

Healing with stories : your casebook collection for using therapeutic metaphors / edited by George W. Burns.
    p. ; cm.
    Includes bibliographical references and index.
    ISBN: 978-0-471-78902-4 (pbk. : alk. paper)
    1. Metaphor—Therapeutic use. 2. Child psychotherapy. I. Burns, George W. (George William)
    [DNLM: 1. Metaphor—Case Reports. 2. Psychotherapy—methods—Case Reports. 3. Narration—Case Reports. WM 420 H4348   2007]
    RJ505.M48H4343   2007
    618.92'8914—dc22

2006025754

Printed in the United States of America
10 9 8 7 6 5 4 3 2 1

This one is for
Oscar, Leah, and Ian.

How much richer and happier my life story is with such a loving family.

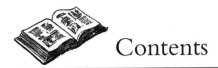

Contents

PART FIVE   DEVELOPING LIFE SKILLS, 211

Acknowledgments

If you were raised in the tiny Himalayan kingdom of Bhutan, one of your earliest memories would most likely be hearing the national story of the four faithful friends. The story tells of a pheasant that found a seed, a rabbit that helped plant and water it, a monkey that fertilized and weeded it, and an elephant that stood guard to protect it. When the tree had grown to maturity, the animals climbed on each other's backs, forming a pyramid, to reach into the high branches so as to collect and share the fruit. Editing this book has made me mindful of this tale of many different beings coming together to work cooperatively on a common, unifying project.

I am deeply honored by all the esteemed and valued colleagues who have so generously contributed, whether as authors, peer reviewers, discussants of the original idea, endorsers, and/or dear friends. They have brought into their contributions, suggestions, and ideas not only a high level of professionalism but also a high level of caring and compassion, which for me is the hallmark of our unique work in these healing and helping professions.

Thank you, thank you, thank you, especially, to all authors who have given of themselves, their time, their clinical experience, and their wisdom. You have enlivened this book with science, humanity, and yourselves.

Julie Nayda continues to be my loyal support, invaluable teammate, and dear friend. You are the Gibraltar of my professional life and practice, Jules.

There are many who have supported this project in many ways though their words may not be on its pages. Liz Sheean of PsychOz Publications and Helen Street, PhD, my coauthor of *Standing Without Shoes,* assisted with early discussions of style and format. Wonderfully creative ideas were offered by Kathleen Donaghy, PhD; Cheryl Bell-Gadsby, MA; Nadia Lalak, MA; Maria Escalante, MA; Deborah Beckman, MS; Rick Whiteside, MSW; and Frances Steinberg, PhD. I am *deeply* grateful for the interest, time, and effort you all contributed.

Peer reviewers are the unsung heroes of many a good book. They give hours and hours of their time with no more recognition than their name appearing on a page that perhaps few readers notice. Stephanie Bennett, MPsych; Teresa Garcia Sanchez, MA, ECP; Valerie Lewis, PhD; and Pam Thompson, DipHealthPsych, your perceptive eyes, critical thinking, and challenging questions have kept all of us contributors on the ball. Pam, your dedication was beyond the call of duty.

For kind words and support in various ways, I also thank Jon Carlson, PsyD, EdD, ABPP; Steven Lankton, MSW; Bill O'Hanlon, MSc; Maggie Phillips, PhD; Rachel Remen, MD; Bernhard Trenkle, DiplPsy; Jeff Zeig, PhD; Lynne and Bryan Kendrick (for the availability of Possum Lodge); and, of course, Suzanne Thomas (for her laughter, loving support, and helpfully critical eye).

I am delighted to have launched this project with my former editor, Tracey Belmont, and even more delighted to welcome Nicholas John. Is this his first mention in a book? Lisa Gebo has helpfully challenged and tuned the manuscript, and, with Sweta Gupta, guided it to completion. Isabel Pratt has been here on each of my Wiley books; Rosa Gonzales has steered my works into Chinese, Spanish, Portuguese, Italian, Korean, and Indonesian; and Susan Dodson has conducted this manuscript into production. The whole team at John Wiley & Sons has once again won my praise and appreciation.

As with the story of the four faithful friends, a book of this nature begins with a seed of an idea that is taken, nurtured, and developed by many who all contribute of their own skills, knowledge, and experience. I hope it has matured into a form that will be helpful and fruitful for you, your work, and your clients.

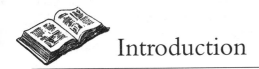

Introduction

As editor of this book, am I permitted to say I am excited by it? Excited by the quality of the contributors who have generously come aboard for the project? Excited by the quality of the contributions they have submitted? Excited by the variety of cases presented and styles of metaphor applications?

Having already written two books on using metaphors in therapy (*101 Healing Stories* and *101 Healing Stories for Kids and Teens*), I thought I had said most of the things I wanted to say about metaphors . . . and then three things happened. The first was an evolving awareness as readers of my books and attendants at my workshops commented that they had found the principles and examples provided in these books helpful and would like to see a greater variety of applications of metaphors in a greater variety of case examples. The second was a request from Tracey Belmont, my Wiley editor at the time, to write another metaphor book. At first I rejected the idea, not wanting to become typecast in the use of metaphors, which are but one aspect of the way I work, albeit an important aspect. There also seemed little point in resaying what had already been said, so Tracey and I began to toss around some ideas about what might be novel, informative, and essentially helpful to practitioners at the coal-face of therapy. As we were engaged in this conversation, the third thing happened. I attended a congress on Ericksonian psychotherapy and hypnotherapy in Phoenix, Arizona, where I was reminded how many practitioners are working with metaphors from theoretically very divergent backgrounds, in divergent ways, and with divergent caseloads. Wouldn't it be interesting, I began to wonder, to bring together the expertise of some of these skilled colleagues, to ask them to provide a case example that clearly represented the ways they work, and to explore the thinking and processing that went on for them as they assessed the client, planned their interventions, and then administered them . . . and put it all in one volume.

I am aware of many books that skillfully outline strategies, techniques, and interventions for *what* to do, but how many seek to get inside the practitioners' thinking, understand their processes of working, and are informed by the choices they made in terms of their therapeutic directions? While many good books have been written about metaphors in therapy, I am not aware of any other that has drawn together such a variety of metaphor practitioners from the well known to the novice, that offers such a range of case examples, that illustrates the use of metaphor in so many theoretic contexts, or that seeks to provide so clear an understanding of the processing of each contributing therapist—something made possible only by the generous efforts of each contributor. I hope you find these contributions as enjoyable and as informative as I did when reading each of them as they flowed in.

WHAT THIS BOOK OFFERS

My aim has been to produce a volume that is an essentially practical and useful clinical tool for practitioners like you and me who sit in our offices on a day-to-day basis seeking to provide the best possible service to the client in front of us. To achieve this aim, I asked the contributing authors to adopt a conversational style as if they were talking with you, a colleague in supervision, answering the questions they thought you might have about what they did and how they did it. My request was meant to allow you, the reader, into their minds, into their thinking, planning, and processing as they decided on, structured, and offered metaphors in a particular case example. I asked that each contribution be a clear explanation of *what, why,* and *how* the therapist did what he or she did, step by step. I wanted their skills to be visible and clearly expounded in such a way that the processes would be replicable by other therapists.

Each author was asked to address a series of specific questions. This guideline proved to be something that we followed, or didn't follow, to varying degrees—thus illustrating the variety of ways in which it is possible to work with metaphors. By setting these questions as guidelines for authors to consider in their writing, I hoped to avoid some of the uneven and inconsistent styles often found in edited books, as well as reach the essence of practice. These are the questions I presented to the contributing authors:

Tell me about the case:
- Who is the client?
- What is the presenting problem?
- What is the context (therapy/training/other)?

How did you go about the assessment? (Describe step by step.)
- What were you looking for in your assessment?
- What were the therapeutic goals you defined?
- How did you arrive at them?

What resources/strengths/skills did you see in the client?
- How did you define these?
- If several, why did you choose what you did to work with?

Why did you choose a story or metaphoric intervention in preference to other interventions for this client?
- What alternatives could you have chosen?

What did you see that your story needed to do?
- What skills to build?
- What resources to strengthen?
- What goals to achieve?

How did you go about constructing the story/stories?
- Take the reader through your thinking step by step.

What was the metaphor or story you used?
- Retell it as you did in therapy.

Was the story the sole intervention?
- If not, what other interventions did you use?
- What was the overall therapeutic plan, and where did metaphor fit in?

What was the outcome/follow-up?

What did you learn from this case?
- Validation of existing ideas
- What *not* to do again
- New discovery about using healing stories
- What you might have done differently in retrospect

"Many good therapists," I found myself telling one contributor in an e-mail—perhaps not surprisingly slipping into metaphor—"are like professional cyclists. After years and years of fine-tuning, they are so good and skilled at what they do that much of it comes almost automatically, without their having to think a lot about how they actually do it. I would like authors to go back to the basics, to let readers into their minds and thought processes. How do you mount the bike without toppling over? How do you keep your balance? How do you coordinate the complex tasks of looking to where you want to go, cycling with your feet, and steering with your hands, simultaneously? How do you go fast enough not to fall off and not so fast as to risk crashing?" This focus on the therapist's thought process, I hope, is what will make this book essentially practical and useful.

THE CONTRIBUTORS

The contributors were invited both on the basis of their skills as therapists working with metaphors and according to their ability to demonstrate the variety of approaches to working with metaphor. I feel particularly honored by those who have come on board, giving so generously of their time, knowledge, and experience. They have approached their contributions with a high level of professionalism that also reflects a depth of caring and compassion. You will find in the following pages contributors whose names are well recognized for devoting much of their professional career to working with, understanding, and writing about the value of metaphors—people like Steven Hayes, Richard Kopp, Carol Hicks-Lankton, Joyce Mills, and Michael Yapko. Roxanna Erickson Klein had the privilege of growing up with the teaching tales of her father, Milton H. Erickson.

Rob McNeilly reminds us in his chapter of what most novice metaphor practitioners experience: "I thought there were two kinds of therapists: those who could tell stories, and those who could not. I had myself pigeonholed in the group that could not. When I read books about therapeutic metaphor, I was further overwhelmed by my relative incompetence compared with the authors." Mindful of this, I also invited contributors whose work I respected yet who were relatively new to the use of metaphor. Richard Kopp incorporates the transcripts of two third-year graduate students, Deanna Guerrero and Heather Demeter. Gregory Smit acknowledges his recent discovery of therapeutic storytelling, and Jana Sutton describes herself as being at the "very beginning" of her career, yet all bravely offer to share their early experiences, provide inspiring examples of their work, and show what is possible, even in the early stages of working with metaphors.

In the following pages you will thus have the chance to closely observe the working styles of novice, mid-career, and highly experienced metaphor practitioners. At the beginning of each chapter, under the heading "Contributor's Story: A Professional and Personal Perspective," the contributors are introduced with some highlights about their professional backgrounds, how they developed an interest in therapeutic storytelling, and sometimes a word or two of a personal nature.

THE CONTRIBUTIONS

Both the contributors and their contributions come from a wide range of theoretical and therapeutic models. Mikaela Hildebrandt, Lindsay Fletcher, and Steven Hayes describe the use of metaphor in acceptance and commitment therapy (ACT). Richard Kopp has a background in Adlerian psychology, and I present metaphor as a means of communicating a cognitive behavioral therapy (CBT) intervention, while Valerie Lewis takes a postmodern, social constructionist perspective. Several authors, such as Rob McNeilly, Carol Hicks-Lankton, and Michael Yapko, incorporate their metaphors into hypnosis. Narrative therapy influences the metaphor work of Christine Perry and Joy Nel, Gregory Smit is a family therapist, and Teresa Garcia-Sanchez works from an Ericksonian approach. Wendel Ray and Jana Sutton come from a brief, solution-focused orientation, while Angela Ebert integrates several models like interpersonal psychology, CBT, and mindfulness training. Some do not define their work by any particular theoretical stance.

While most contributors follow the traditional, oral presentation of metaphors, others show us this is not the only way to communicate. Julie Linden and Joyce Mills employ dolls, toys, and other objects that belong to their child clients. Christine Perry has her client draw his stories on a whiteboard; Teresa Garcia-Sanchez offers experiential, "two-minute" metaphors; Joy Nel's child clients create their own storybooks; and I work with nature-based experiential metaphors. Children's storybooks and a pet bird form the basis of Roxanna Erickson Klein's therapy with a child in hospice care.

Some have listened attentively for the story inherent in the client's use of language (such as Richard Kopp, Christine Perry, Wendel Ray, and Jana Sutton); some have actively elicited the story from the client (Rubin Battino); some have explored the client's cultural background for stories (Angela Ebert); some have sought to build stories collaboratively (Rob McNeilly); some have created metaphoric learning experiences (George Burns and Teresa Garcia-Sanchez); some have used play as a source (Julie Linden and Joyce Mills); some have generated the story themselves (George Burns, Carol Hicks-Lankton, Gregory Smit, and Michael Yapko); some have utilized what experience brings their way (Roxanna Erickson Klein); and some have told tales of other clients (Valerie Lewis).

In the following pages you also will find a broad spectrum of styles. At one end of the continuum, Rubin Battino and Richard Kopp advocate prescribed protocols, with Richard recommending that therapists have the protocol in front of them as they work with the client. Most contributors appear to have some broad model in mind around which they can elicit and/or structure a story, whether generated by the client, by the therapist, or in collaboration. Carol Hicks-Lankton, for example, has an outline for multiple embedded metaphors around which stories can be constructed to meet the needs of the client. I describe the PRO (Problem, Resource, and Outcome) approach as a loose guide with which to structure and present therapeutic tales. At the other end of the spectrum are those with a postmodern perspective who resist the concept of structure altogether. Valerie Lewis argues against being formulaic, asserting that there are "no rules."

This diversity means there are likely to be approaches in the following pages that fit comfortably with the way you work already, that perhaps feel as familiar as slipping into a favorite pair of shoes. By the same token, there are likely to be approaches and styles that are different from, or strange in comparison to, the way you currently work. Difference can provide us with the opportunity to examine our own ideas, challenge our thinking, experiment with something novel, and explore possible new options.

THE STRUCTURE OF THIS BOOK

Following the opening chapter that covers some of the key concepts of metaphor in therapy, the main part of the book is structured around five thematic outcome-oriented therapeutic goals. Part One, "Improving Mood," has four chapters addressing affective problems with cases of depression and anxiety. Deciding whether to separate from a marriage, struggling with the role of responsibility, dealing with an abusive relationship, and coping with a parental divorce are the relationship-based subjects of chapters in Part Two, "Building Positive Relationships." In Part Three, "Changing Patterns of Behavior," contributors cover processes of change relating to work stress, childhood abuse, global lifestyle, and psychogenic symptoms. A dying child, a self-mutilating young woman, a child with insomnia, and a girl facing invasive, painful surgery form the case base for metaphors in Part Four, "Enhancing Health and Well-Being." Part Five, "Developing Life Skills," looks at offering skills that will enhance future coping for a case of Posttraumatic Stress Disorder, a depressed adolescent goth, and a disruptive group participant with existential questions.

Each chapter opens with some brief biographical information about the contributor in a section entitled "Contributor's Story: A Professional and Personal Perspective." This is followed by "Preview the Chapter," a section designed to give a synopsis of what is to follow, outline the therapeutic characteristics of the case and metaphor, and provide some consistency and continuity across the book. As editor, I have added this section, and I acknowledge that it fits my way of conceptualizing, creating, and structuring metaphors along the PRO approach, which views metaphors, like all stories, as having a beginning (the problem), a middle (the resources), and an end (the outcome). I have attempted to draw the therapeutic characteristics from the actual words and concepts of the authors to represent their approach as accurately as possible.

As one peer reviewer commented, "This is not just a book that you read from cover to cover but also a reference book that readers will want to delve back into for dealing with a particular case." To help you do this I have included a Resource Section, in which you will find further reading resources, including major publications by the contributors (if you wish to extend your exploration of their work) and the contributors' favorite sources of metaphors.

As the contributions for this book flowed in I began to enjoy their diversity: the diversity of cases, the diversity of metaphor use, and the diversity of writing styles. During the book's compilation, one contributor asked me, "Have you learned new things about metaphor from the contributions?" I certainly have. She then astutely asked, "Have you applied those things in your work?" Again I could reply I certainly had. The contributions in this book celebrate the professional, caring, creative work of therapists, the amazingly diverse power of stories in the healing process, and the spirit of our clients to overcome the most challenging adversities. My hope is that you will be able to appreciate the variety, observe the commonality, and ponder how these approaches might be applied in your own work.

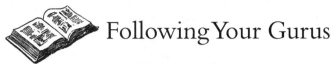

Following Your Gurus

An Opening Story

In one of the hundreds of e-mails that went back and forth between myself and contributors in the course of editing this book, Carol Hicks-Lankton made a comment that I thought was important enough not to lose in a piece of personal correspondence. As we were discussing our favorite metaphor books, she said, "Life is the big book of metaphors—a new story every day."

Therapeutic stories are there in our day-to-day living. They can be found everywhere, as will be discussed further in Chapter 1. We might observe them in everyday experiences, such as seeing a young child develop a new set of skills or watching the interaction between people in a shopping center. They may be present in a book you read, a movie you watch, or the way a client learns to cope with a challenging set of circumstances. They may, as in this story, be a conversation that speaks of one person's experience in a way that could help another.

At a national conference, I met up with an interstate colleague I had known over the years yet not seen for some time—and was surprised by her appearance. It was not surprising that she now had her head shaven and wore the maroon and yellow robes of a Buddhist nun, for I had known that she was studying Buddhism and had been planning to take the vows of a monastic order. What did surprise me was the very dark, swollen bruising of a black eye that she wore on the left side of her face, as if she had not long stepped out of a barroom brawl.

Curiously, I asked, "What's happened to you?"

"Well," she replied, "it is sort of funny and sort of embarrassing and sort of profound."

Now I was even more curious.

She went on to explain, "I was following my guru along the street, absentmindedly watching his tan shoes moving below his robes, distractedly preoccupied in my own thoughts, not being very present in the moment, when suddenly he stepped aside. By the time I realized what he had done and looked up, I walked straight into the lamppost he had avoided. Hence the black eye."

Then she looked at me, as if she had been embarrassed in recounting her tale, and added with a twinkle in the one eye that was not bloodshot and partially closed, "But I guess there is a lesson in the story: Don't blindly follow in your guru's footsteps."

CHAPTER I

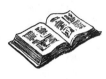

Metaphor and Therapy

Clarifying Some Confusing Concepts

George W. Burns

"Metaphors work," claims Stephen Lankton, "because the mind is metaphoric" (Lankton, 2002, p. xiii). He explains, "There is something about stories and metaphors that has a profound effect on listeners: they teach, inspire, guide, communicate, are remembered, and, most of all, are everywhere" (p. v). In fact, I continue to be amazed by the ways in which clients find metaphors everywhere to describe and resolve their problems. Vanessa, a 33-year-old single mother of three young children subjected to horrific and unprovoked violence, revealed very clearly how metaphors might be discovered in the most unlikely places. The background to her story was that one day when out shopping she had been seen and followed home by a young male, who then lurked around her house until after dark. When her children had gone to bed, and as she sat up studying, he entered the house and attacked her, beating her into semiconsciousness with a baseball bat before violently raping her. Sixteen days later, when I first met her, her physical injuries were still visible: a bandaged, fractured nose; bloodshot eyes; a bruised and lacerated face. The emotional scars were not initially so apparent. In seeking therapy, she positively said her goals were to be free of the feelings of panic that were overwhelming her, to cease being scared, and to lose her intense feelings of self-doubt.

During our second session, Vanessa expressed a need to "get away," spend some time meditating in a peaceful environment, and "become centered again"—a desire I encouraged. With her parents looking after the children, she booked herself into a coastal farm retreat for five days. This provided an opportunity to set up an experiential metaphor. Before she departed, I suggested she take a walk in an area that was safe and pleasant, simply experiencing what there was to experience. I relayed a couple of outcome-oriented metaphors about how other clients had benefited from such experiences, and asked her, in a very general way, to observe what might be helpful to her.

When she returned for her third therapeutic session a week later, there was a marked improvement not only in her physical healing but also in her emotional and mental state. She told me how she had spent time walking along the beach, beside the banks of the river, and through neighboring woodlands. Two experiences in particular stood out.

While taking a walk along a riverbank one day, she paused to sit and look at the reflections in the still water. She started to contemplate how one image was real and one was an illusion. She thought about how reality and illusion could look so alike that, at times, they could be hard to differentiate. She wondered whether, if you took a photograph, you could tell which was the illusion and which was the reality. Picking up a stone, she threw it in the water, and watched the illusion shatter. Tears filled her eyes as she later told me, using metaphor, that her "past blocks" were shattered with the illusion in the river. She began to experience a sense of peacefulness, as at that moment things again "came together."

The second metaphoric experience occurred while Vanessa was walking through 500 acres of woods. Absorbed in her thoughts, she became lost. It was late in the day, she was fearful of being out in the woods alone at night, and she felt panicky about being in an unplanned and unexpected situation. As she described the situation, she noted that the feelings it evoked paralleled those she had felt as a result of her assault. Thinking about what she needed to do, she reached the conclusion that she had to rely on her own intuition and trust her sense of direction to make the right choices. She found her way back to the farmhouse just as the last rays of sunlight were disappearing below the horizon. The metaphoric parallel she saw between this experience and her previous trauma helped her to reestablish a sense of self-confidence and trust that had been "lost" following the assault. Vanessa carried something across from one experience (watching reflections in the water) to another (freeing past blocks). She transferred a meaning from finding her way out of being lost in the woods to regaining confidence after trauma.

WHAT IS METAPHOR?

In the original Greek, the term *metaphor* meant "to carry something across" or "to transfer." In communication it refers to carrying one image or concept across to another, just as Vanessa did. Most dictionaries or textbooks define *metaphor* as a comparison between two things, based on resemblance or similarity. For Aristotle it meant the act of giving a thing a name that belongs to something else, such as by saying, "His vulture eyes followed their every move." *Vulture* is imaginative and thus not literal if we are talking about another human being, but it does imply characteristics, images, and meaning not present if one had simply stated, "His eyes followed their every move." For this reason, Diomedes described metaphor as the transferring of things and words from their proper signification to an improper similitude—something that was and is done in language and literature for the sake of beauty, necessity, polish, or emphasis.

Metaphor is thus a form of language, a means of communication, that is expressive, creative, perhaps challenging, and powerful. As therapy is a language-based process of healing, heavily reliant on the effectiveness of communication between client and therapist, it behooves the therapist to be familiar with language structures, such as metaphor, that best facilitate the client's process of change.

WHY USE METAPHORS IN THERAPY?

In Chapter 10 of this volume, Christine Perry draws our attention to a study that found an average of three metaphors per 100 words in a single hour of therapy (Ferrara, 1994). Metaphors are so common that they *fall* into our everyday conversations. They *enliven* ordinary language. They add *color* to our communication. They *open our eyes* to new ideas and possibilities. As the italicized words in the previous sentences show, metaphors *slip* into our language with such commonality that they frequently go unnoticed. If our clients are using such frequent figurative language to express their experience then it seems only appropriate, logical, and practical that the therapist join that language, meet the client in his or her mode of communication, and facilitate both figurative and pragmatic processes of change. There are several ways metaphor can facilitate that.

Metaphors Are Interactive

Unlike other forms of communication, such as a lecture, where the presenter is active and the listener may be so distracted, passive, or uninvolved as to not even be listening, metaphor requires an active involvement on the listener's part. If you hear someone say, "It's hot outside" or "I am feeling tense," there is nothing more for you to do as a listener. You have heard it and acknowledged it, and that is it. If, however, someone says, "I'm facing an Everest" or "I'm running blind" you are suddenly confronted by a new image. You need to think about it and choose from many possible meanings inherent in the metaphor. The ambiguous links demand attention if meaning is to be found, the listener has to en-gage with the teller, and a form of interactive communication is established between both teller and listener. As you read the following chapters, it may be interesting to observe how the use of therapeutic metaphors engages the client, to varying degrees, in this interactive process of learning.

Metaphors Teach by Attraction

Everyone loves a good story. Look at the way children sit wide-eyed listening to a teacher read from a storybook, or beg for a bedtime tale. Observe how adults flock to movies, devour a novel, or delight over stories shared around the table at a dinner party. Notice what happens as you begin to tell clients a therapeutic metaphor. What changes are there in their indexes of attention? What happens to their eye contact with you, their rate of respiration, and the amount of bodily movement? Metaphors and stories attract, with the result that listeners are drawn to both the tale and the message or learning embedded in the tale.

Metaphors Bypass Resistance

By the time many clients get to therapy, many well-meaning people have often offered them some sound and helpful advice. That this advice has not been accepted means that any similar approach in therapy is also likely to be met with resistance. Metaphor can be helpful in bypassing this resistance, particularly when the therapeutic metaphors are generated by the client (see Chapters 3 and 10), come from the client's own story (see Chapters 9 and 11), or are built collaboratively with the client (see Chapters 16 and 18). If the idea, metaphor, analogy, or story comes from the client, there is simply nothing for the client to resist.

Metaphors Engage and Nurture Imagination

In Chapter 5, Mikaela Hildebrandt, Lindsay B. Fletcher, and Steven C. Hayes describe metaphor as "a bridge between the world created by language and the experience of the world that transcends language." They go on to add, "Metaphors intentionally disorient clients so that they must discover what works and what doesn't based on their experience rather than literal, linear rules." Engaging and nurturing processes of imagination and figurative thought, metaphors require a level of processing that tends to bypass the linear, logical, and cognitive ruts in which clients may have become stuck during their struggle to resolve an issue or problem.

Metaphors Engage a Search Process

When Zurich psychiatrist Hermann Rorschach devised his famous inkblots, he may not have created an objectively validated test but he did hit on something important: that as a species we are not good at tolerating ambiguity and have a strong desire to search for meaning, even in something as abstract as an inkblot. Like a projective test, metaphors offer the listener a somewhat ambiguous stimulus—even though the teller may have deliberately structured the metaphor with a defined purpose. If a woman in an abusive relationship is told a story of a mountain climber (see Chapter 8), or a person who has lost her voice hears a tale of marching penguins (see Chapter 13), or a child insomniac is engaged in a conversation about Harry Potter and biting sharks (see Chapter 16), there is uncertainty and perhaps even confusion. The listener engages in a search: Why am I being told this? What relevance does this have for me? What purpose does my therapist have in relating this tale?

This search for meaning is the very basis of the therapeutic value of metaphor. For that reason, there is no correct or right way for a client to interpret a metaphorical story. The most meaningful interpretation a client gives to a therapeutic tale is usually the one he or she ascribes to it. Different people are likely to see different meanings in the same story. The art of the good therapist is to be flexible enough to utilize the client's understanding and build on his or her meaning in a way that will constructively facilitate the client's move toward the therapeutic goal. An example of this search process is presented in Chapter 2.

Metaphors Develop Problem-Solving Skills

We all encounter problems throughout life. Learning how to solve them effectively is one of those essential life skills that prevent us from slipping into debilitating states of anxiety or depression, and contribute to our living a contented, happy existence. A good story usually begins with a problem or challenge faced by the main character, whose task is to find the means to reach an appropriate resolution. Becoming engaged with the character or problem of the tale, the listener also becomes involved in the process of how to resolve the problem or how to develop appropriate problem-solving skills that may not have existed before. Learning the problem-solving skills required by a mountaineer's solo ascent of the steepest summit on earth may carry over to developing skills for coping with an abusive relationship (see Chapter 8), or discovering how Mr. Pasta coped with the trauma of being cooked may transfer to managing the pain of invasive surgery (see Chapter 17).

Metaphors Create Outcome Possibilities

If therapy is about one thing, it is hopefully about creating new possibilities and providing means for those possibilities to be achieved. Often the initiating factor that leads people to seek therapy is the sense that possibilities are at an end. A metaphoric story has the power to allow the listener to step out of the frame of reference in which he or she has become stuck and, in a different realm of experience, reexamine the possibilities. Examples of this can be found extensively throughout the following chapters, including the discovery of what options there are when you are 61 years old and bogged down with the question of whether to divorce (see Chapter 6), of what possible ways you might reframe your experience when you are 8 years old and dying of an incurable disease (see Chapter 14), or of how you could possibly cope with the personal and peer challenges of your parents' divorcing and still living together (see Chapter 9).

Metaphors Invite Independent Decision Making

Because they offer options or possibilities, metaphors invite the listener to make decisions about those choices. As the old saying goes, if you give a person a fish he will eat for a day, but if you teach him how to fish he can eat for a lifetime. The same holds true for how we do therapy. If you give a person an answer he may cope with the current situation, but if you teach him the skills of using imaginative thinking, developing problem-solving strategies, finding new possibilities, and making independent decisions, he has the means to creatively cope with not just present but also future challenges. The value of metaphors in this therapeutic process again can be found across all chapters, as they invite, for example, a child to make the choices that will free her from separation anxiety (see Chapter 4), a depressed adolescent goth to make decisions about styles of thinking more likely to enhance her happiness (see Chapter 19), and a highly responsible mother to choose to engage in a little self-nurturing (see Chapter 7).

IS METAPHOR THERAPY OR COMMUNICATION OF THERAPY?

It is not just *what* you say to a client (the therapeutic intervention), but also *how* you say it (the communication of that therapeutic intervention) that determines whether the therapeutic message is going to be heard, accepted, and acted upon. Let us take the example of two teachers who are teaching their mathematics classes about subtraction. The first teacher writes on the board: $4 - 2 = 2$. The second teacher tells the class a story: Johnny was good at playing marbles; in fact, he was so good that he won four new marbles. Having won the four new marbles he kept playing, and in the next game lost one of the marbles. He played another game and lost another marble. While Johnny began with four marbles, he lost two, meaning that he now had only two marbles left.

The content that each teacher wanted to communicate to the class was exactly the same. When we look at how they communicated it, we see that there is a marked difference. It may be interesting to observe, as you read the preceding paragraph, which approach you felt the greater affinity with. With which did you identify more, and which, if you were still back in elementary school, would have better helped you learn that new concept?

Therapeutically, we have choices similar to those of the two teachers in communicating their message. We can communicate therapy directly or we can communicate it indirectly. Take the example of working with a client who has a phobia of heights. Having chosen the therapeutic model with which we are going to work, we then need to select what strategy or intervention we might use within that model. Are we going to work with systematic desensitization or exposure therapy for example? Having made that choice the next question becomes: how do we communicate that intervention most effectively for this particular client? Our first alternative could be to take a direct approach that tells our client what to do: learn a relaxation technique and then, having done that, start to gradually climb up a place where you previously felt uneasy, taking time to pause and relax along the way. Second, we could accompany our client in that exercise, doing an *in vivo* desensitization, coaching and encouraging him as he gradually steps through the previously anxiety-arousing experience. Third, we could also do that in covert imagery, teaching our client an effective strategy for relaxing and then walking him through successive approximations with guided imagery. A fourth alternative might be to tell a story: I once saw another client who experienced similar feelings to yourself who whenever faced with the prospect of ascending a flight of open steps or standing close to a window in a tall building, felt so scared that he avoided doing things that he would dearly have loved to do. The story can then step that client through the stages and processes of systematic desensitization to a satisfactory outcome. In all of these approaches the therapeutic intervention is the same. The difference is in the way that therapeutic intervention is communicated and metaphor is just *one* way of communicating the contents and processes of an effective therapeutic intervention.

As you read the literature you will find that at times metaphor has been described as therapy, however, as we look at the above examples of learning subtraction or overcoming a phobia, it is perhaps more appropriate and more functional to see metaphor as a form of communication rather than a therapy in itself. In Chapter 6, Michael Yapko makes the point that hypnosis is generally not considered to be an independent therapy (American Psychological Association, 1999). The reasons that he offers for using hypnosis in therapy are equally applicable for metaphor. That is metaphor, like hypnosis, can create a readiness and context for therapeutic learning as well as enhance the delivery of the therapeutic message. With the example of the mathematics teachers wanting to teach their students about subtraction, there are ways of doing it that may get the message across, and ways of doing it that may get the message across more effectively. Metaphor can thus help to describe a psychodynamic understanding, reflect a client's own story of their situation, offer a strategic intervention, present an evidence-based intervention, explore solution-focused outcomes, or communicate any of the psychotherapeutic modalities with which you work.

If a teacher says "Four minus two equals two" and the student grasps that concept, then obviously that is the simplest and perhaps most effective way of communicating for that particular student. If the student has never come across the concept of subtraction, has difficulty understanding it when it is presented, or doesn't yet have the means to adequately process it, then the teacher may need to look for other means of communicating the premise. Even if the student does understand the concept, the use of story is a richer way of learning, permeates more the processes of thinking and remembering, and empowers the listener to find his or her own conclusions. Herein lies the parallel with therapy. If we can say to compulsive gamblers, "You are ruining your life and the life of your family; go home and stop gambling," and they do it, that similarly is the simplest and most effective intervention to offer. If we can say to a depressed person, "Get out and socialize more, engage in more physical activity, or look at the positive things that are happening in your life," and that person does it, again, we have provided the simplest and most effective assistance. A problem often encountered in therapy is that most times when clients arrive at our office they have already been offered the direct approach on many previous occasions from well-meaning family members, friends, physicians, counselors, and therapists. If the direct approach has not worked, we know something very important: Taking the direct approach again is not likely to work. It is in such situations that metaphor, along with other forms of indirect suggestion, begins to have its place.

WHAT TYPE OF METAPHOR IS THAT?

As you read the literature on metaphors, you will encounter a confusing array of descriptive titles, with different authors employing different categories for metaphors that reflect the way they perceive and structure them. You will find goal-oriented metaphors (Lankton & Lankton, 1989) and outcome-oriented metaphors (Burns, 2001, 2005); embedded metaphors (Lankton & Lankton, 1986) and embodied metaphors (Bell-Gadsby & Donaghy, 2004); artistic metaphors (Mills, 2001) and affect metaphors (Lankton & Lankton, 1989); linguistic metaphors (Kopp, 1995) and guided metaphors (Battino, 2002), to name just a few. In fact, some authors have even coined their own words, like *metaphorms* (Kopp, 1995) and *metaphoria* (Battino, 2002). As there is no absolute way for categorizing the types of metaphors in therapy, let me review some of those varying labels in an attempt to bring some clarity to this confusion, and propose a classification that will provide a structure for viewing metaphors throughout the remainder of this book.

In broad terms, metaphors tend to be defined by one of two characteristics. The first classification defines them by their *function* or the purpose they serve. Stephen Lankton and Carol Hicks-Lankton's writings (Lankton & Lankton, 1983, 1986, 1989), for example, generally refer to types of metaphors defined by their function. In their writing, a matching metaphor serves the purpose of matching the character and problem of the client so as to engage that person in the process of therapy and the attainment of an outcome. A resource metaphor has the function of retrieving therapeutically useful resources and making them available for the resolution of the problem. An embedded metaphor is one whose function is to embed the direct therapeutic work within a story (within a story within a story), on the assumption that such embedded messages are less susceptible to critical analysis and conscious rejection (Lankton & Lankton, 1983). Affect, attitude, and behavior metaphors (Lankton & Lankton, 1989) have the function of offering mechanisms for change within those particular areas.

A large percentage of other therapists writing about metaphors have opted to classify them according to the second characteristic, defining metaphors by their *source* or origin. Joyce Mills (2001; Mills & Crowley, 1986), who works primarily with children, refers to storytelling metaphors, which, as the name implies, have their source in the tradition of orally presented stories; artistic metaphors, which are sourced from drawing strategies; board games and healing books created by the child; and living metaphors, which are based on out-of-the-office assignments.

Similarly, for Corydon Hammond (1990), there are "three basic styles of metaphors," each with a different source. The first he refers to are the metaphoric stories therapists tell from their own background of experience, whether they be previous case examples or personal life experiences. The second type is the "truism metaphor," whose origins lie in such common, universal themes "that the patient cannot deny them," while his final category is "make up metaphoric stories," imaginary tales the therapist creates to parallel aspects of the client's current and desired circumstances. While he acknowledges that there is no research to indicate that one metaphor type is more effective than another, he expresses a preference for the first two, feeling that the third type may cast doubt on therapist authenticity and appear condescending to some clients. While recognizing the important place of metaphors, he also adds the appropriate precaution that "we must keep a balanced perspective and realize that therapy is more than storytelling" (p. 37).

Richard Kopp identifies what he calls "two broad categories" of metaphors, namely client-generated metaphors and therapist-generated metaphors (1995, p. xvi). In the case of the former, the therapist listens for the metaphors used by the client to describe his or her situation: "I feel like I'm stuck in a maze and can't find my way out," or "I can't see a light at the end of the tunnel," or "I'm a rudderless ship." The therapeutic task, for which Kopp provides a step-by-step process, is then to join clients in *their* metaphor and invite them to start exploring possible resolutions (see Chapter 3 in this volume). Conversely, with the latter type of metaphor it is the therapist who is the source of the story, who creates the character and tale to match the client's problem, processes for resolution, and desired outcome. Within the area of client-generated metaphors, Kopp includes subgroups that he refers to as "early memory metaphors" and "linguistic metaphors."

Of course, there are many other possibilities. We could think of metaphors in terms of the source by which they are communicated: oral metaphors, book-sourced metaphors, drama metaphors, video or DVD metaphors, toy-based metaphors, humorous metaphors, or playful metaphors (Burns, 2005). We could categorize them in terms of the therapeutic basis on which they are built or constructed: evidence-based metaphors, strategic metaphors, psychodynamic metaphors, solution-focused metaphors, and so on. Or we could classify them as client case metaphors, everyday experience metaphors, cross-cultural metaphors, and life experience metaphors (Burns, 2001, 2005).

It is important to remember that all such classifications are simply a useful way of thinking about metaphors rather than an absolute. One of the first questions for a therapist to ask him- or herself, if deciding on using metaphor as a means to communicate the therapeutic directive, is "What will be helpful for the metaphor to provide for my client? Is its purpose to allow him to identify with the story and feel that his problem is heard and understood, as in a matching metaphor? Is the function to access and utilize existing or new resources and skills that are necessary to achieve the therapeutic goal, as in a resource metaphor? Is it to provide her with hope, to open up the possibility for change and attainment of a realistic goal?"

Having decided on the *function* of the metaphor, the therapist may then find it helpful to ask about its *source:* "From where am I going to acquire an appropriate metaphor? Has my client come up with a workable metaphor to describe his situation, and can that metaphor be utilized to reach an appropriate outcome? Is it more desirable for me as the therapist to generate a metaphor that can introduce means and strategies of which the client may not yet be aware? Will it be better for my client and me to work on the story collaboratively, or can I set up an experiential activity that may have metaphoric meaning?" These questions form a convenient and useful structure in which to think about the best way to work with metaphors for a particular client.

For convenience, I have used four source-based categories throughout this book, which you will commonly find mentioned in the preview of each chapter, simply to give some common ground to how we view and discuss them. I have sought to give a definition of each, an idea of their advantages, and some ways in which they are used, but would caution that they are not mutually exclusive and the boundaries may be more merged than defined. Different contributors may describe their metaphors in different ways . . . or want to avoid any classification at all.

Group 1: Client-Generated Metaphors

Client-generated metaphors are by definition those that come from the client. The more the therapist begins to listen for these, the more he or she is likely to hear metaphors such as "I'm stuck in a hole," "I've reached the end of my tether," "My life is at a crossroads."

When working with client-generated metaphors the therapist usually identifies the main metaphor that describes the client's problem, begins to explore the meaning or experiences the client associates with it, and helps the client start to shape that metaphor toward a more satisfactory outcome. Some, like Richard Kopp (Chapter 3) and Rubin Battino (Chapter 8), follow a prescribed protocol or guidelines for working with client-generated metaphors, while others, like Christine Perry (Chapter 10), take a less prescribed approach.

The advantages are that these metaphors are the clients' own stories of their experience, such as those presented at the beginning of the chapter in Vanessa's image of a shattered illusion and a feeling of being lost. The therapist can join clients in using their imagery, there is nothing for the client to resist, there is no need for the therapist to generate some creative story, and change comes about within the client's model of the world.

Group 2: Therapist-Generated Metaphors

Most of the literature tends to deal with therapist-generated metaphors, those created by the therapist to match the client's circumstances and desired outcome.

These are commonly told as a tale or tales in therapy, presenting a problem with which the client is likely to identify, building the resources, skills, and means to resolve that problem before reaching an appropriate outcome.

Times to use therapist-generated metaphors may be when clients are stuck for ways to resolve their problems and the therapist's professional training has made available strategies, techniques, or methods from which the clients may benefit. Examples of therapist-generated metaphors can be found in Chapters 6, 8, 13, 19, and 20.

Group 3: Collaborative Metaphors

By "collaborative metaphors," I refer to those that do not originate predominantly from either the client or the therapist but are constructed and utilized by both client and therapist actively working together on the story.

They combine the advantages of the two previous categories in that they actively work with clients' stories and allow for input by the therapist. By nature they are less protocol based than some client-generated approaches, yet they put fewer demands on the therapist to produce a story. The client is a more active participant in the creation of the story, the resolution of the problem, and the attainment of the outcome than in therapist-generated metaphors. Chapters 9, 10, 11, 15, 16, and 17 all give examples of working collaboratively with metaphors.

Group 4: Experiential Metaphors

Metaphors need not exist only in the *telling* of a tale but may also lie in the *doing* of an experiential assignment with metaphoric intent. One important way of helping clients grow in skills, competence, and confidence is to create and facilitate the opportunities for them to have a broader range of novel experiences from which meaning or understanding may "carry over" to help them reach their therapeutic goal.

By their nature, experiential metaphors invite a client to discover something in one realm of experience (such as watching reflections in a stream, as Vanessa did at the beginning of this chapter) that may be applicable to another (such as dealing with a traumatic attack). They create the opportunity for self-discovery and the learning of essential life skills, and thus provide a sense of empowerment. Such metaphors ground or anchor the therapeutic message in an actual experience.

Experiential metaphors may be created by utilizing a journey a client is undertaking (see Chapter 2), having a client care for a pet parrot (see Chapter 14), or presenting a challenging visual task (see Chapter 20).

ARE THERE TIMES *NOT* TO USE METAPHOR?

The answer to that question is simply yes. All of us who have contributed to this book have done so in the hope that it will help build your skills as a therapist and, ultimately, benefit the clients you work with. I invite you to work and experiment with the approaches we have offered, but also caution that having a new tool in the therapeutic tool kit does not mean it will work for every client in every situation. While stories have a universal appeal and have long formed a basis for human interactions and learning, metaphor is not necessarily for everyone. First, as mentioned, if you can directly communicate to a person what to do in such a way that he or she will do it, there is no point in wasting your time or that person's by constructing elaborate, indirect forms of communication, such as metaphors. Second, there are clients who may see storytelling as condescending or evasive, in which case it is inappropriate and possibly even demeaning to use them. Third, because using metaphors in therapy is an ambiguous, indirect approach to treatment it may not be appropriate for clients who have more concrete cognitive styles. Fourth, there may be times when someone is so depressed that he or she has difficulty engaging in the active and interactive processes required by metaphors. And, finally, as the brief therapy school has taught us, if something is not working, there is no point in persisting. Give up and try something different.

Just having a well-honed tool—no matter how good it is—does not mean that it is the most appropriate or relevant for every job you encounter. With every single case, we need to assess which tool is best for which task. Hopefully, from the array of approaches presented here, metaphor will be *one* of the tools in your well-equipped therapeutic toolbox, but bear in mind, too, that there is nothing biblical about how any one therapist views metaphors as compared to another. My motivation in creating this book has been to allow you to see some of the diversity with which metaphor practitioners perceive and practice their therapeutic art of storytelling, and to assess which of those approaches may be most helpful for you and the clients with whom you work.

REFERENCES

American Psychological Association, Division of Psychological Hypnosis. (1999). *Policy and procedures manual.* Washington, DC: Author.

Battino, R. (2002). *Metaphoria: Metaphor and guided metaphor for psychotherapy and healing.* Williston, VT: Crown House.

Bell-Gadsby, C., & Donaghy, K. (2004, December). *Embodied metaphors.* Workshop presented at the ninth International Congress on Ericksonian Approaches to Hypnosis and Psychotherapy, Phoenix, AZ.

Burns, G. W. (2001). *101 healing stories: Using metaphors in therapy.* New York: Wiley.

Burns, G. W. (2005). *101 healing stories for kids and teens: Using metaphors in therapy.* Hoboken, NJ: Wiley.

Ferrara, K. W. (1994). *Therapeutic ways with words.* New York: Oxford University Press.

Hammond, D. C. (Ed.). (1990). *Handbook of hypnotic suggestions and metaphors.* New York: Norton.

Kopp, R. R. (1995). *Metaphor therapy: Using client-generated metaphors in psychotherapy.* New York: Brunner/Mazel.

Lankton, C., & Lankton, S. R. (1989). *Tales of enchantment: Goal-oriented metaphors for adults and children in therapy.* New York: Brunner/Mazel.

Lankton, S. R. (2002). Foreword. In R. Battino (Ed.), *Metaphoria: Metaphor and guided metaphor for psychotherapy and healing* (pp. v–xv). Williston, VT: Crown House.

Lankton, S. R., & Lankton, C. (1983). *The answer within: A clinical framework of Ericksonian hypnotherapy.* New York: Brunner/Mazel.

Lankton, S. R., & Lankton, C. (1986). *Enchantment and intervention in family therapy: Training in Ericksonian hypnosis.* New York: Brunner/Mazel.

Mills, J. C. (2001). Ericksonian play therapy: The spirit of healing with children and adolescents. In B. B. Geary & J. K. Zeig (Eds.), *The handbook of Ericksonian psychotherapy* (pp. 506–521). Phoenix, AZ: Milton H. Erickson Foundation Press.

Mills, J. C., & Crowley, R. J. (1986). *Therapeutic metaphors for children and the child within.* New York: Brunner/Mazel.

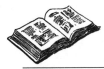

PART ONE

Improving Mood

CHAPTER 2

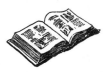

The Healing Is Complete

Outcome-Oriented Experiential Metaphors in a Case of
Major Depression

George W. Burns

CONTRIBUTOR'S STORY:
A PROFESSIONAL AND PERSONAL PERSPECTIVE

George Burns is an Australian clinical psychologist whose innovative work as a practitioner, teacher, and writer is recognized nationally and internationally. The author of numerous articles and book chapters, he has published six books available in seven languages (see Resource Section).

He is director of the Milton H. Erickson Institute of Western Australia and the Hypnotherapy Centre of Western Australia, is an adjunct senior lecturer at Edith Cowan University, and has a busy private practice with a brief, solution-focused, positive psychology orientation that reflects a love of nature, enjoyment of life, and depth of care.

From bedtime tales read by his mother and stories of life told by his father, a storytelling tradition of communication easily passed on to his children and grandchildren and into his therapeutic communication. A keen traveler, George enjoys combining his passions for nature, culture tales, and psychotherapy into workshop/study tours for colleagues that venture into remote areas such as the Himalayan kingdom of Bhutan.

PREVIEW THE CHAPTER

What do you do when a client tells an overwhelming story of largely unchangeable events? Where do you begin when that client has symptoms of major depression and sees no light at the end of the tunnel? These are some of the questions George faced with Mary. In answer, he steps you through the questions he asked himself, the therapeutic options he considered, the choices he made, and some of the interventions he used. Initially, he listens empathically to Mary's story while keeping his focus on her desired outcome. This he explores with outcome-oriented questions, narrowing his enquiries to attain her specific, workable therapeutic goals. Using the information gained in this process, along with attention to Mary's resources, he explains how he structured two experiential metaphors and one therapist-generated metaphor. The therapeutic intentions he had in developing each metaphor, how it was presented to the client, and what was the outcome, are described in detail.

Therapeutic Characteristics

Problems Addressed

- Major depression
- Memory/concentration
- Unchangeable circumstances
- Inadequate coping skills
- Hopelessness
- Powerlessness
- Unhappiness

Resources Developed

- Learning to relax
- Enhancing positive, pleasurable experiences
- Focusing on sensory experiences
- Discriminating between the changeable and unchangeable
- Developing acceptance
- Learning to make choices
- Developing empowerment

Outcomes Offered

- Enjoyment
- Discrimination
- Acceptance
- Choices
- Hopefulness
- Empowerment

The story that Mary told about her life was one of major depression. Diffuse symptoms, lack of joy, obesity, a gambling problem, ruminative worries, avoidant behaviors, an unhappy marriage, and recent concerns about memory and concentration had led her on a journey from her physician to a neurologist to a neuropsychologist and, finally, to my office. At 50 years of age, Mary had a life story that she needed to be sure was heard, yet her story was so overwhelmingly complex and complicated that I found myself asking, "Where do I begin?"

As I read the neuropsychological report, I was assured there were no indications of an early dementia. While her higher cognitive functioning appeared sound for her age and IQ levels, her score on the Beck Depression Inventory (Beck, Steer, & Brown, 1996) suggested a "potentially serious" level of depression, with significantly depressed affect and high levels of both self-denigration and self-criticism. Mary described herself as indecisive, withdrawn, irritable, and fatigued. She ruminated over most things she did, was burdened with guilt, and described passive suicidal ideation. These symptoms had been present for so many years they had become second nature to her. What triggered her search for assistance were her more recent concerns about memory, as she found herself becoming increasingly forgetful of things she set out to do, appointments she should have kept, and names she should have remembered.

Whoever coined the expression "bad things happen to good people" could have been using Mary as the role model. Chronologically she reported being sexually abused as a younger child by her father and a close family friend. She suffered a growth disorder that resulted in a short, rotund physique and was consequently the butt of other kids' jokes at school. Neither academic nor athletic, she could not excel where her peers did. Her marriage was difficult and unhappy, but she held it together. Two of her four children developed the same congenital growth disorder as Mary and, not wanting them to suffer as she had, she put them on a treatment program of growth hormones, only to discover years later that some batches had been contaminated and her kids were now at risk of developing the fatal Creutzfeldt-Jakob Disease (CJD). Doing what she thought was best, she joined a CJD society, received their typically depressing newsletters, and generously volunteered to counsel other affected families, but this further fueled her ruminative worries about whether her children would be next to die.

Around the same time, her widowed father was diagnosed with cancer. She dutifully moved with her husband into the father's home to nurse him, giving her own home to her daughter and family as they were in financial difficulties and could not afford a house of their own. Mary did not want to be with a father who, she said, she hated because of his abuse of her as a child, but she felt it her duty to care for him and could not return to her own home without making her daughter homeless. I could also mention her two automobile accidents, her volunteer hospice work, and the death and illness of several family members and friends who she supported, but this is enough to show that Mary's problems were clearly very complex, long-standing, and real. Yet, even given the extent of her own problems, she was always caring for everyone else's problems, like a universal mother.

WHERE TO BEGIN?

It may help to explain that as I sit with a client in my office, my approach tends to be based on questions I ask myself: What is the therapeutic outcome this client is seeking? What is helpful for me to know about her? What resources does she have that may be utilized productively? What interventions are likely to be the most effective? How can I engage her and her resources in that process? Through this chapter I will pose the type of questions I asked myself while working with Mary and the type of answers that I came up with, hoping to permit you to observe the processes I worked through and how these shaped the interventions and outcomes. While I have previously told aspects of Mary's story, this chapter allows me the opportunity to bring together those aspects, place them in the context of the overall therapeutic plan, and present the thinking and rationale behind the therapeutic strategies I employed (Burns, 1998, 2005b, 2006).

On hearing Mary's overwhelming story, the initial question I asked myself was "Where to begin?" Here are the thoughts that followed.

First, it is perhaps obvious but also important to be aware that it is not helpful for the therapist to be as overwhelmed by the client's depressive story as the client. While we need to hear the client's story, it may not be therapeutically beneficial for the therapist to reach the same conclusion as the client, particularly if the client's conclusions are ones of helplessness, powerlessness, and hopelessness. Second, if the therapist can hold some realistic and genuinely hopeful belief about the client's outcome, there is a greater chance the client will be able to modify the processes for managing his or her experiences, build better coping skills, and thus reach a satisfactory outcome. Much has been written about hope, with some describing it as the most crucial ingredient in, or determinant of, therapeutic outcome (Frank, 1968, 1975; Hubble & Miller, 2004; Snyder, 1989, 1994, 2000, 2002). Third, with the complex and diffuse nature of problems in cases such as Mary's it is generally helpful to break the desired outcome down to specific goals, then break it down some more, and then break it down further still. Finally, once a specific goal or goals have been defined the processes for achieving them can more easily be defined and communicated to the client.

WHAT DID MARY WANT FROM THERAPY?

"What is going to be helpful for you to gain from this session?" I asked Mary after having heard her story. This clearly and unashamedly outcome-oriented question is based on the assumptions that (1) Mary had enough depression in her tale without me asking her to explore it any further and (2) her taking the effort to make an appointment, show up, walk into my office, and tell her story indicated she was seeking a change in her experience, and a change for the better. My question was thus designed to specifically seek how she wanted life to improve as a result of just this first session. If Mary had replied with something like "I want to know why I am feeling so depressed," it might have been useful to explore with her whether her more important objective was to have an understanding of her problems or to develop the skills and strategies necessary to bring about a desired change.

"I don't want to be feeling so forgetful, irritable, or withdrawn," she responded. Her statement of what she *didn't* want rather than what she did highlights how, perhaps particularly in the area of depression, the therapist can expect answers to be worded in a negative or avoidant style. Avoidance is one of the common coping styles associated with depression (Yapko, 2001; Seligman, 2002), and orientation toward avoidance goals (i.e., trying to avoid what you do *not* want) rather than approach goals (i.e., seeking what you *do* want) has a similar correlation with depressive symptoms (Emmons, 1991, 2003; Street, 1999, 2000, 2001, 2002). Therefore, accepting an avoidance goal as your therapeutic contract may unintentionally reinforce this aspect of depressive cognitions and behavior because it does not provide the client with effective strategies for either the direction of therapy or the direction of life.

Acceptance of a negatively expressed outcome can also be frightening for the client. What happens if she does stop feeling irritable and withdrawn? What happens if you take away a person's only or major coping skills, even though they may not be the most functional? How does she then cope with life's challenging situations? Conversely, if you have a positive goal and an outcome that can realistically be achieved, the client is offered both hope and skills to function in a healthier manner.

So if, like Mary, a client expresses a negative or avoidant goal, it may be practical and beneficial to gently question and guide him or her toward ways to shape it into an approach goal: "If you don't want to feel so irritable, how do you want to feel?" or "If you don't want to be so withdrawn, what would you rather be doing?"

Mary replied that she wanted to feel more relaxed and be more outgoing. As global, inclusive thinking is also characteristic of depressive cognitions, I was keen to assist her to explore her generally stated therapeutic goals more specifically. What did being more relaxed mean, specifically, for this particular client? When were the times she relaxed, or could imagine herself relaxing? How did she manage to do that? And what did being more outgoing mean? Did it mean Mary wanted to build better skills in social communication, learn how to relax in the company of others, join appropriate interest groups, shift focus away from her own worries, go out visiting more often, or initiate phone conversations with friends more frequently? The bottom line here is that the more specific the goal, the greater the probability of attaining it.

"I feel most relaxed and happiest when gardening," came the response. Pushing for the specifics was beginning to reveal possible specific interventions. But still I wanted her to be more specific.

"What is it specifically about the gardening that helps you feel relaxed and happy?"

"Tending my roses," she answered.

"And what is it about the roses you find so enjoyable and relaxing?" I asked. When Mary described her sensory experiences of the sights and smells among the roses, I still wanted to know more. "What are the particular sights you enjoy?" "What are the fragrances you associate with pleasure and comfort?" Such detailed questions were, first, opening possibilities for Mary to explore her own specific pleasurable experiences and, second, providing me with possible intervention opportunities. For a more detailed account of how to undertake an Outcome-Oriented Assessment with adults see Burns (2001, pp. 233–237) and with children and adolescents see Burns (2005a, pp. 256–258).

WHAT WAS USEFUL TO KNOW ABOUT MARY?

First and foremost, while life had seemed to deal Mary an unfair proportion of challenges, I was reminded that what matters is not *what* happens to a person so much as *how* that person perceives those events and *how* they manage those events. Mary was not on antidepressant medication, was not in a psychiatric institution, had not committed suicide, and, in fact, had survived all these challenges until the recent concerns about her memory and concentration. Obviously, there were some things, perhaps many, that she had been doing well, things that had enabled her to cope with some very challenging circumstances.

Mary had shown she was a caring person, deeply concerned about the well-being of her daughters, willing to go out of her way to help others through her voluntary hospital work, and available to family members and friends in their times of trouble. When focused on assisting others she was less focused on her own worries and concerns.

I had learned from the assessment that there were some specific situations (such as tending roses) where Mary found it easier to relax and experience pleasure. Relaxation and pleasure were possible, and if they were possible in this context, they might be possible for her in other contexts. Barbara Fredrickson talks of what she calls her broaden-and-build model, based on the well-documented premise that people cope well when they have good access to a range of strong, positive emotional responses (Fredrickson, 2000, 2005). Maybe it would assist Mary to build on those positive experiences she was already capable of knowing, help her develop a broader range of positive responses, and strengthen them further.

Something I discovered in subsequent sessions was that Mary had an amazing and somewhat idiosyncratic sense of humor. This will become apparent as you read some of the letters she wrote to me. It was a strategy through which she had coped in the past and which she could be assisted to continue to employ in the future.

WHAT INTERVENTIONS WERE LIKELY TO HELP?

A therapist may select, adapt, and abandon many interventions in the course of therapy. Working with Mary was no exception. I spent time listening, as she needed to know that her story was heard. I worked with various suggestions (Hammond, 1990), solution-focused interventions (Berg & Dolan, 2001), cognitive strategies for depression (Segal, Williams, & Teasdale, 2002), hypnosis (Yapko, 2001, 2006), and nature-guided therapy (Burns, 1998, 2005b) depending on Mary's immediate circumstances and long-term goals. Among the interventions offered, Mary was asked to complete the Sensory Awareness Inventory, an inventory that requests clients to list 10 to 20 items under headings for their five basic senses from which they gain, have gained, or could gain pleasure and relaxation, and also contains a section for the activities from which they derive pleasure (Burns, 1998). Not surprisingly, the sight and smell of roses along with the activity of gardening featured on Mary's inventory, and there was much more. Not all of the information supplied by the inventory nor all the interventions used to help broaden and build Mary's experiences and skills can be covered in this chapter, so I have provided a detailed explanation of just three of the metaphor interventions offered to her.

Intervention One: Stopping to Smell the Roses

The Therapeutic Intention

Given that Mary had described many negative feelings and undesired symptoms, my first objective was to help her create at least some positive experiences. To know that once, in one set of circumstances, it was possible to feel better would open the possibility for her to experience similar feelings in other circumstances at other times. It would provide her with a glimmer of hope, a light at the end of a long, dark tunnel.

Fortunately, Mary had already described specific positive feelings associated with tending her roses. My initial therapeutic intention was to draw her attention to her capability for experiencing positive emotions—at least in some situations—utilize that helpful resource, and assist her to broaden and build her own capacity to feel better. With this capacity would come the opportunity to develop further positive feelings in other areas of her life.

Mary associated relaxation and happiness with a nature-based experience of gardening among the roses, and this I wanted to utilize as well. Research shows us that during contact with nature levels of stress diminish rapidly (Ulrich, 1981; Ulrich et al., 1991), depression can lift (Burns, 1998; Burns & Street, 2003), and overall functioning is enhanced (Kaplan & Kaplan, 1996). From the assessment it was obvious there was a mismatch between what contributed to Mary's sense of well-being and what she was actually doing. She was not doing the things that enhanced her comfort and pleasure, such as gardening, but was doing what exacerbated her stress and distress, such as ruminating over unresolved and, in many ways, unsolvable family issues.

Finally, because so many of the circumstances that Mary described were outside her area of control (the history of abuse, the risk of her daughters developing CJD, her father's diagnosis of cancer, the two automobile accidents, the death of people close to her) I considered it would be beneficial if she could take from our first session an awareness that there were some things (such as her feelings) that were potentially in the realm of her control. I hoped that both the awareness and the ability to exercise some control would be empowering.

The Intervention

An experiential metaphor is more than just a homework assignment. It is a homework assignment with metaphoric intention, which means that it creates an experience with an imaginative, but not literal, relationship to the client's problem and desired outcome. To this end, Mary was asked to spend time each day over the week before her next appointment among the roses in the garden of her father's home, where she was staying. In gardening there are many potential metaphors: planting, nurturing, pruning to facilitate growth, thorns (pain) and flowers (pleasure), seasons of change, and so on. Moreover, Mary was asked to attend specifically to her senses and the various sensory experiences she noticed. The metaphoric suggestion came in the request for her to observe what she learned, implying that there was something to be gained beyond just being among the roses, something from which she might learn, something that could be related to her goals of greater relaxation and happiness.

The Outcome

Mary was a prolific letter writer. After that first session, in which we did little more than explore her specific outcome goals and set up the intervention with the roses, she wrote to me, saying,

> Yesterday I was so embarrassed. I got such a shock that I wished myself anywhere but there [a reference to her suicidal ideation]. But, it was so funny when I was on the train later. I was sitting there visualizing making my husband rose petal sandwiches, marinating his meat in rose perfume, rose petals in the stew, lighting rose candles, sprinkling rose petals all around the room, some other ideas that I won't write down. I started to giggle, people next to and

opposite me moved and put a lot of space between us, all were giving me funny glances. By the time I got off the train I was laughing out loud while walking down the street. I found a freedom of spirit that hasn't been there for a long time. Thanks for letting me find my own way through it. The rose petals are a great idea.

Simply setting up a basic experiential metaphor provided the opportunity for Mary to create a new story for herself and a new set of responses. It opened the way for her to giggle, laugh out loud, and express her sense of humor—responses that had not been present for a long time. Of course, "stopping to smell the roses" did not resolve all the complex issues with which Mary was dealing, but it did remind her of some of her resources and that there were other, more positive ways of dealing with those issues. Instead of thinking ruminatively about her worries, she could be mindful of positive experiences. Instead of being negative and avoidant, she could be more positive and outcome-oriented. Instead of thinking globally, she could think in more specific terms. She discovered skills and methods of coping different from those she had been using, and, by acknowledging that she had found her own way through her depression, she was taking ownership of the skills she had discovered.

Intervention Two: A Tale of Acceptance

The Therapeutic Intention

When people are faced with life events outside of their control, as Mary was, and wish they would magically change, it is an almost guaranteed formula for disappointment, frustration, and even despair. If I plan a weekend barbecue with friends and it pours with rain, my wish for it to be fine is not going to alter the weather. If I go on wishing for something that will not be, complaining how unfair it is, and failing to adapt to the reality, the probability is that I will feel decidedly unhappy. If, alternatively, I accept that despite my wishes this is the way things are, then I am in a position to adjust to them and thus feel better. Given this knowledge, I considered that offering Mary some practical information through therapist-generated stories about acceptance might assist her in discriminating between the things that she could change and the things she could not, as well as teach her ways to adapt to the unalterable and, thus, feel more empowered.

The Intervention

I love stories and am a collector of them, many of which have been compiled in *101 Healing Stories* (Burns, 2001) and *101 Healing Stories for Kids and Teens* (Burns, 2005a). There are times in therapy when it is useful to have such a repertoire of tales from which you can draw, a collection of story ideas in your head that can be drawn on and adapted for a particular client. Wanting a story of acceptance for Mary, I chose one from my collection about a stonecutter who felt powerless and unhappy with his lot in life, constantly wanting things that he was unlikely to attain. One day on his way home from work he looked through the window of the home of a wealthy merchant. Seeing the house filled with luxurious furniture, the walls decorated with expensive artwork, and the table laid with exotic food, he wished he were the merchant. Magically, he became the merchant, owner of the home and furnishings, sitting at the head of the table, but it wasn't long before he realized that not everything is as it seems. Life as a wealthy merchant had its positive side but also its downside. His new possessions came at a cost. Dissatisfied with this lot, as he had been with his lot as a stonecutter, he saw the emperor passing and, thinking he would be happier and more powerful as the emperor, he magically became the emperor . . . and so the story goes until eventually he returns to being the stonecutter, accepting his lot, and discovering in it a new sense of empowerment. A fuller version of this story, "Learning to Accept Our Circumstances," can be found in Burns, 2001, p. 59).

As Mary appeared to be making good progress, we started to reduce the frequency of sessions, and for several weeks she was handling her challenging circumstances better. Later she suffered a relapse when several new uncontrollable events occurred, and she began to reexperience feelings of powerlessness, wishing for miraculous solutions that would never be. Again it occurred to me that a story of acceptance seemed relevant and, completely forgetting that I had already told her a version of "Learning to Accept Our Circumstances," I retold it with applicability to her current situation. Mary sat quietly, seemingly absorbed in the story, and left the session without making any comment about the tale.

The Outcome

Before our next session she wrote me another letter. In it she said, "I have worked out the story about the stonecutter [as she referred to it]. It is told once while the person is sick, then again when they are feeling better. It stops them from relapsing, because they know that if they do you will tell them the damn thing a third time!"

Her response highlights several aspects of metaphor work. First, it further revealed a valuable resource of Mary's, her sense of humor. Twice now she had expressed it, revealing a therapeutic potential to both reinforce it and further employ it as a coping strategy.

Second, while it was an act of pure forgetfulness on my part and with no deliberate intention that I told the story to her a second time, my doing so stimulated a search in her for some meaning or purpose in the second recounting of the story. This is often referred to in the literature as a "search phenomenon" or "search process," terms that describe the typical search for meaning a person engages in when presented with an ambiguous stimulus such as a metaphor. The conclusion that Mary reached was so important that she needed to put it in writing. And this is where something both common and fascinating can occur when using metaphors: The therapeutic intention I had as a therapist in telling the tale was very different from the meaning Mary attributed to it. What she found, however, was both constructive and therapeutic for her, namely that if she didn't get "better" she would have to listen to "the damn thing" for a third time.

At the end of therapy Mary wrote another letter, which she entitled, "The final letter of the series." In it she said,

> I do know you reached out and took my hand at a time when I had no strength. You demanded I hold on and trust in you. [Again her perception was different from mine, in that I did not see myself as "demanding" anything of her.] I am aware that there were times when you did not understand where I was coming from. How could you? I didn't know myself. I appreciate you didn't pretend. You just were still, listened with the ear of your heart or told a story. George, I really like the stories, especially The Stone Cutter. It was great.

Intervention Three: Promising Much for the Future

The Therapeutic Intention

Toward the end of our sessions, Mary told me that she and her husband were planning a vacation to the world's largest single monolith in Central Australia. Long called Ayer's Rock by European settlers, it has been known even longer as Uluru to the indigenous Aboriginal residents. Her planned visit afforded a therapeutic opportunity: I could simply wish her a happy vacation, or utilize the holiday as a resource to further her therapeutic gain. I chose the latter.

Mary suffered from a heart condition and consulted her cardiologist prior to departure to seek his advice about climbing Uluru. He categorically forbade it, which she appeared somewhat dejected by and which posed a dilemma for me. My work with Mary had largely been aimed at facilitating her skills in discriminating between the things she could change and the things she couldn't, at building her perception of choices available, at selecting appropriate coping skills for the particular situation, and at feeling empowerment in her choices and action. She saw that the cardiologist's directive undermined her choice and left her feeling powerless. I wanted to encourage her choices, but safely and with regard for her physical health.

The Uluru trip was an opportunity to further expand Mary's sensory awareness of stimuli that might further enhance her relaxation and happiness. Knowing what we know about the positive role of the natural environment in human well-being (Burns, 1998, 2005b), combined with the fact that Mary had already demonstrated a beneficial response to nature-based assignments, my intention included helping her broaden and build her repertoire of positive, pleasurable experiences.

In addition, I hoped she could utilize the journey metaphorically. Our language is rich in metaphors about travel, journeys, and movement: Life is a journey; it is better to journey than arrive; we move on from a bad experience; we leave things behind; the road can be rough or easy; we journey into a new experience. An open-ended suggestion could invite her to look at her experience of Uluru metaphorically.

The Intervention

In discussing her forthcoming trip, wanting to encourage her well-discriminated choices and invite her to look at it metaphorically, I said, "I think it is important that *you* make up your mind if you want to climb or not. Making any choice involves weighing the information available to us, looking at the advantages and disadvantages. Part of that information, of course, comes from your cardiologist, who you employed to give you his professional opinion, which I am sure he did out of his care and concern for your health. That is part of the information to consider in deciding what is best for your well-being."

To help direct her awareness toward the positive and pleasurable, to focus on each sensory modality, I continued, "Once you have made that decision, you may like to focus on what a unique pleasure it is to be in such a special place, allowing yourself some quiet time to tune in to your senses, to enjoy the sights of all the colors and shapes, the sounds of the many things around you, the smell of the different fragrances in the air, and the feel of the things you touch."

Inviting her to experience her time there metaphorically, I added, "Uluru has long been seen as a special place with special meaning by the local Aboriginals, and it is woven into their dreamtime stories. I look forward to hearing what meaning it may have for you, or what stories you may have to tell of your experience there when you return."

The Outcome

Again, in her prolific writing style, Mary put pen to paper about her experience. She described how her husband and others started to climb Uluru at 5:30 A.M. so as to be at the summit for the sunrise, three-quarters of an hour later. After considering the information available and weighing the options, Mary chose not to make the climb. She wrote,

> Instead, I walked around the base. I was on my own. I could neither see nor hear anyone else and in the expectant stillness of the dawn, it was like the beginning of time. The Rock seemed to be alive and it was as if it was whispering the secrets of the past, promising much for the future. I felt blessed to have had that time just there alone in such a spiritual place. Time stood still. Later I learnt the traditional owners prefer visitors not to climb Uluru. I am glad I chose not to climb. The experience of standing alone in the vastness was truly a spiritual experience. The healing is complete.

Mary created her own healing story in a very personal journey as she walked around the base of Uluru. She established a relationship with "the Rock," as intimate as if it were whispering secrets to her. These activities facilitated a therapeutic change more rapid and more effective than what I think she would have gained from sitting in a consulting room exploring the traumas of her past. She was able to look forward to a promise of the future and sense that her own healing was complete. With her letter she enclosed a photograph of a golden sunrise emerging from behind the dark silhouette of Uluru. She had the photograph blown up to poster size and hung it on the kitchen wall as a constant reminder of her metaphor of healing.

WHAT WAS THE LONG-TERM OUTCOME?

It is almost a decade since Mary visited Uluru. Over that time she has occasionally sent me a letter, telephoned, or made an appointment to see me. She still has problems, and some of them won't go away. What has changed is the way Mary feels about, thinks about, and manages them. She can now choose to create experiences that are likely to enhance greater feelings of happiness and pleasure. Simply thinking of roses brings a smile to her face. Looking at the poster-size photograph of an Uluru sunrise in her kitchen is an opportunity for her to be in touch with a sense of healing and spirituality. She is better able to discriminate between the changeable and unchangeable aspects of her life, and is more accepting of what cannot be altered. She is empowered in the knowledge that she can make choices about acceptance and change. And she still maintains her sense of humor.

Recently, Mary phoned me after a friend told her she had heard from another psychologist that I was retiring. I assured her, "I have no plans to retire while I still enjoy what I am doing and while the marbles are still rattling around." The next week she came into my office and left a gift-wrapped parcel with my secretary. When I opened it I found a bag of marbles with a note that simply said, "May you never lose your marbles!"

REFERENCES

Beck, A. T., Steer, R., & Brown, G. (1996). *Beck depression inventory* (2nd ed.). San Antonio, TX: Harcourt Assessment.

Berg, I. K., & Dolan, Y. (2001). *Tales of solutions: A collection of hope-inspiring stories.* New York: Norton.

Burns, G. W. (1998). *Nature-guided therapy: Brief integrative strategies for health and wellbeing.* New York: Brunner/Mazel.

Burns, G. W. (2001). *101 healing stories: Using metaphors in therapy.* New York: Wiley.

Burns, G. W. (2005a). *101 healing stories for kids and teens: Using metaphors in therapy.* Hoboken, NJ: Wiley,

Burns, G. W. (2005b). Naturally happy, naturally healthy: The role of the natural environment in well-being. In F. Huppert, B. Keverne, & N. Baylis (Eds.), *The science of well-being* (pp. 405–431). Oxford: Oxford University Press.

Burns, G. W. (2006). Building coping skills with metaphors. In M. D. Yapko (Ed.), *Hypnosis and treating depression: Applications in clinical practice* (pp. 49–69). New York: Routledge.

Burns, G. W., & Street, H. (2003). *Standing without shoes: Creating happiness, relieving depression, enhancing life.* Sydney, Australia: Prentice Hall.

Emmons, R. A. (1991). Personal strivings, daily life events, and psychological and physical well-being. *Journal of Personality, 59,* 453–472.

Emmons, R. A. (2003). Personal goals, life meaning, and virtue: Wellsprings of a positive life. In C. L. M. Keyes & J. Haidt (Eds.), *Flourishing: Positive psychology and the life well-lived* (pp. 105–128). Washington, DC: American Psychological Association.

Frank, J. D. (1968). The role of hope in psychotherapy. *International Journal of Psychiatry, 5,* 383–395.

Frank, J. D. (1975). The faith that heals. *John Hopkins Medical Journal, 137,* 127–131.

Fredrickson, B. L. (1998). What good are positive emotions? *Review of General Psychology, 2,* 300–319.

Fredrickson, B. L. (2000, March 7). Cultivating positive emotions to optimize health and well-being. *Prevention and Treatment, 3,* article 0001a. Retrieved November 20, 2000, from http://journals.apa.org/prevention/volume3/pre0030001a.html

Fredrickson, B. L. (2005). The broaden-and-build theory of positive emotions. In F. Huppert, B. Keverne, & N. Baylis (Eds.), *The science of well-being* (pp. 217–238). Oxford: Oxford University Press.

Hammond, D. C. (Ed.). (1990). *Handbook of hypnotic suggestions and metaphors.* New York: Norton.

Hubble, M. A., & Miller, S. D. (2004). The client: Psychotherapy's missing link for promoting a positive psychology. In P. A. Linley & S. Joseph (Eds.), *Positive psychology in practice* (pp. 335–353). Hoboken, NJ: Wiley.

Kaplan, R., & Kaplan, S. (1996). *The experience of nature: A psychological perspective.* Ann Arbor, MI: Ulrich's Bookstore.

Seligman, M. (2002). *Authentic happiness.* New York: Free Press.

Segal, Z. V., Williams, J. M. G., & Teasdale, J. D. (2002). *Mindfulness-based cognitive therapy for depression: A new approach to preventing relapse.* New York: Guilford Press.

Snyder, C. R. (1989). Reality negotiation: From excuses to hope and beyond. *Journal of Social and Clinical Psychology, 8,* 130–157.

Snyder, C. R. (1994). *The psychology of hope: You can get from there to here.* New York: Free Press.

Snyder, C. R. (Ed.). (2000). *Handbook of hope: Theory, measures and applications.* San Diego, CA: Academic Press.

Snyder, C. R. (2002). Hope theory: Rainbows in the mind. *Psychological Inquiry, 13,* 249–275.

Street, H. (1999). Depression and the pursuit of happiness: An investigation into the relationship between goal setting, goal pursuit and vulnerability to depression. *Clinical Psychologist, 4,* 18–25.

Street, H. (2000). Exploring relationships between conditional goal setting, rumination and depression. *Australian Journal of Psychology, 52,* 113.

Street, H. (2001). Exploring the role of conditional goal setting in the aetiology and maintenance of depression. *Clinical Psychologist, 6,* 6–23.

Street, H. (2002). Exploring relationships between goal setting, goal pursuit and a depression: A review. *Australian Psychologist, 37*(2), 95–103.

Ulrich, R. S. (1981). Natural versus urban scenes: Some psychophysiological effects. *The Environment and Behaviour, 13,* 523–556.

Ulrich, R. S., Simons, R. F., Losito, B. D., Fiorito, E., Miles, M. A., & Zelson, M. (1991). Stress recovery during exposure to natural and urban environments. *Journal Environmental Psychology, 11*(3), 201–230.

Yapko, M. D. (2001). *Treating depression with hypnosis: Integrating cognitive-behavioral and strategic approaches.* New York: Brunner/Routledge.

Yapko, M. D. (Ed.). (2006). *Hypnosis and treating depression: Applications in clinical practice.* New York: Routledge.

CHAPTER 3

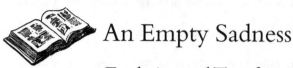

An Empty Sadness

Exploring and Transforming
Client-Generated Metaphors

Richard R. Kopp

CONTRIBUTOR'S STORY:
A PROFESSIONAL AND PERSONAL PERSPECTIVE

Richard Kopp, PhD, ABPP, is distinguished professor at the California School of Professional Psychology at Alliant International University, Los Angeles; a faculty member of the Rudolf Dreikurs Summer School; a diplomate in clinical psychology (the American Board of Professional Psychology); and a diplomate in Adlerian psychology (North American Society for Adlerian Psychology). He is a consulting editor for the *Journal of Individual Psychology* and has published over 25 articles and book chapters on Adlerian psychology and metaphor therapy.

Richard first became interested in metaphor as a source of data for identifying the Adlerian concept of lifestyle. Upon reading *Metaphors We Live By* (Lakoff & Johnson, 1980), he began to think that an individual's metaphoric language may be a direct expression and indicator of his or her metaphoric structure of personal reality. He says that "this led to a figure-ground shift in how I viewed metaphor" and resulted in a major therapeutic reorientation from the more traditional therapist-generated metaphors to client-generated.

PREVIEW THE CHAPTER

Richard set out to develop new interventions that he perceived were needed to access, explore, and change clients' own metaphors, as well as to help them create their own healing metaphoric images. In the following pages he provides the step-by-step interview protocol he developed, guiding you through the exploratory processes, providing the style of questions useful in each stage of that process, and leading to the client's application of his or her own healing story. He discusses how the therapist can listen for and identify the many metaphors in the client's story that often go unheard and, once these have been identified, how to select a core metaphor with which to work. To illustrate the application of client-generated metaphor therapy, Richard provides the transcripts of two cases with *Diagnostical and Statistical Manual of Mental Disorders* diagnoses of Major Depressive Disorder in which the therapists were third-year graduate students. The first case is that of a 30-year-old woman with the metaphor of "an empty sadness," and the second that of a 37-year-old man who "blew up."[1]

Therapeutic Characteristics

Problems Addressed

- Major depression
- Relationship breakup
- Sadness
- Fatigue
- Feelings of worthlessness
- Hostility
- Anger

Resources Developed

- Becoming aware of problem metaphors
- Exploring those metaphors
- Changing problem metaphors
- Creating new metaphors
- Applying the changed stories
- Taking control

Outcomes Offered

- Empowerment to change stories
- Better understanding of relationships
- Forgiveness
- Exploration of ways to love
- Setting of appropriate boundaries

"The greatest thing by far is to be the master of metaphor."
—ARISTOTLE, *Poetics*

How can we help our clients unlock the healing power of their own metaphoric stories? How can we tap the power of spontaneously spoken client metaphors to evoke deep feelings and reveal the hidden meanings that lie beyond the veil of everyday awareness? In this chapter, I describe and illustrate how therapists can use a structured protocol for exploring and transforming client-generated metaphors that can facilitate insight and accelerate the process of therapeutic change. After discussing the relationship between stories and metaphor, I will describe the intervention procedure in more specific terms. Finally, I will present two transcripts of therapy sessions that illustrate the healing power of exploring and transforming client metaphors.

Like the opening of a story, the client's metaphor "is a compressed emotional promise of things to come . . . [that] contains the seed of everything that will grow from it" (Boles, 1984, p. 8). The "vehicle" of the metaphor is the image. It is the metaphoric image that conveys the emotional experience to which the metaphor refers. At the moment of its creation the metaphor is mainly unconscious. For example, when a client says, "I'm sinking in quicksand" or "I keep beating myself over the head with a hammer," his or her attention is focused on the life situation represented by the image of sinking in quicksand or the experience of self-criticism referred to by the image of beating oneself over the head with a hammer.

The emotional promise of the metaphor lies in its image, not in the topic or content to which it refers. To allow this seed to grow the therapist must pluck it from the ground of logical verbal discourse and place it as a figure before the client's awareness. The client becomes the storyteller, thinking in pictures—which, in Freud's view, are nearer to unconscious processes than thinking in words (Freud, 1923 / 1960). He or she thus weaves a tapestry or, more accurately, follows the unspooling threads of associated images evoked by the therapist's questions. Like the yellow brick road that stretched out before Dorothy and Toto in *The Wizard of Oz,* the cascading images provoked by the therapist's sequence of questions lead the client down a path whose destination is unknown to both the client and the therapist. The client's unconscious is the storyteller, crafting the story in a series of images that often surprise and inform both client and therapist. The client then chooses words to describe the images he or she sees, allowing them to be communicated to the therapist as the client's left hemisphere processes linguistically what the right hemisphere has created in sensory-affective imagery. Enabling the right hemisphere to "speak" to the left fosters bilateral integration and more coordinated interhemispheric functioning (Siegel, 1999). In this way, what was beyond sensation and feeling is sensed and felt, and what was hidden is brought to light.

The therapist must be skillful in helping the client stay in the domain of the client's metaphoric imagery so that the client can continue to develop the story authored by his or her creative imagination. Once the client has developed the new story the therapist guides the client to create a resolution of the story. Now the client is ready to create and discover the ways in which his or her invented story is a metaphor for the current life problem to which the original client-generated metaphor referred. In the final phase of the process, the therapist guides the client in creating connections between the changed metaphor and the current issue, thus empowering the client to use the changed metaphor as a source of new possibilities, directions, and solutions to the current problem. The client returns to the place where he or she began, but experiences and understands it in a new and different way.

EXPLORING AND TRANSFORMING CLIENT-GENERATED METAPHORS: THEORY AND TECHNIQUE

The protocol for exploring and transforming clients' linguistic metaphors consists of three phases (see Figure 3.1).

In Phase I therapists ask questions to elicit a personal description of the problem. The first question, "In what way is this a problem for you?" is useful when clients talk in a general way about the situation or when clients' attention is directed toward others rather than themselves. This question helps clients focus on their personal reactions and feelings about their problem situation. Clinically relevant metaphors are more likely to emerge when clients describe their personal experience. The next three questions help clients focus on the aspect of their problem that is most difficult for them. Asking "Which part of this is most difficult for you?" or "What's the biggest problem?" or "Where in all of this are you most stuck?" focuses clients' attention on the issue that is most important for them.

The questions in Phase II help clients move from a factual description to their feelings and their subjective experience of the problem or issue they are describing. Asking "What are your feelings?" "How do you feel?" "What is this (it) like for you?" "What is your experience of this?" or "How does it feel to you?" is important because people use metaphors to express their subjective experience and feelings. They may respond by saying things like "I'm sinking in quicksand," "I'm running around in circles," or "I'm between a rock and a hard place." A Vietnam veteran complained that he was under "constant pressure," stating, "I feel like a tea kettle that can't let the steam out" (Kopp, 1995, p. 102). A woman who was angry with her estranged husband for repeatedly coming over to her house without calling in advance in spite of her persistent requests exclaimed, "He barges into the house like a locomotive" (Kopp, 1995, p. xiv).

If a client is already describing his or her feelings and is spontaneously generating metaphors in the session, the therapist may omit Phases I and II of the protocol and begin the intervention with Phase III, exploring and transforming the client-generated metaphor.

In Step 1 of Phase III, the therapist tunes in to the client's use of metaphors. This skill requires practice because we typically listen and attend to the topic or content of what is communicated. By using a metaphor log to record metaphors that others use (e.g., in meetings, on TV, in lectures and discussions, etc.), therapists learn to notice metaphors. It is necessary to write down the metaphor at the moment one hears it because it is difficult, if not impossible, to remember metaphors used in conversation even several minutes after they occur. It appears that, like dreams, metaphors are lost in the flood of verbal logical meanings that dominate our conversations and thought patterns.

The Four Stages of Learning to Identify Client-Generated Metaphors

Four stages characterize learning to listen and attend to metaphoric speech. At first, you can expect that the habit of attending to the content of your clients' verbal communication will continue and that you will miss most spoken metaphors. For example, therapists at this stage would not pick up on the metaphor used in the previous sentence ("miss") or in the present sentence ("pick up on"). In the second stage, therapists begin to hear and identify metaphors. You know you have "arrived at" the third stage when you hear metaphors "all over the place," perhaps even to "the point" where you

Figure 3.1   Exploring and Transforming Client-Generated Metaphors: Interview Protocol—Short Form   By Richard R. Kopp, PhD, ABPP

Phase I: Moving from General to Personal (Find the Person in the Problem)

---

   1. In what way is this a problem for you?
   2. (a) Which part of this is most difficult for you? *or*
       (b) What is the biggest problem? *or*
       (c) Where in all of this are you most stuck?

Phase II: Moving from Facts to Feelings (Find the Feelings behind the Facts)

   What are your feelings? *or* How do you feel? *and/or* What is this (it) like for you? *or* What is your experience of this? How does it feel to you?

Phase III: Exploring and Transforming Client Metaphors

Step 1: Noticing Metaphors (especially in the client's response to the preceding questions)

Step 2: Focusing on the Metaphor Image
   When you say [the metaphor] what image/picture comes to mind?" *or* What image/picture do you see in your mind's eye? *or* What does the [metaphor] look like?

Step 3: Exploring the Metaphor as a Sensory Image
   1. Setting (e.g., What else do you see? *or* Describe the scene or an aspect of the scene [associated with the metaphoric image]?)
   2. Action/interaction (e.g., What else is going on in [the metaphoric image]? *or* What are the other people [in the metaphoric image] saying/thinking/doing?)
   3. Time (e.g., What led up to this? *or* What was happening [just] before [the situation in the metaphor]?)

Step 4: Exploring Feelings Associated with the Metaphor Image
   What's it like to be [the metaphoric image]? *or* What's your experience of [the metaphoric image]? *or* What are you feeling as you [the metaphoric image]?

Step 5: Changing the Metaphor Image
   If you could change the image in any way, how would you change it?

Step 6: Creating Connections (i.e., Metaphors) and "In-Sight"
   What connections (parallels) do you see between your original image that you explored and the original situation?

Step 7: Healing Metaphors: Applying the Changed Image to the Current Situation
   How might the way you changed the image apply to your current situation?

Note: You should have these steps in front of you when you use this intervention with clients.

have difficulty "paying" attention to the content of the conversation. With practice, this stage yields to the final stage, when you can note and quickly jot down psychologically relevant metaphors while continuing to track and respond to the topic and content of the conversation.

How to Select a Metaphor

Several factors play an especially important role in determining which of the many metaphors you hear is the best to explore in therapy.

1. Clinical experience and knowledge of the client guide the therapist in choosing metaphors that convey key issues and core dynamics unique to the client.

2. Metaphors that include a representation of self, such as "I feel like I'm hitting my head against a wall," "I feel like I am walking on eggshells," or "I feel like I'm sinking in quicksand," are more helpful than metaphors that represent only the situation, like "Life is a jungle," or only others, such as "He's a snake in the grass." If a metaphor in which the self is not represented seems significant, the therapist can begin by asking the client to create a metaphoric image that represents the client in relation to the situation or to the other. For example, in the case of a client who said that her husband "barges into the house like a locomotive," the therapist asked her, "If your husband is a locomotive, how do you picture yourself?" After some thought, the client said, "I guess I'm the tunnel." One might be tempted to interpret this metaphor, but doing so would shift the focus away from the client's subjective imagery and disrupt the client's inner exploration and discovery. Also, theoretical interpretations (e.g., the locomotive represents a phallus and the tunnel a vagina) replace the client's personal metaphoric representations with metaphoric representations rooted in the symbolic language of the theory. By staying with the client's metaphoric image, and avoiding the temptation to interpret, the therapist can now continue the intervention with Phase III, Step 2 in the protocol.

3. Metaphors expressing a client's wish or desire should be avoided because they do not represent the client's view of the current situation or problem. Such metaphors invariably suggest an ideal state which is not attainable. Also, metaphors that express what the client does *not* want are not usually productive. For example, "I wish my mother would boost me up" expresses what the client's mother isn't doing. Since the client cannot control her mother's behavior, exploring and transforming this metaphor is unlikely to lead to productive insight or change in the client's relationship with her mother.

4. Expressions like "I can't seem to get a handle on things" are not good candidates for exploration and transformation because they represent what the client is not able to do. Asking "What is it like for you when you can't get a handle on things?" may help the client describe what he or she *is* experiencing.

Steps 2–4 in Phase III isolate the metaphor from the surrounding sentence in which it appears and help the client shift from the actual situation to the metaphoric image. The therapist knows that the client has entered the domain of creative imagination when the client associates new imagery with the metaphor. If the client continues to talk about the actual situation and the actual people involved in their current issue, the therapist continues helping the client shift his or her attention and cognitive process from *description* to *depiction*, that is, from describing the problem to creating new imagery associated with the metaphoric image.

Step 5 invites the client to use his or her creative imagination to change the metaphoric story. The question must be asked in the open-ended format stated in the protocol. Therapists learning this technique must be vigilant lest they allow their own projections and imagery to leak into their questions. Doing so would derail the process and disrupt the client's flow of inner imagery. For example, a client told her therapist that she felt like she was sinking in quicksand. Instead of asking the client to describe what image came to mind as she pictured herself sinking in quicksand, the therapist asked, "How deep is the quicksand?" thus inadvertently projecting her own concerns. This required the client to think about the depth of the quicksand, and interrupted the client's inner exploration and elaboration of her metaphor.

Step 6 invites the client to create metaphoric connections between the metaphoric images and the current issue or problem. The client creates a new metaphor each time he or she creates a connection (resemblance) between an image created when exploring the metaphor and an aspect of the current life situation.

Finally, in Step 7, the client explores how his or her changed metaphor story might offer new meanings, directions, actions, and solutions regarding the actual problem or issue.

METAPHOR THERAPY AND DIVERSITY

Developing therapeutic approaches that are responsive to race, ethnicity, sexual orientation, and gender have gained increasing importance. Therapists' knowledge of characteristics typical of various large cultural and ethnic groups may or may not impact the outcome of psychotherapy (Sue & Zane, 1987). The meanings of ethnicity are more important than ethnicity itself because they are more likely to influence therapy outcomes (Sue, 1988). Thus, a client's problems must be understood by the therapist in a manner that is congruent with the client's belief system (Sue & Zane, 1987). Exploring and transforming client-generated metaphors help both therapist and client expand and deepen their understanding of the client's subjective experience and organizing principles (Stolorow & Atwood, 1992).

Dwairy (1997) suggests that therapists who have adopted traditional western beliefs and who work with nonwestern clients need to develop intervention techniques that fit their clients' metaphoric-physical language characteristics of nonwestern cultures that have a non–dualistic, holistic view of reality. Dwairy uses metaphor therapy methods described here. He concludes that this type of metaphoric work influences the mind-body system and helps clients from nonwestern cultures find solutions within their own sociocultural beliefs.

The two case examples described below were conducted by two third-year graduate students enrolled in my course on metaphor therapy at the California School of Professional Psychology at Alliant International University. The therapy took place in each student's clinical internship. Students in the class participate in a sequence of learning experiences: (1) reading *Metaphor Therapy: Using Client-Generated Metaphors in Psychotherapy* (Kopp, 1995), (2) reading case examples, (3) observing the instructor's in-class, unrehearsed demonstration of using the protocol with a student volunteer, (4) a "coached role-play" in which the instructor coaches a volunteer student "therapist" using the protocol with a volunteer student "client," and (5) three weeks of experiential learning using the protocol in which students, in groups of three, rotate playing the roles of therapist, client, and observer.

"AN EMPTY SADNESS": CASE EXAMPLE #1

Presenting Problem

Barbara is a 30-year-old woman who reported experiencing multiple losses resulting from a breakup with her boyfriend of five years. She described being extremely depressed after the breakup. She said she was now determined to change this pattern. Her *Diagnostic and Statistical Manual* (*DSM-IV*) diagnosis was Major Depressive Disorder, Recurrent, Severe without Psychotic Features (American Psychiatric Association, 2000). Her symptoms included sadness most of the day, every day; loss of appetite; insomnia; fatigue and loss of energy; and feelings of worthlessness.

Goals

The client and therapist agreed on three goals of treatment: (1) decreasing her depressive symptoms, (2) recognizing and understanding her relationship problems, and (3) increasing her self-esteem. Therapy was provided on a sliding fee scale at a nonprofit outpatient mental health center.

Phase I: Moving from General to Personal

At the beginning of our tenth session, Barbara was talking about her relationship difficulties. I asked her what part of it is the most difficult for her. She replied, "It's difficult to believe someone is really going to love me."

Phase II: Moving from Facts to Feelings

I asked, "What's this like for you, how do you feel?"
    Barbara responded, "Sad."

Phase III: Exploring and Transforming Client Metaphors

Step 1: Noticing Metaphors

She then said, "I feel empty. It's an empty sadness." She did not say anything else, and the sadness showed in her face, so I chose this metaphor to explore.

Step 2: Focusing on the Metaphor Image

I said, "When you say 'empty,' what image comes to mind . . . what do you see in your mind's eye?"
    She replied, "Dark. Black. Just dark. There's nothing there. Everything's dark." She began to cry.

I was unsure where she was in the image, so I asked, "Where are you?"

She said, "It's inside my body. All I see is dark inside. No emotion. Hollow." I waited to see if she would elaborate, but she sat quietly.

Step 3: Exploring the Metaphor as a Sensory Image

"What else do you see?" I continued.

Her response was, "I'm crying . . . wanting love."

I asked, "What else is going on?"

She stopped describing her image and began to talk about how the men in her life did not ever really love her. As the effectiveness of this technique requires that the therapist keep the client's focus on the imagery and not on the current "real" life situation, I said, "Let me bring you back to the image you just described, the dark, the 'dark inside.' What else is going on in this image you see?"

She said, "All I see is dark. There's nothing." So I asked if there was anything else, to which she said no.

Step 4: Feelings Associated with the Metaphoric Image

I ventured, "What's it like to be dark inside?"

Crying a little harder, Barbara said, "You feel nothing. No senses. Like you can't see anything, or hear anything. There's nothing." I paused to give her time to say more, and then, after a moment of silence, moved on to the next step.

Step 5: Changing the Metaphor Image

I said, "If you could change the image in any way, how would you change it?"

Still teary, she said, "Lots of light. Bright light. All around me. It's everywhere."

She paused, so I asked, "Anything else?"

"There are arms around me, giving me hugs. They're not attached to anyone, just arms. I see the words *I love you* . . . and I'm smiling." I asked if there was anything else, and she said no.

Step 6: Creating Connections (i.e., Metaphors) and "In-Sight"

I asked, "What connections do you see between your original image of the dark and your difficulty believing someone's really going to love you?"

Barbara replied, "I portray it on them. I show them the glass half empty, not half full. I push them away to not love me. I give them too much power and control—to determine my happiness. [The rest was spoken through heavy sobs.] It's too hard of a fall. Like at the top of a roller coaster, straight down." I gave her time to cry before moving on.

Step 7: Healing Metaphors: Applying the Changed Image to the Current Situation

When I asked the final question, "How might the way you changed the image apply to your difficulty believing someone's going to love you?" she continued to talk about her roller coaster metaphor, so I emphasized the changed image and repeated her words back to her. She struggled with this step because she felt she should be at the point of the changed image, "But I'm not there yet, that isn't me yet." Once I reassured her that it did not matter, all she was doing was making connections, she was able to continue.

"I don't love them as much as they love me. [Crying again] I can't love anything right now. [Gasp of realization, eyes widening] I don't feel like I could love someone. There's just nothing there. It's been drained out of me." She continued to shake her head in bewilderment and talked about how she had gotten to this point of feeling she could not love someone.

Results

In the Session

This intervention had a clear impact on the client. She began crying with the visualization of her metaphor, and at one point could not talk through the sobs. She gasped with realization, and her eyes widened as she formed connections and gained understanding about herself. At the end, she kept shaking her head, saying, "wow!" I acknowledged that it was a powerful process, and she gave an enthusiastic "yeah!" Prior to this intervention she had been focused on her fear that no one would love her and her question of how she could tell if a guy truly loved her. Now she was exploring her ability to let go and love another, to be vulnerable and trusting.

In Subsequent Therapy

Barbara has reported that she knew these things about herself but that nothing really "sank in" until this intervention, which helped her realize how the men in her life are similar to her abusive mother. She has begun to understand how her childhood has impacted her adult relationships, and what her role in that process has been. She also noted that she needs to forgive her mother, not for her mother's sake, but for her own.

The atmosphere in the room seems lighter, as if a weight has been lifted. Barbara feels she has accomplished something significant. I also experience a stronger therapeutic bond between us.

Although Barbara was often insightful, she seemed to struggle with connecting her childhood experiences with her adult life patterns. Exploring her metaphor enabled her to make these connections, and her self-esteem has increased. She is now actively exploring ways to love, such as being a "cuddler" for the newborn babies at a hospital where volunteers hold babies in the nursery who are unable to be held enough by the mothers and fathers.

"I'M THE ONE WHO BLEW UP": CASE EXAMPLE #2

Presenting Problem

Tom is a 37-year-old male who has been in treatment for three months. He presented with symptoms of depression (depressed mood, anhedonia, decreased appetite, insomnia, and fatigue) that began six weeks prior to intake, and "lifelong" feelings of hostility and anger. He was given a diagnosis of Major Depressive Disorder (moderate, single episode; American Psychiatric Association, 2000) and has been taking 10mg of Lexapro daily.

Goals

The treatment goals are: to (1) improve the ability to cope with current emotional and financial crisis, (2) explore early developmental history and how current coping skills and defenses may have emerged, (3) increase feelings of connection with others, (4) improve interpersonal relationships, and (5) reduce inner conflict.

Phase I: Movement from General to Personal

Tom began the session by saying, "So last week I was telling you about my friend Greg and how I'm uncomfortable accepting money from him for the work I'm doing for him. We've worked together before when he asked me to do him a favor and work with him without getting paid. It felt really awkward, so I got up in the middle and left because I felt it was really inappropriate. We had a big fight in the hallway. I felt like I was getting screwed over. I was completely taken aback and mad. I couldn't believe he would actually do that."

"So how does this history between you two affect what's happening now?" I asked.

"It brings up the same feelings basically. I don't want to . . . I feel guilty on some level. I feel like I've done something wrong," replied Tom.

"Those sound like different feelings," I reflected.

"Well, I feel like I didn't handle it well, that I should have done something different in the hallway. It feels awkward and complicated, too complicated. I keep replaying it in my head. I'm getting worried about it. It feels too heavy, much heavier than it should be, I guess. I feel like the complication is coming from me and I'm not sure how to move forward and handle the situation."

I echoed, "It feels so heavy."

"Yeah," said Tom.

"What other feelings come up?"

"Guilt," he responded. "I feel guilt for when he was working on that project and he asked me for help. I never handled it the way I feel I should have. I chose not to be honest about the whole thing and instead I pushed it to a situation where it just blew up in the hallway. So I feel guilty about it."

Being somewhat directive here, because the client wanted to stay in this past event instead of discussing his current problem, I asked, "So in your current situation . . . ?"

Tom answered, "So now I don't want to take money from him because of what happened. I feel like he doesn't owe me anything and I owe him a lot. I'm the one that blew up even though he did do something inappropriate. And I used it to stop being friends with him, the final straw. It was like I was collecting evidence as to why he shouldn't be my friend even though I'm the one that blew up."

Phase II: Movement from Facts to Feelings

"What did it feel like when you blew up?"

"I was furious," he said. "I felt like I was better than him and better than what he had written and that the project was stupid. I was so angry."

Phase III: Exploring and Transforming Client Metaphors

Steps 1 and 2: Noticing Metaphors and Exploring the Metaphoric Image

Seeking to explore the metaphor further, I asked, "So when you say 'blew up' what image comes to mind?"

Tom spontaneously moved on to Steps 3 and 4, creating the following story using a series of metaphoric images. "When I think of blowing up I see a big explosion, something just being completely obliterated. I see a wooden box on the ground," he said, laughing and appearing uncomfortable. "It's outside and lit up, like there's a spotlight on it. People are watching it. I can't actually see any people but there's just a sense that they're there. It feels like it's at an old dirt track . . . a racetrack with a light on it."

Step 5: Changing the Metaphor Image

I could have invited Tom to explore these images further but chose instead to ask how he might change the image. "If you could change the image in any way, how would you change it?"

"It wouldn't blow up," he answered. "The people wouldn't be watching. Also, I'd change the surroundings so that the box is in the forest. It's green and calm. There's a brook. It's small, gurgling. The box is the same. It's just not being watched. It's not under pressure to do anything."

Step 6: Creating Connections (i.e., Metaphors) and "In-Sight"

"What parallels do you see between your original image and your current situation with Greg?" I inquired.

"It feels like the same pressure because it feels like a test. Like a test to see if we can work together again," answered Tom. "I feel like I'm being watched, like it's a performance."

Step 7: Healing Metaphors: Applying the Changed Image to the Current Situation

Seeking to help Tom apply the changes, I asked, "How might the way you changed the image apply to your current situation?"

"To feel more supported and not to have so much pressure on me. I don't want this all to be on me. The box in the other image becomes part of the forest. It's like the box belongs there. It's just comfortable there."

"What does this mean in relation to your current situation?" I pressed.

"I could tell Greg my fear that there was too much pressure on me before because he asked me to do too much work for him. Before, I could never express my feelings and it would lead to me just blowing up."

Results

In the Session

Once we completed the intervention, Tom immediately commented on the sensation he experienced while he saw the original image in his mind. He stated, "I felt like I had no legs, it was the weirdest sensation. It was so bizarre." He described feeling as if his whole body consisted only of his torso.

I had never observed Tom to be as calm and introspective as he was in this moment immediately following the intervention.

We discussed how the fear in his current situation and in the metaphor was the anticipation of the explosion, not the explosion itself. He stated that he realized the important part for him wasn't even the anticipation of the explosion but the audience, the sense of being watched. He felt the intervention was really helpful in understanding that he wants to feel a part of the work with Greg, as opposed to Greg telling him to do all the work and then monitoring and scrutinizing him.

It is interesting how his exploration in his imagination revealed, or brought into consciousness, central issues that were lurking behind his verbalized, conscious concerns. I remarked that the "explosion" that happened in the past seemed to emerge from not feeling connected to others and from being under a spotlight and being judged. The rest of the session centered around discussing how people feel a part of their environment by expressing their hopes and fears and how expressing himself could be more rewarding for him.

In the Client's Life and Relationships and Subsequent Therapy

In the next session, Tom reported speaking to Greg about his remorse over the past incident and how it left him feeling anxious about working together again. He was able to set appropriate boundaries about what he felt comfortable taking on in their upcoming work together. He felt relieved by their discussion and believed that Greg understood how he felt.

The intervention helped Tom move toward several therapy goals: improving his ability to cope with his current emotional crisis, increasing his feeling of connection with others, improving interpersonal relationships, and reducing inner conflict. The goals of coping with his current financial crisis and exploring his early developmental history were not directly addressed.

CONCLUSION

These case examples highlight the importance of the client's shift from a verbal/descriptive/logical/mainly secondary process representation of a current issue or conflict to an imaginal/pictorial/predominantly primary process representation that reveals and brings underlying dynamics into focus and encourages clients to initiate action to resolve their problems.

1. The author would like to thank Deanna Guerrero, who was the therapist in the case example of Barbara ("An Empty Sadness"), and Heather Demeter, who was the therapist in the case example of Tom ("I'm the One Who Blew Up").

REFERENCES

American Psychiatric Association. (2000). *Diagnostic and statistical manual of mental disorders* (4th ed., text rev.). Washington, DC: Author.

Boles, P. D. (1984). *Story-crafting: A master storyteller teaches the art and craft of writing fine short stories.* Cincinnati, OH: Writers Digest Books.

Dwairy, M. (1997). A biopsychosocial model of metaphor therapy with holistic cultures. *Clinical Psychology Review, 17,* 719–732.

Freud, S. (1960). *The ego and the id* (I. Riviere, Trans., J. Strachey, Ed.). New York: Norton. (Original work published 1923)

Kopp, R. (1995). *Metaphor therapy: Using client-generated metaphors in psychotherapy.* New York: Brunner/Routledge/Taylor & Francis.

Lakoff, G., & Johnson, M. (1980). *Metaphors we live by.* Chicago: University of Chicago Press.

Siegel, D. (1999). *The developing mind.* New York: Guilford Press.

Stolorow, R., & Atwood, G. (1992). *Contexts of being: The intersubjective foundations of psychological life.* Hillsdale, NJ: Analytic Press.

Sue, S. (1988). Psychotherapeutic services for ethnic minorities: Two decades of research findings. *American Psychologist, 43,* 301–308.

Sue, S., & Zane, N. (1987). The role of culture and cultural techniques in psychotherapy: A critique and reformulation. *American Psychologist, 42,* 37–45.

CHAPTER 4

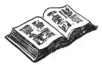 And This Little Piggy Stayed Home

Playful Metaphors in Treating Childhood
Separation Anxiety

Julie H. Linden

CONTRIBUTOR'S STORY:
A PROFESSIONAL AND PERSONAL PERSPECTIVE

Julie Linden, PhD, is a psychologist in private practice, specializing in children of all ages. She has worked in various hospital settings, developing and expanding her expertise to utilize hypnosis, guided imagery, and play therapy with children suffering from pain, trauma, and chronic illnesses. She has also volunteered psychological services on Acute and Posttraumatic Stress Disorders and conflict resolution to student refugees from the Balkan war.

Julie is the 2006–2007 president of the American Society of Clinical Hypnosis (ASCH), associate editor of *Psychological Hypnosis* (published by the American Psychological Association), recipient of the 1993 Special Award from ASCH "for promoting the greater involvement of women in teaching and leadership and for facilitating sensitivity to women's issues," and recipient of the 2003 Josephine Hilgard Award from the *American Journal of Clinical Hypnosis* for her paper "Playful Metaphors."

When at play outside the office, Julie can be found creatively cooking in the kitchen, snowshoeing in the mountains, and traveling around the globe in pursuit of new metaphors for her work.

PREVIEW THE CHAPTER

"I do not just do play therapy; I do therapy that is full of play," says Julie of her work, and in this chapter she sets out to show us how that may be done. Using the example of the case of an eight-year-old child, Emily, with separation anxiety, limited peer relationships, and thumb sucking, Julie describes the clinical framework from which she operates and the learning and developmental benefits of using play and playfulness in therapy. Focusing on the dissociation induced by play, metaphors, and playful metaphors, she carefully employs language to facilitate change. In this case, we have the opportunity to observe how a therapist can join the child in his or her world, incorporate the child's toys, and build a collaborative metaphoric process of therapy through an object such as a doll. Here you will not find a story that is told as a single tale from the beginning through the middle to the end. Instead, Emily's doll matches the child's problems, develops the resources for individuation, evolves with the client, and communicates the therapeutic interventions. "At some level," says Julie, "all of play therapy is metaphorical work."

Therapeutic Characteristics

Problems Addressed

- Anxiety
- Separation anxiety
- Parent-child relationships
- Limited peer relationships
- Thumb sucking

Resources Developed

- Understanding how to make things happen
- Learning to make choices
- Taking control
- Learning to relax
- Developing playful learning
- Enhancing positive relationships
- Enhancing pleasurable experiences

Outcomes Offered

- Reduced anxiety
- Greater independence
- New friendships
- Freedom from thumb sucking

This is a story about Emily, a vivacious, talented eight-year-old. When I first met Emily I was struck by her wonderful red-brown curly hair, which hung in a long braid down her back. She was comfortably dressed in corduroys and clogs, and her tee shirt blazed with sparkles that matched her smile and seemed to say, "watch out world, here I come." I was sure I was meeting a future performer. The presence that Emily exuded surprised me, since it did not fit with the way her parents had described her.

Emily's parents initially consulted me, without Emily, because of concerns that their daughter was showing excessive signs of anxiety. Her mother said over the phone, "I don't know if this is to help me manage my daughter better, or for Emily to help reduce her fears." Her parents appeared to be young, bright, highly energetic individuals who live a very full life. Her father was a medical doctor, her mother a stay-at-home mom who enjoyed sports and was physically active. Emily had a younger brother, age six. The parents reported that Emily had always appeared to be highly sensitive. She didn't like loud noises, was particular about the texture of clothing, was a very finicky eater, and never liked to be separated from her mother. At age seven, during her second year of grade school, she went to a clinic to learn ways to reduce anxiety. Her mother reported that this was helpful, but now, eight months later, the old anxious behaviors had returned.

During the history taking, the parents mentioned that Emily still sucked her thumb at night, saying it soothed her but also embarrassed her. She did not want her friends to see that habit. Her parents reported that she had "major meltdowns," at which times she went to her room. They would just let the meltdowns happen and not engage with her. The only significant item reported in the extended family was that her father said he had "little worries" (a sleeping problem and a bleeding ulcer when he was unhappy at his job).

Both parents had many things to say about what they liked about their daughter—a question I like to ask parents. This helps to assess the perceived strengths of the child as well as the level of attunement the parents have to their offspring. They described her as sweet, smart, full of depth when conversing; fun to be with when she was happy and not determined to have her way (she could be unflinchingly demanding); and with an amazing singing voice. What they didn't like was her fearfulness and stubborn refusal to try new things. Both parents felt they had a good relationship with Emily.

The reason for the timing of seeking help for Emily was that the family was anticipating a ski vacation, and her mother knew that it would be hard to ski because Emily would want to be with her, and would not be open to taking lessons with other children. This was not presented as a narcissistic need but with what seemed to be a real wish for her daughter to enjoy herself and learn more skills in skiing. Emily was described as quite competent on the slopes.

A CLINICAL FRAMEWORK

Before proceeding with the story of Emily, I would like to briefly outline the framework I use for my clinical work. Over many years I have developed a style of therapy that incorporates several principles. The first of these is that healthy relationships are healing. They are nurturing, safe, and supportive. The literature on attachment has reinforced how important the infant's early relationships are to development (James, 1994). Relationships are not limited to those with *real* people. The child's inner world is a community of archetypes (Kalsched, 1996), each one potentially available for the child's healthy ego development, a resource within. As you will see in the story that follows, Emily owned some favorite dolls, and each one represented a part of her developing personality traits. One was the archetype of the caregiver; another was the archetype of determination and independence.

My second principle is that the source of all human suffering is some kind of trauma. This is a bold assertion and requires some explanation. Many people prefer to reserve the use of the word *trauma* for very big events in a human's life, such as the decimation of a town by a hurricane or the loss of family in a serious car accident. I, on the other hand, prefer the definition that trauma is the emotional response to both the sudden cessation of human interaction and the meaning we give to an event (Gil, 1998; Lindemann, 1944). The process, context, and depth of trauma also affect both the meaning we give it and the outcome of the trauma (Linley, 2003). For example, if Emily had lost her mommy in the supermarket she might have been *traumatized* by that experience. She might say that she believed mommy was gone forever, that there would be nobody to take care of her, and that it was the end of her life.

In fact, at a young age Emily had lost a caregiver to whom she had been quite close. Sound dramatic? Yes. But treatment of adults who recount their childhood fears, nightmares, and worries has taught me that even the incidents that seem smallest from the adult perspective look quite different from the child's perspective. The meaning we give to a highly emotional event in our lives and the impact of that highly charged event on our nervous system determine whether we experience it as traumatic. The developmental stage at which a trauma occurs is critically important. Infants, we assume, do not have the same "meaning-making" apparatus as a toddler, a five-year-old, or an adult, so the developmental stage of a person is extremely important to the way in which an event is processed and becomes traumatic.

Most of the literature on trauma agrees that the particular sensitivity of the individual's nervous system, as well as the environmental context in which we grow up, may increase or decrease our vulnerability to an event (Herman, 1992; Perry, 2000; Pynoos, 1994; Van der Kolk, 1987). Parents, family, community, and society all have an influence on our experience and interpretation of what we call traumatic (Bloom & Reichert, 1998; Bonnano, 2004; Self-Brown, LeBlanc, & Kelley, 2004). So what is traumatic for one child may have no effect on another.

Third, dissociation is both the source of our suffering and the resource for our healing. Dissociation is the process by which we remove ourselves from painful, discomforting feelings and experiences (Cardeña, 2000; Putnam, 1997). We distance through repression, suppression, and denial. We can repress feelings, suppress thoughts and behavior, and deny that an experience ever happened. The numbing of affect, the removal from our sensory experiences, and depersonalization are all normal dissociative symptoms that the mind and body exhibit in the face of trauma. These symptoms, which are useful in the short term for helping us to manage a traumatic experience, may become harmful in the long term.

When I first met Emily I watched her push away her anxiety by suppressing tears. Some minutes later she complained of a tummy ache. I asked her if she knew what had caused the upset stomach. She had no idea. She was unaware that there might be a connection between the suppressed tears and the now painful tummy. Observing this dissociation, I saw both strength in her ability to remove herself from discomfort (in this case the tears) and the liability that comes when emotions end up in tense muscles. I had a hunch her thumb sucking was a similar dissociative mechanism, a way her psychological upsets were transformed into bodily movements rather than the release of words.

A FAMILY OF PORCUPINES

After the initial information gathering with Emily's parents my clinical picture was one of a stay-at-home gal, "joined at the hip" to mom, and consequently separation anxiety was the working diagnosis. I was already thinking metaphorically about how to turn being close to someone into a positive and mastery-filled experience for Emily. Being close can be loving, caretaking, warm, and nurturing. Emily's closeness to mom was all those things, but it also left her feeling afraid to venture out on her own. I trusted that some metaphor would emerge if I watched the images that floated through my mind, and very soon I found myself thinking about an example of a family of porcupines. They huddle together for closeness but don't get too close, lest someone be hurt by the quills (M. Linden, n.d.). I knew I would look for places in Emily's life where she was "close," but not so close that she was getting hurt, and for places where she was in charge.

The metaphor of the porcupine is one I had learned in my youth and had always connected to psychological issues of closeness or separation. I often tell it to clients who are dealing with issues of separation or independence. In Emily's case, her world of dolls was a similar metaphor, and I chose to work just with that since I have found the client's personal metaphors to be far more effective and evocative than those I introduce.

At the second session, I met Emily for the first time. Her mother was unsure how she would get Emily to the session, believing that Emily's fears would emerge and she would fight doing anything new. I had instructed her to remind Emily of how the previous work at the anxiety clinic had helped her. This was an implicit suggestion that because something had helped before, something could help again. Our use of language is critical in treatment. I had also asked her mother *not* to do anything different, and to allow me the opportunity to observe the separation behaviors she was worried about.

I greeted Emily at the door to my office. She immediately threw her arms around her mother and clung to her. After I introduced myself I told her to hang on tightly to mom so she wouldn't lose her when entering my office. Emily looked at me as though I was strange and pulled mom into the office. This was a suggestion that she had control over the behavior; if she controlled holding on, she also controlled letting go. The strange look told me she was surprised, I had captured her attention, and she was open to suggestion.

She sat on the sofa so close to her mom that she looked like she was trying to crawl back into the womb. I said, "It's good you are sitting so close to mom; that way you won't lose her until you are ready to have her leave the room." Again, she looked at me strangely and held her mom closer. Her mother didn't like this and told her it was too tight, and Emily softened her hold. This brief initial encounter established that Emily was in charge of her own change, but not in charge of her mother. It also left open the suggestion that she would at some point be ready to let her mom leave the room. As we discussed why Emily was here and her relationships at home, she described her father as "ferocious," which really surprised her mother. Emily's mother said he could be a little prickly, but she had no idea why her daughter used such an evocative word. Again, I thought about porcupines. They can be prickly creatures when they are too close. I inferred that Emily understood at some level that the closeness was hurting her.

When there is a discrepancy in perception such as this, it is often a projection. I guessed that Emily was communicating to me that the way her mother handled things was different from the way her father handled things. I stored this away for future exploration. When Emily was leaving her first meeting with me, I wondered out loud if she would be ready the next time she came to leave her mom outside of the office part of the time. This suggestion was meant to motivate her, to embed a suggestion that it was just a matter of time, and that she could titrate the separating, do it a little at a time.

PLAY AND PLAYFUL THERAPY

Play, for children, may be thought of as a form of dissociation. It is characterized by absorption in the sensory, imaginal, or emotional experience. At play a child may be firmly and happily in the moment. Conversely, play can provide a way to escape the moment, the body, the emotions, and/or the thoughts. The child can use play to create an inner world that is safer or better than the outside world. Or the child can get locked into posttraumatic play that is repetitive or compulsive and fails to relieve anxiety (Gil, 1998). It is because of the importance of dissociation in my thinking that I have found working metaphorically, with *playful* metaphors (J. Linden, 2003), to be so valuable in therapy. I do not just do play therapy; I do therapy that is full of play (J. Linden, 1996).

My work with children is through their play, because I see play as metaphoric in itself. The careful choice of language in therapy is timed to match their absorbed states of concentration. This is when the unconscious is most likely to accept the suggestions for change hidden in the metaphors (J. Linden, 2003).

There are many functions that normal play provides for children (Schaefer & O'Connor, 1983). First, there is the biological function. Play is a way to relax, to release energy, to exercise, and to learn basic skills. Swinging and climbing, biking and running, jumping rope and wrestling with playmates are common forms of play. Emily, as I was to discover, liked to horseback ride and ski.

A second function is the intrapersonal. Through play the child develops and explores the mind-body connection, learns mastery of situations, and learns mastery of conflicts through internal symbolism, fantasy, imaginings, and wish fulfillment. Daydreams and imaginary friends are the mind's creative pathways for emotional development. My awareness of this fact enabled me to utilize a doll Emily called M to facilitate her creative development in managing the anxiety of separation.

Third, the interpersonal function of play fosters the development of social skills, the development of identity, and ultimately the important achievement of separation–individuation. Because separation and individuation were indeed the very therapeutic goals we had for Emily, it seemed appropriate to utilize and develop this interpersonal function of play with her. Because make-believe and pretend play with playmates, board games, and team sports all provide opportunities for learning the rules of social interactions, I also employed some of these forms of play as interventions with Emily.

Finally, play functions to teach the sociocultural schemas wherein children learn the desired roles for their particular culture. This is often through imitative play, such as playing house, detectives, or combat, or, for older children, being actors in a theatrical production. Normal play sometimes is not enough for healthy development. *How* we come into the world (the genetics and temperament the child brings), *where* (the sociocultural context), and into *what* situation (the psychodynamic context) may either assist children to develop to their potential or put them at risk of less than optimal development. Therapeutic play can help children to heal from whatever interruptions they have experienced in their development.

In *playful* therapy, dissociation can be recreated. It can be used to assess the nature of the trauma experience. And it can also be used to create a new pathway to the nervous system, to the unconscious where resources can be mobilized for healing (Perry, 2000). When we are in deep concentration, absorbed attentionally, we are more open to suggestion. Whether our parents are yelling and telling us what a failure we are (a negative suggestion) or our teachers are telling us what a good reader we are (a positive suggestion), how we take in suggestions depends on the state of mind we are in. I refer to the absorbed state of mind, a kind of dissociative state, as the place where suggestions can do their damage or do their healing. Thus, a goal of my work is to identify or induce this state of mind and utilize it therapeutically. I work with metaphors most of the time because direct talk with the conscious mind rarely produces results (Anbar, 2001; LeBaron & Hilgard, 1984). Just suggest to someone that they stop a behavior that is dangerous to their health, like smoking, overeating, or drinking, and you know what happens: nothing. However, when we work metaphorically, we often bypass the conscious thoughts and behaviors, activate the imaginative part of the brain, and unearth inner resources. In the case of Emily, you will see each of these principles at work.

FINDING STRENGTHS AND EXCEPTIONS

Wanting to learn more about Emily's relationship with her father, I asked her if she would bring her ferocious father with her for the next session. She smiled. That indicated to me that she felt I had heard her, and that maybe her dad was not all that ferocious. Unlike with her mother, Emily was not holding on to her father when she came to the office, and I was not sure if this was because she knew he was coming in and they would not be separated or because she typically behaved differently with him than with her mother. Together we played a board game, called Trouble, which Emily chose. Board games provide a number of therapeutic functions. First, they can offer a window into the social interactions of children, and in this case into family interactions. Second, the particular game a child chooses also provides a clue to his or her unconscious thinking. Third, the name of the game and the style in which it is played (e.g., competitive, strategizing, etc.) can both have psychodynamic significance. Finally, board games can teach developmental skills as the child experiences being in charge and having control when permitted to choose the game. Emily's attention to the game was erratic. She was easily distracted when it was not her turn, but it was clear she liked to win and was highly competitive.

Her dad received a cell phone call and left the room. Emily showed no sign that this was uncomfortable for her. In fact, she acted as if this happened all the time and returned to the game.

I asked her, "How did you do that?"

"Do what?" she asked.

"Stay in the room without dad being here."

"I don't know," she said, once again with that strange look.

My reasons for this interchange was to give the implicit suggestion that she had strengths and had control over her separation behaviors. I asked her if it made her nervous, and how she knew when she was nervous. She said she could be nervous, she could get tummy aches and could have throwing-up tummy aches. I asked how they were different and learned there was a hierarchy to her affective responses. Meeting me for the first time caused nervousness, a relatively small thing.

Starting school on the first day was bigger; it caused tummy aches. And going away on vacation to a strange place, especially if she would be separated from her mother for any length of time, caused throwing-up tummy aches. She was feeling none of that. The only trouble that day was the game. Meanwhile I was concluding that Emily's dynamics with her mother and vice versa were somehow feeding her anxious behaviors.

Emily arrived at the third session with a new doll she simply called M. She had just gotten the doll that day, and it was a gift for agreeing to see me. While I had been unaware of that deal, it provided an opportunity to use M and Emily's relationship with her metaphorically. First, it seemed to me that the doll was full of transference power since it was intimately connected with her being in treatment with me. Second, Emily was engrossed with her doll. She combed its hair, played with the doll's pet cat, and held the doll the whole session. Several times while we talked she whispered to the doll, rather than answering me. Third, the way in which Emily was relating to M exhibited certain information about her experience of closeness. The doll was at times receiving abundant loving attention from Emily and at other times was held as if it was an ignored appendage, just something that was there but disregarded, like traces of food around a child's mouth that she doesn't bother to lick away. As a result, I imagined Emily's relationship with the doll would both inform me about what she needed to be less fearful and provide the metaphoric avenue for her to practice being more confident and less anxious.

She had arranged that her mom would spend half the time in the session with her and wait outside during the other half. I knew that her internal attention would be on when that separation would take place, so I asked Emily to watch the clock and tell me when half the session was over. This directed her anxious energy and gave her control. At the halfway mark, her mom got up to leave, and Emily let her go reluctantly with tons of kisses and hugs.

When her mother had left I asked, as I had with her father, "How'd you do that?" This is a strategy designed to draw children's attention to their self-efficacy, to show that they have, in fact, just accomplished something. I use it when I want to make them consciously aware of some behavior. It gets them thinking about how they did what they did. This process teaches self-reflection in a nonjudgmental manner.

She answered, "I don't know."

I countered, "Well, that would be a really interesting thing to know. It seems like the hugs and kisses help."

I then looked at her doll and asked M if she knew how Emily had done that. This playful engagement with her doll moved us into imaginary play, where the element of dissociation may permit a bridge to unconscious motives. Emily said, talking for the doll, "She just did it." I was impressed by this show of ego strength, and began to wonder how many of Emily's anxious behaviors had become empty habits, old patterns that no longer actually served the need they originally had. I talked further with the doll and told her how lucky she was to have such good mothering from Emily. "She brushes your hair so beautifully, and has picked out such a beautiful outfit for you to wear. And she really knows how to take care of your cat," I said, reiterating what I had observed. In this way Emily knew I was "listening" to her behavior and I was establishing Emily's role of caretaker/mother.

At the fourth session, Emily entered the room easily with her doll, after lots of hugs and kisses for her mother, and settled right in. I treat the toys that children bring as metaphoric representatives of some part of themselves, like an ego state but externalized onto an object. "Hello, M," I said to the doll, "so glad you came with Emily." I asked the doll if she was interested in learning some relaxation techniques that I was going to teach Emily, and told her she was to just follow along. I then taught Emily a simple imaging technique for relaxing the muscles in her body. I offered her a choice of imagery related to how she felt after vigorous activity in her favorite sports of horseback riding or skiing. It was the middle of winter, and Emily wasn't riding, so it was easier for her to think about skiing, which I had been hoping for.

I consider it important to provide choice, in order for a child to feel in control while making choices that move us in the direction of a positive outcome. Our goal at this time was to have Emily go skiing on the family vacation with confidence and without anxiety. She imagined herself just after skiing down a challenging slope, "but not the advanced one," she said. "I am not ready for that."

"Yet," I added.

A DOLL AS METAPHOR AND COTHERAPIST

When it was time to leave, and Emily was talking about what we could play with M next time, I knew she was now fully engaged in treatment, with M as my cotherapist. We had discussed whether Emily was taking M on her vacation, and I had strongly urged her to do so. "She will feel lonely if she stays at home by herself," I cajoled, "and she'll miss all the fun." I talked to this dissociated part of Emily by using M to metaphorically state the variety of thoughts that might be there. Then addressing M, I continued, "You know Emily can put you in a backpack so you can even ski down the slopes with her. I will be really interested in hearing all about your vacation when you return."

Two weeks later, Emily was back from her trip. M was also present. Her mother was very complimentary of Emily's success on the vacation. She had taken some ski lessons, had skied with her mother and cousins, and had had no meltdowns or tummy aches the entire vacation.

Emily came to the sixth session without M. Instead she was with her little brother and had a terrible time separating from her mother. She started fighting with her brother, who was patiently waiting for their mother to read to him. This time I began to see that some of her mother's behavior was ambiguous to Emily. She would accept all of the hugs and kisses and tell her it was time to go into the office, but show no nonverbal cues to do so, such as letting go of her. I was reminded of Emily's absentminded holding of her doll in an earlier session.

"Emily, you'll miss all of your play time with me if you spend it fighting with mom and your brother," I said. This was a message to both Emily and her mother. While her mother understood she was to forcefully separate, Emily had the carrot of playtime. Once in the office, she gravitated toward some new toys. Previously, she had been very constricted about exploring the playroom. This time she took out the doctor's kit, set up the toys to mimic a hospital, and had a little girl with a broken leg go through surgery. Emily's mother had had minor knee surgery some weeks prior to the ski trip, which may have accounted for Emily's choice of the leg injury. I decided that Emily was feeling somewhat broken that day, and she insisted that the little girl would need at least a week in the hospital before she was better. (That was the amount of time between our sessions.)

Before the seventh session I spoke with Emily's mom about how to separate from her with a clear message of her intentions, both verbally and nonverbally. The session allowed her to practice that, with mother separating lovingly but firmly and Emily separating easily.

"THANK YOU, M"

My clinical framework for therapy, which I discussed at the beginning of this story, has three principles: Healthy relationships are healing; the source of all human suffering is some kind of trauma; and dissociation is both the source of our suffering and the resource for our healing. I have illustrated these principles in my story about Emily and her dolls. Emily's relationship with me was a healthy one in which I was able to mirror for her the internal strengths she already exhibited in her preexisting relationships with her dolls and toys. This mirroring reinforced her healthy behaviors. While past traumas are often indeterminable with youngsters, it was clear that Emily's anxiety in new situations was in itself traumatic for her. She was motivated to feel better, to feel stronger, and to be more like her peers (as some of her dolls were). Her dissociation had caused her tummy aches and allowed her to project parts of herself onto her dolls, both strong parts and scared parts. Using the natural dissociation of play, I was able to build on the elements Emily gave me to work with—her relationships with her dolls, her peers, and her family—to help her create the perfect distance (and the perfect closeness) so that she grew strong and overcame much of her separation anxiety.

By the tenth session, both parents were reporting that overall Emily was much less anxious. She was eager to give up thumb sucking, and they had promised to get her ears pierced if she did. She had accomplished her ski trip and was working on going to friends' houses and developing a few new friendships. She had even agreed to go to a party and be left there without her mother. These were all terrific accomplishments in a relatively short time. She complained that her sleep had gotten worse when she couldn't find the stuffed toy she held while sucking her thumb, but decided that she was ready to stop so maybe it was a good thing that the toy was missing. I asked if M sucked her thumb. "No, she doesn't need to," was her reply.

When the metaphor has been established, it is easy to move between imaginary play and reality, checking for the readiness of the unconscious. I was confident that Emily was ready to give her thumb a new lease on life. She wanted to learn some more imagery techniques to help herself get to sleep. She did, and by the next session had stopped sucking her thumb and set the appointment for her ears to be pierced. She was exhibiting lots of strengths, had decided her dad was not ferocious anymore, and had decided that maybe visits with me could be removed from the list of "hard" things. I thought, "Thank you, M."

A POSTSCRIPT

While M was a central playful metaphor in Emily's therapy, interests, contexts, and themes can change rapidly in your work with children. Part of the art of the therapist is to adapt to those changes, utilize what your young client brings into therapy, and help shape that into a useful outcome-oriented metaphor. The skiing season passed, Emily resumed horseback riding, and our metaphorical work shifted to toy horses. M no longer attended sessions. Instead Emily constructed elaborate stables, equipped with horses and all of their gear. She gave pretend lessons to dolls, in effect teaching them to separate from parents, form new relationships (with their ponies), and develop a range of new skills. In our last session, her six-year-old brother asked me, in the way that kids often have of simply getting to the core of an issue, "How can *playing* with horses help you with your fears?" Responding to him, and conscious that both Emily and their mother were listening, I gave an answer that, on reflection, summarizes much about my concepts and approach to working with playful metaphors, and much about what I have hoped to communicate in the chapter. I replied, "The same way riding *real* horses helps you to be brave."

REFERENCES

Anbar, R. (2001). Automatic word processing: A new forum for hypnotic expression. *American Journal of Clinical Hypnosis, 44*(1), 27–36.

Bloom, S., & Reichert, M. (1998). *Bearing witness: Violence and collective responsibility.* Binghamton, NY: Haworth Press.

Bonanno, G. A. (2004). Loss, trauma, and human resilience: Have we underestimated the human capacity to thrive after extremely aversive events? *American Psychologist, 50*(1), 20–28.

Cardeña, E. (2000). Hypnosis in the treatment of trauma. *International Journal of Clinical and Experimental Hypnosis, 48*(2), 225–238.

Gil, E. (1998). *Play therapy for severe psychological trauma* [Videotape and manual]. New York: Guilford Press.

Herman, J. (1992). *Trauma and recovery.* New York: Basic Books.

James, B. (1994). *Handbook for the treatment of attachment-trauma problems in children.* New York: Free Press.

Kalsched, D. (1996). *The inner world of trauma: Archetypal defense of the personal spirit.* New York: Routledge.

LeBaron, S., & Hilgard, J. R. (1984). *Hypnotherapy of pain in children with cancer.* Los Altos, CA: William Kaufmann.

Lindemann, E. (1944). Symptomology and management of acute grief. *American Journal of Psychiatry, 101,* 141–148.

Linden, J. (1996). Trauma prevention: Hypnoidal techniques with the chronically ill child. In B. Peter, B. Trenkle, F. C. Kinzel, C. Duffner, & A. Isot-Pter (Eds.), *Munich lectures on hypnosis and psychotherapy* (pp. 15–26). Hypnosis International Monographs No. 2. Munich, Germany.

Linden, J. (2003). Playful metaphors. *American Journal of Clinical Hypnosis, 45*(3), 245–250.

Linden, M. (n.d.). *Lesson of the porcupine.* Retrieved August 27, 2005, from http://www.uwec.edu/counsel/pubs/lessonPorc.htm

Linley, A. (2003). Positive adaptation to trauma: Wisdom as both process and outcome. *Journal of Traumatic Stress, 16*(6), 601–610.

Perry, B. (2000). *Violence and childhood: How persisting fear can alter the developing child's brain.* Retrieved July 23, 2000, from http://www.childtrauma.org

Putnam, F. W. (1997). *Dissociation in children and adolescents: A developmental perspective.* New York: Guilford Press.

Pynoos, R. (1994). Traumatic stress and developmental psychopathology in children and adolescents. In R. Pynoos (Ed.), *Posttraumatic stress disorder: A clinical review* (pp. 65–98). Lutherville, MD: Sidran Press.

Self-Brown, S., LeBlanc, M., & Kelley, M. (2004). Effects of violence exposure and daily stressors on psychological outcomes in urban adolescents. *Journal of Traumatic Stress, 17*(6), 509–528.

Schaefer, C. E., & O'Connor, K. J. (Eds.). (1983). *Handbook of play therapy.* New York: Wiley.

Van der Kolk, B. (1987). *Psychological trauma.* Washington, DC: American Psychiatric Press.

CHAPTER 5

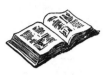

Climbing Anxiety Mountain

Generating Metaphors in Acceptance and Commitment Therapy

Mikaela J. Hildebrandt, Lindsay B. Fletcher, and Steven C. Hayes

CONTRIBUTORS' STORY:
A PROFESSIONAL AND PERSONAL PERSPECTIVE

Mikaela Hildebrandt is currently a doctoral student in clinical psychology at the University of Nevada, Reno. She uses metaphors clinically in acceptance and commitment therapy (ACT) and has always enjoyed parables and short stories, especially those that encourage individuals to live according to valued principles.

Lindsay Fletcher is a graduate student in clinical psychology at the University of Nevada, Reno, researching the efficacy of ACT for insomnia. Her interest is in how metaphors in therapy, like Zen koans and stories told in other Buddhist traditions, provide a way of using language to communicate concepts that transcend language.

Steven Hayes is foundation professor of psychology at the University of Nevada and author of 27 books and 360 scientific articles (see Resource Section). His career has focused on developing a new approach to the nature of human language and cognition, relational frame theory (RFT), and its application to the understanding and alleviation of human suffering, particularly through ACT, which is heavily based on the use of metaphor. He spends his days writing, teaching, researching, helping his students, answering e-mails, playing with his new baby, hanging out with his older children, and supporting the ACT and RFT work of others worldwide.

PREVIEW THE CHAPTER

A passionate mountain climber has become too anxious to climb, his enjoyment of life has given way to fear, and every reasonable effort he has made to control it has failed. In this case Steven Hayes was the therapist, while Mikaela Hildebrandt and Lindsay Fletcher are principal authors of the chapter. Together they describe the use of various metaphors in the framework of acceptance and commitment therapy (ACT). Claiming that metaphors transcend language and point clients to processes that cannot be fully explained using language, they walk us through the mindfulness processes of ACT and discuss the importance of integrating the client's values into the therapeutic agenda. Clear examples are provided of how process-focused metaphors can be employed to enhance acceptance, shift control, notice the process of thinking, observe the self-as-context, contact the present moment, and make decisions in accord with life values. Overall, metaphors assist in the facilitation of the essential life skills of greater psychological flexibility.

Therapeutic Characteristics

Problems Addressed

- Anxiety
- Panic attacks
- Fear of losing bladder control
- Somatic symptoms
- Experiential avoidance

Resources Developed

- Acceptance
- Defusion
- Self-as-context
- Being present
- Mindfulness skills
- Clarification of values
- Committed action to valued living
- Psychological flexibility

Outcomes Offered

- Valued living
- Psychological flexibility
- Confidence
- Acceptance

While hanging onto a vertical rock wall and looking for his next hold, Aaron found his mind busy with thoughts: *I can't do it; I'm feeling too tired; this is impossible; oh no, I'm getting anxious.* Aaron felt weak and shaky, and his palms began to sweat. A moment later, he lost his grip and fell off the wall. As he hung in the air from the climbing harness, Aaron looked up and wondered what was happening to him. He wondered how he had lost the ability to climb the mountain. He wished he were standing at the top.

Aaron recalled struggling with his anxiety since the first grade, particularly in situations where he felt he was being evaluated. He developed a compulsive fear of losing bladder control in public, which waxed and waned throughout his school years. By the time he reached college this anxiety had expanded into many social situations. He felt as though he might be urinating during class presentations, and felt that it was visible to others. He avoided social interactions, even with family, and particularly if they might involve drinking liquids. He felt panicky when away from home. His grades dropped, and he was considering leaving school.

"Recently," Aaron said, "anxiety has been creeping into other areas of my life." Although an excellent rock climber, he was climbing less and anxiety was visiting him even there. He was now experiencing many somatic symptoms, such as a racing heart and sweaty palms. He began to fear the panic attacks that came more frequently now, and had begun avoiding the situations in which he had experienced them. It seemed that the more he tried to get rid of anxiety, the more it invaded his life.

DEFINING THE PROBLEM

Aaron sought treatment from a university psychological service center. After a brief assessment of his presenting problem and history, he was referred to a treatment team that specialized in acceptance and commitment therapy (ACT, pronounced as one word). Because the goal of ACT is to help clients behave effectively in the presence of unpleasant private events (thoughts, feelings, bodily sensations, memories, and so on), this approach to therapy seemed appropriate for Aaron (Hayes, Strosahl, & Wilson, 1999).

In accord with a standard ACT assessment, I wanted to examine the possible role of experiential avoidance in Aaron's behavior. By experiential avoidance, I refer to the client's unwillingness to re- main in contact with particular thoughts, feelings, memories or bodily sensations even when attempts to avoid them only seemed to exacerbate the problem. I asked Aaron to list all the ways he had tried to reduce his anxiety. He replied, "I've tried not thinking about it, taking medication, or distracting myself by watching TV. I try to make the thoughts go away. Whenever I think *I'm going to have a panic attack* I try telling myself *it's okay to feel this way* or *everything will work out* instead. Sometimes I won't go out to dinner with friends or to a party, so I don't have to feel anxious. And when I know I am going to have a panic attack, I take really deep breaths to keep my heart from racing and rush to the bathroom so I don't have to worry about having an accident." Together, we came up with a list of about twenty different ways that Aaron had tried to reduce his anxiety or make it go away.

The assessment process revealed that Aaron exhibited a high degree of experiential avoidance in both his public and private behavior. During the first few sessions, it became apparent that although some of these strategies were effective in the short term, attempting to control his anxiety seemed to have a paradoxical effect in the longer term. In other words, the energy exerted to control or suppress the experience of anxiety wasn't helping to reduce his anxiety overall. As he tried more ways to run away from his private experience, he was gradually participating less in the life he wished to live. Therefore, the goal of therapy was to give up the war with anxiety and instead to focus on engaging in a meaningful, values-based life. Aaron agreed that it was time to try something different. Radically different. I suggested, "You've tried all the reasonable ways to deal with your anxiety. And yet it seems like the thought 'I can't do X until I get rid of anxiety' is really controlling your life. Maybe it's the case that trying to control it is the problem."

To further illustrate the problem, I introduced a metaphor. Aaron had treated the anxiety like a hungry baby tiger, feeding it to keep it from crying. Like a fed tiger, his anxiety was placated by avoidance but grew in strength and appetite. Although Aaron came to therapy thinking he just needed to get better at controlling his anxiety, from an ACT perspective the problem was *trying* to control the unpleasant feelings. Aaron felt relieved that it was not his fault he couldn't make anxiety go away, but that the strategy of control itself is flawed.

To help Aaron contact the problem of control, I told him the "Man in a Hole" metaphor.

> One day a long time ago you were walking around and you fell in a hole. When you found yourself at the bottom of this hole, the only thing you had with you was a shovel. Not knowing what else to do, you started digging. You tried digging quickly, then slowly, big shovelfuls and small ones. But the hole only got deeper and wider. Is that like your experience? Now you're down here, and you may be hoping that I will give you a golden shovel that will finally get you out of there. . . . Well, I don't have a golden shovel, and even if I did I wouldn't use it, because digging is not the way out of this hole. We may need to give up on the whole agenda.

THE FUNCTION OF METAPHOR IN ACT

In working with Aaron, I considered the use of metaphors to be beneficial in helping him to identify control and avoidance as the problem, as well as to illustrate the unworkability of the previously attempted "solutions." Metaphors functioned to highlight the psychological processes occurring within the client's struggle with his anxiety that can serve to entangle or trap a person in maladaptive patterns. Unlike short stories or examples, which are often proscriptive in nature and are usually specific to the content of the problem, ACT metaphors speak to psychological processes that are applicable across situations. Whether a person is presenting with social anxiety (like our client) or depressed mood with suicidal ideation, ACT metaphors help clients view their *struggle* with their pain as the problem rather than seeing the anxiety, depression, or pain itself as the problem. For example, I told Aaron the "Tug-of-War" metaphor in order to draw attention to his struggle with anxiety.

> Imagine yourself in a tug-of-war with a big ugly monster. In between you and the monster is a dark, deep pit. If you fall into the pit you will die. So you pull and pull as hard as you can, but the monster is very strong and you are inching closer to the edge of the pit. While you are caught in this struggle, it is difficult to see that your job is to drop the rope.

My therapeutic aim in telling Aaron this metaphor was to encourage a new perspective on the problem. For Aaron, seeing anxiety itself as the problem called for trying to change it or get rid of it. This metaphor illustrates the struggle with anxiety as the problem and choosing to "drop the rope" as the solution.

In ACT, metaphor is a bridge between the world created by language and the experience of the world that transcends language. Metaphors are used repeatedly, creatively, and spontaneously so that both client and therapist are continually pointing to processes that cannot be fully explained using language. Metaphors are like the signs pointing the way to a mountain. They direct us toward the experience itself.

Metaphors intentionally disorient clients so that they must discover what works and what doesn't based on their experience rather than literal, linear rules. For example, the "Man in the Hole" metaphor I told to Aaron may leave the client without an answer for how to get out of the hole. This confusion encourages clients to think about the problem in a different way and eventually come to an answer on their own. Additionally, the "solution" of dropping the rope is vague and lacks explicit instructions in order to encourage the client to find an answer by noticing what works according to his or her own experience. One goal of this approach is to create flexibility in clients' behavior based on learning to attend to their experience rather than to what their mind is saying about their experience: *You shouldn't be feeling this way; if I could make anxiety go away, I could do the thing I care about; there must be something wrong with me.*

One way that clients demonstrate increased flexibility is by generating their own metaphors. Stepping out of the ongoing verbal struggle allows choices to open up that were not previously considered. Based on their own experience, clients can then evaluate the effectiveness of the choices they make. Metaphors help to shift clients from aversive control, or avoiding unwanted internal experiences, to appetitive control, by defining values and experiencing the rewards of living a life that is consistent with those values.

THE THERAPEUTIC RELATIONSHIP

I wanted to communicate to Aaron that my role as a therapist was not to provide the answers to his problems ("I don't have the golden shovel that will get you out of this hole") but, rather, to be a guide and fellow traveler. I did not want to be seen as an expert as much as a person with a different perspective.

Imagine you are making your way up a mountain. Your route is sometimes difficult and treacherous, with steep cliffs and overhangs. At other times you come to a place with a path and you walk along easily. I am on another mountain, and I can see you over on yours. When you get to a tricky part, I can see some ways to get over an overhang or up a steep section that you may not be able to see so easily. From my vantage point, I can act as your guide by pointing these out. Meanwhile, I am climbing my mountain and have my own path with its own difficulties.

GENERATING ACT-CONSISTENT METAPHORS

Within ACT, mindfulness is conceptualized as the interaction of four psychological processes: defusion, acceptance, a transcendent sense of self, and contact with the present moment. These processes are interrelated and interdependent. With clients, these processes are discussed in a fluid manner as they relate to the topic at hand. In session, a significant portion of therapy is also spent discussing the client's values and making commitments to act according to those values. As in other successful ACT cases, you will see that the outcome for Aaron was the ability to respond to difficult situations (including undesirable thoughts and the feelings occasioned by them) with psychological flexibility.

Because Aaron had extensive experience with rock climbing, metaphors were frequently generated in session to connect the parallel processes that occurred in the therapy context and on climbing trips. For this reason, the most reasonable place to start illustrating Aaron's progression through therapy is at the bottom of the mountain, where the journey begins.

Mindfulness Processes

Defusion

Defusion is the ability to recognize thoughts as thoughts. In other words, when an individual is defused from thoughts, he or she sees the process of thinking instead of merely the products of thinking. This mindfulness process allows for contact with previously avoided feelings, bodily sensations, and memories.

Because understanding defusion at the level of cognition is full of traps similar to the ones clients have already found themselves in, I used the "Leaves on a Stream" metaphor to communicate this skill to Aaron.

> Imagine a stream in front of you, with leaves floating by on the surface of the water. As a certain thought occurs to you, I want you to carefully place it on a leaf and watch it float by until the thought naturally fades away. Notice how as it disappears, another one shows up. Like with the first, I want you to place that thought on a leaf and watch it pass. Continue to do this with the next thought, and the next.

In this way, Aaron could practice noticing his thoughts with some space between himself as an observer and the content of the thoughts.

To demonstrate the process of defusion in yet another way, I asked Aaron to visualize his thoughts as a pair of blue-colored glasses. "If you hold the pair of blue-colored glasses at arm's length you can see the world colored blue, but you can also see what colors it. If you were wearing the glasses on your face you would perceive a blue-colored world without being aware of the process that colors it. Every experience would be tinted by the color lenses you wore."

As Aaron began to understand the process of defusion from an experiential perspective, he generated metaphors that captured the process on his own. "While standing at the base of the mountain, my mind generates all sorts of stories regarding my ability to climb on a particular day: *I may slip from a hold because of the rain; maybe I didn't get enough sleep last night; what might other climbers think of me; what would they think of me if I fall near the base; what if I get so anxious that I pee and everyone laughs?*"

When this multitude of evaluations presented themselves, Aaron's temptation was to buy into them as truths and disregard his experience of what is in front of him: the rock and his history as a rock climber. Recounting these few moments in session, Aaron commented, "My mind is a doubting Thomas. It generates all sorts of ideas."

I sought to further facilitate the process of defusion by responding to Aaron's observation that "Nothing in thought is going to help you do what you need to do. In other words, deciding that you can or cannot climb the mountain does not affect your actual ability to climb. It's the training and experience of climbing that predicts your performance on these tasks. However, buying into the content of your doubts will certainly affect your ability to climb, due to the fact that it interferes with your ability to attend to the task."

Acceptance

Acceptance means unconditionally allowing whatever thoughts, feelings, memories, or bodily sensations that arise in the present moment to do so without trying to change them. Acceptance in ACT is not based on a belief that accepting internal states is "better" but on the evidence that trying to change or control them does not seem to work. In Aaron's case, this meant noticing uncomfortable sensations, such as tightness in his chest, shaking of his hands, and unpleasant thoughts like *I might pee on myself,* and fully allowing these thoughts and feelings to occur instead of pushing them away. This involves a profound change in the relationship to these thoughts and feelings. As the "Tug-of-War" metaphor illustrated, dropping the rope instead of fighting with the monster is the psychological move needed to accept things as they are. From this nondefensive stance, Aaron is able to contact the unwanted experiences he had been previously avoiding, as well as the pleasurable ones he had been missing.

Once he had defused from the content of thoughts, it was easier for Aaron to accept the thoughts as they showed up for him. Suggesting that we revisit the rock-climbing metaphor, I asked Aaron to apply acceptance as a process to the journey of climbing. He stated, "It is not unusual when climbing to come across some unexpected obstacle, such as an overhang. When this occurs, it is natural for the best of climbers to wish it were not there, fret about how much trouble it may cause them, and wonder if they should just give up." I added, "However, navigating the overhang requires the climber to accept its presence. No wishing or fretting on the climber's part is going to make it disappear. Rather, the experienced climber notices the characteristics of the overhang and makes an informed decision based on his climbing experience about how to proceed up the mountain."

The example of the overhang was used in session to illustrate how the process of acceptance could be applied to Aaron's life. Aaron often spent a considerable amount of time trying to reduce the occurrence and frequency of his anxious thoughts. Paradoxically, when Aaron practiced acceptance of his thoughts and feelings and engaged in a meaningful life, the anxiety and tension became less bothersome. Only by completely accepting his experience in the moment did the frequency of difficult private events actually decrease, just as maneuvering an overhang requires acceptance of the challenge before one can successfully find a way over it.

A Transcendent Sense of Self

Self-as-context refers to observing one's experience from the position of I/Here/Now. It is a reference to a transcendent sense of self that is aware of what is happening both inside and outside the skin, in the present moment. This so-called self-as-context is distinct from a self that is defined by content: *I am anxious; I am a bad rock climber; I am a total loser.*

To help convey this mindfulness process to Aaron, I told him the "Chessboard" metaphor.

> Imagine a chessboard. It has white pieces and black pieces. These are your thoughts, feelings, memories, and so on. The black pieces are negative thoughts, like *I'm anxious; I might pee on myself; I will be so embarrassed,* and the white pieces argue with these thoughts, saying things like *It will be okay; you haven't peed on yourself in a long time; people will understand.* So where are you in all this? Consider the possibility that you are more like the chessboard that holds the pieces than the pieces themselves.

My aim in using this metaphor was that when a person experiences self-as-context rather than self-as-content, they can see that the thought *I am a bad climber* is just a dark piece on the chessboard. I explained to Aaron, "Like the chessboard, you are the space where these events are occurring. You are able to watch the 'players' move as they always do without getting caught up in the war."

To help Aaron defuse from self-referent thoughts, I reutilized the metaphor of thoughts as glasses, thus improving contact with self-as-context. "When glasses are unconsciously on your face, it feels like the thought is 'true' and represents who you are. So, when you have the thought *I am a bad climber,* it is hard to act in a way that is contradictory to that thought. However, when defused from thoughts of self, you can notice your experience of climbing as an observer in the moment without any tint of color. You can notice what it feels like to grip the rock and move toward the next hold. You can notice the strength required, the stretch in your legs, and your motion in space."

Contact with the Present Moment

Being in contact with the present moment is the awareness of internal and external experiences as they occur. Contact with *now* is vital to strengthening the other mindfulness processes. Thus, metaphors use language to point to the experience of contacting the present moment, defused from thoughts, taking the view of the self as an observer unconfined by content, and fully accepting whatever arises.

To promote contact with the present moment, I asked Aaron to apply the defusion metaphors to the thoughts and anxiety he was currently experiencing. When the thought *I'm anxious* appeared, it was followed by *Maybe I'll get more anxious* and then *I don't want to feel this.* Aaron allowed each of these thoughts to be a pair of colored glasses and noticed what it was like to hold these in front of him. The practice of contacting the present moment in session demonstrated to Aaron how he could remain in contact with the present moment while climbing.

Values and Committed Action

Values are chosen qualities of action. They are life directions. They are not specific, concrete goals that can be achieved or completed. They are not nouns. Rather, they are qualities of patterns of living. They are adverbs. Defining values in therapy serves to connect clients with the long-term implications of their behavior in the present moment. Metaphorically, these desired qualities are like a point on a compass—they are a direction to be pursued. As clients start to make decisions in their lives in accord with their values, as opposed to trying to avoid certain feelings or thoughts, they come in contact with increasing feelings of satisfaction with their life. In Aaron's case, attempts to control his anxiety were getting in the way of engaging in his values of learning, spending time with friends, and participating in physical activity, such as rock climbing.

Clients' clarifying their values would not lead to successful outcomes without committed action. Until a leap is taken, a commitment made, life is hesitant and self-focused. When larger and larger patterns of effective values-based action are built, the historical nature of human action begins to work for people instead of against them.

Choosing a path up the mountain and reaching for the next hold with vigor was used as a metaphor for Aaron's values and committed action. Choices about the path to be followed allow the process of climbing to occur. If "up" was not more important than "down," then the joy of mountain climbing would be impossible. The true goal is to climb—to live. But having a direction enables that process.

Aaron has learned repeatedly that new moves half done would be certain to fail. In order to learn a new move, one had to *do* it—fully. This became the metaphor for commitment, and each new therapy exercise was linked to "going for the new hold." This metaphor was useful when barriers and issues were confronted. Aaron had said that he wanted to climb with confidence and complained that his anxiety was interfering. This statement could be a seed from which a new version of experiential avoidance could grow. I related this observation to the therapeutic agenda by explaining, "The word *confidence* is made up of two parts: *con,* which means "with," and *-fidence,* which means "fidelity" or "faith." In this manner, climbing with confidence is similar to climbing with faith or according to one's values. This does not necessarily mean feeling confident, at least at first. It means being true to yourself—acting with faith. That is con-fidence."

Identifying his value to climb with confidence freed Aaron up to commit to each move in service of heading in his chosen life direction. Now when Aaron's mind is busy with old thoughts like *I can't do this; I'm feeling too tired; this is impossible; oh no, I'm getting anxious again,* he can defuse from those thoughts, notice them in the moment as they are, and accept them without reservation from the standpoint of the observer self. When he confronts an overhang unexpectedly, he can navigate it without resisting its presence. By committing to act according to his values as a climber, as opposed to what his mind would dictate, Aaron can reach the top of his real and metaphoric mountain.

Psychological Flexibility

Clients demonstrate psychological flexibility when they use the mindfulness processes to make values-based choices and commit to act accordingly. As Aaron progressed through therapy, he began describing experiences he had while rock climbing that exemplify psychological flexibility. He introduced this strategy as "learning how to rest en route," and described the difference between "resting" and the previous strategies he had tried in attempts to get rid of the tension in his arms and hands. "I used to shake my arms, but recently I realized that I am actually wearing myself out, expending energy I need for climbing." Resting, he discovered, was more of a mindful approach to doing nothing. Rather than "doing something in order not to do something," like shaking his arms in order to relax, he learned to hold himself against the rock with just enough tension to prevent falling in order to regain his strength before resuming the journey.

This discussion enabled us to use resting as a metaphor for learning how to let go of the struggle with anxiety. I stated, "Like muscles doing relaxation, if you are doing *anything,* it is not acceptance." Aaron added, "Just like knowing how to let your arm hang is something you know how to do without thinking about it." I responded, "There is a connection between what you're doing there and what is going on here with your anxiety." He concluded, "If I could do this kind of letting go with my life, that would be it, right there. I've started to experience what that would feel like."

CASE OUTCOME

The use of metaphors for effectively communicating the various processes of ACT was highly successful for Aaron. Anxiety receded as a focus in his life. He began to climb more frequently, traveling farther and farther away from home, regardless of anticipated anxiety. Finally, he joined a troop of international climbers, and raised the money needed for a world climbing tour. Therapy concluded after 18 sessions, shortly before this wonderful endeavor began. For the next year postcards periodically arrived from around the world, showing one mountain after another being confronted, embraced, and climbed. It was obvious, from both his words and the look on his face, that the mountains being climbed were not just physical. One of the cards showed Aaron standing near the top of a high peak, and bore a simple phrase for a caption: Anxiety Mountain.

REFERENCE

Hayes, S. C., Strosahl, K., & Wilson, K. G. (1999). *Acceptance and commitment therapy: An experiential approach to behavior change.* New York: Guilford Press.

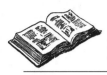

PART TWO

Building Positive Relationships

CHAPTER 6

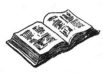

The Case of Carol

Empowering Decision-Making through Metaphor and Hypnosis

Michael D. Yapko

CONTRIBUTOR'S STORY:
A PROFESSIONAL AND PERSONAL PERSPECTIVE

Michael Yapko, PhD, is a clinical psychologist and marriage and family therapist residing in Fallbrook, California. He is internationally recognized for his special interest in brief therapy, clinical hypnosis, and the treatment of major depression, authoring numerous books, book chapters, and articles on these topics (see Resource Section).

He is a member of the American Psychological Association, a clinical member of the American Association for Marriage and Family Therapy, a member of the International Society of Hypnosis, a fellow of the American Society of Clinical Hypnosis, and a recipient of the Milton H. Erickson Award of Scientific Excellence for Writing in Hypnosis and the 2003 Pierre Janet Award for Clinical Excellence.

Michael is happily married to Diane, a pediatric speech-language pathologist. Together, they enjoy hiking in the great outdoors in their spare time. He has long recognized how a good story can captivate and educate people, just as effective therapy must do.

PREVIEW THE CHAPTER

In this case, Michael describes a single-session treatment in which he offers a therapist-generated metaphor in the broader context of an hypnotic intervention for Carol, a client racked with indecision about whether to get a divorce from a long-standing marriage. With typical Yapko clarity, he outlines the processes he used to access the client's resources and goals, while focusing on her processes for handling the challenging task of decision-making. We see the thinking involved in his assessment and planning of treatment, the basis of his therapeutic constructions, and the rationale for incorporating metaphor in the session. The metaphor presented in this chapter is just one of the "interventions" offered to Carol during the therapy session. The session in its entirety was filmed professionally and is available on Dr. Yapko's web site: www.yapko.com.

Therapeutic Characteristics

Problems Addressed

- Indecision
- Ruminative thinking
- Ambivalence
- An unhappy marriage
- Fear of leaving
- An "approach-avoidance" conflict

Resources Developed

- A compelling, positive vision
- Positive coping mechanisms
- Follow-through on a decision
- Acceptance of doubt and mixed feelings
- A sense of progress
- Increased confidence
- Acceptance that there is no "right" decision

Outcomes Offered

- Empowered decision-making
- Sense of purpose
- Self-development and evolution
- Stepping forward
- Acceptance of the cost factors

THE CONTEXT OF THE SESSION

In December 2003, I had the privilege of serving as a faculty member at the Brief Therapy Congress sponsored by the Milton H. Erickson Foundation. The meeting was held in San Francisco, California, and was attended by more than a thousand therapists who all shared a common interest in doing psychotherapy more briefly as well as more effectively.

During that meeting, I was asked to conduct a live clinical demonstration that might illuminate some aspects of my clinical approach. I titled the demonstration "Possibilities and Probabilities in Hypnosis," a title general enough to encompass whatever kind of problem I might be asked to address during this session, since I had no idea who might volunteer from the audience to serve as my partner in the endeavor, much less what kind of problem he or she might ask me to address. My general intention was to demonstrate the potential merits of hypnosis in clinical interventions.

INTERVIEWING CAROL: DETERMINING GOALS AND ASSESSING RESOURCES

Following a short presentation on ways that hypnosis can enhance problem solving, I asked the audience whether anyone present would be interested in volunteering to be my client in the demonstration. From the corner of my eye I saw a hand go up, and I immediately acknowledged it and nodded an assent to the woman who had raised her hand before I realized there was something familiar about her. As it turned out, my volunteer was a woman who had been in a workshop of mine approximately seven years earlier, and who had also served as a demonstration subject in that workshop. Beyond that one contact years earlier, I'd had no other contact with her.

My volunteer was a woman named Carol, who began by reminding me of when and how we had previously met. I began the therapy session by asking Carol whether there was some particular goal or issue that she wanted to address that day. She said, "I'm at sort of a juncture in my life, actually a rather important one. I'm trying to decide whether I should become a single woman at sixty-one, or whether I should remain married." She went on to say, "I've been deciding for a very long time, and I thought it might be something good to work on."

I asked Carol the following question: "How are you going about making this all-important decision in your life?" To clarify that I was seeking to understand the process of her decision-making, I reiterated: "I'm not asking what the decision is as much as I'm asking how you're going about deciding."

Carol responded, "Well, I've been thinking about it for some time, and there have been some events that have happened which have spurred this decision to . . . more of a point of decision. I've been talking to colleagues, very dear friends, not a lot of people, but really trying also, I think, to be more inside myself and really see myself in a different way or see the possibilities in myself being, living a different life. And that has both been exciting and . . . scary. But I've noticed that, in some ways, [it's] more exciting than scary lately, and I feel kind of curious about that. I've been alone, and I've actually enjoyed it." She went on to say she felt she was "seeing myself as an individual more, rather than a part of a family or a part of a marital couple."

In listening to Carol describe the huge, potentially life-changing, decision she wanted to make, my focus was on trying to understand the process by which Carol approached making such a decision. After all, a flawed decision-making process is unlikely to yield a sound decision. Thus, I wanted to know what factors Carol was considering, which ones she might be giving too much weight, and which ones, if any, were being overlooked or underrepresented.

WHY USE METAPHOR IN CAROL'S CASE?

In working with Carol in the unusual context of a single-session intervention performed before hundreds of strangers, my approach needed to be supportive and nonthreatening. I didn't want to ask too much and make her feel vulnerable in front of the group, nor did I need much information beyond what I asked for. More details and more examples of her process would only have told me more of what I already knew. Indirect suggestions, including the use of metaphor, are ideal in such situations—that is, when someone is potentially vulnerable—and with clients who both want and resist direct advice, preferring to get where they want to go independently (B. Erickson, 2001; M. Erickson, 1958; Erickson & Rossi, 1976; Haley, 1973). Thus, the use of metaphor seemed a respectful way of simultaneously challenging and supporting Carol. Furthermore, because Carol, by her very nature, tends to think more deeply about things than other people might, it was apparent to me that I could employ metaphors and rely on Carol's natural tendency to engage in a personally meaningful search for relevance. It was not all indirect, however: I provided Carol a direct framing of the key issue when I questioned how she was going about the process of decision-making. By the time I introduced the principal metaphor at the heart of her therapy session, Carol was already attuned to the issue I was addressing: making and implementing a difficult decision despite mixed feelings in the present by focusing on eventual benefits. Consequently, she was easily able to absorb herself in the cognitive and perceptual frame provided by the story.

GENERAL POINTS ABOUT HYPNOSIS, INDIRECT SUGGESTION, AND METAPHOR

As a longtime practitioner of clinical hypnosis, and a writer and teacher on the subject, I have been deeply committed to advancing a more widespread application of hypnosis among clinicians. There is certainly substantial evidence that hypnosis enhances psychotherapy in general, and cognitive behavioral therapies in particular (Lynn, Kirsch, Barabasz, Cardeña, & Patterson, 2000; Schoenberger, 2000; Yapko, 2003). Integrating hypnosis with cognitive behavioral therapy (CBT) and strategic approaches to treatment has been a strong professional focus throughout my career, particularly in the treatment of Major Depressive Disorder (MDD; Yapko, 1992, 2001, 2006).

Hypnosis is generally not considered to be a therapy in its own right (American Psychological Association, 1999). Instead, hypnosis is considered to be a means of delivering therapeutic concepts to the client as well as a means of creating an appropriate environment (i.e., client's internal readiness and supportive context) for the client to better absorb key therapeutic messages. When one studies the scientific and clinical literature regarding hypnosis, one learns a great deal about human information processing, perception, suggestibility, dynamics of interpersonal influence, the relationship between the brain and the mind, the power of expectations in influencing therapeutic results, the power of ideas in shaping emotional and behavioral responses, and many other variables that singly, and in combination, directly affect one individual's response to the communications of another (Yapko, 2003).

The field of clinical hypnosis has been particularly interested in the potential of therapeutic metaphors as a communication device (B. Erickson, 2001; Haley, 1973; Lankton & Lankton, 1989). In the formulation of hypnotic suggestions, there is a range of possible ways to package and deliver a communication intending to have a therapeutic value. The range is from direct suggestions at one end of the suggestion structure continuum to indirect suggestions at the other end of the continuum. Thus, it has been an ongoing area of interest among clinicians and researchers to examine the strengths and weaknesses of both direct and indirect approaches to communication in the context of psychotherapy (Lynn, Neufeld, & Mare, 1993; Yapko, 1983, 2003).

Metaphor is clearly an indirect form of communication. Instead of speaking directly to someone about his or her concerns, or instead of directly suggesting to someone that he or she respond in a particular way, therapists who employ metaphor use indirection as a means of stimulating the subjective associations of the listener. The listener is told a story about someone else in some other circumstance, or is provided an elaborate analogy that only indirectly relates to the concerns he or she has.

The potential benefits in employing metaphors have been well described in a variety of places. These include:

1. The advantages of being able to learn from someone else's experience
2. The decreased potential for arousing resistance or defensiveness on the part of the client by offering suggestions in a one-step-removed fashion
3. The greater flexibility in allowing the client the opportunity to interpret the meaning of the metaphor in his or her own unique way
4. The adaptability of metaphors that allows them to be applied to a single or any combination of dimensions of experience that one wishes (i.e., physiological, behavioral, cognitive, etc.)
5. Their potential for bringing important therapeutic learnings to life in a memorable way (thereby associating the learnings with specific contexts; Burns, 2001, 2005; Zeig, 1980)

The therapeutic potential of metaphors may easily be negated, however, if the conditions in which they are used are not appropriate. There are limitations associated with the use of metaphors:

1. Metaphors are an abstract form of communication, yet many, if not most, people are quite concrete in their cognitive style, potentially missing the teaching points of the story.
2. Metaphors require the listener to engage in what is called a "search for relevance," a proactive process that passive people (particularly depressed ones) may not strive to perform.
3. Metaphors may be seen as evasive in their lack of direct relationship to the client's concerns and thereby devalued if the client prefers a more direct style (Burns, 2001; Yapko, 2003).

Any clinical hypnosis session, like any therapy session, will inevitably involve many different forms and levels of communication. When initiating and then conducting this live clinical demonstration, I assumed that some of my communication with my demonstration partner would be quite direct and some would be quite indirect. If one were to watch the entire clinical demonstration, one would observe a full range of suggestions employed in the service of achieving the larger therapeutic goals. In this chapter, however, I will focus primarily on the use of metaphor as it was applied in this demonstration of hypnosis.

IDENTIFYING GOALS OF TREATMENT

When I am interviewing a client, most often I find it easy to align with the client's goals. My clinical experience suggests that most of the time people know what they want but are unsure how to obtain it. Sometimes, however, people find themselves in a forced-choice situation, where they need to make a decision but none of the alternatives are attractive. Worse still is when people feel they must choose between alternatives that are not only unattractive but maybe even painful. This is Carol's dilemma: She is unhappy in her marriage and doesn't want to stay, and she is afraid to leave her marriage. Neither choice is desirable for her, and both choices carry with them the potential for considerable emotional pain. This is a classic "approach-avoidance" conflict. Carol needs to be able to make a decision and implement it, realistically knowing that whatever decision she makes will have some negative consequences for her, but none she can't manage if she knows what she's doing and why she's doing it.

What allows someone to endure the pain of a divorce? What allows someone to cope with and eventually transcend painful life episodes? In my experience, there are several factors that determine whether someone will be able to make a hard decision and carry it out. First, and foremost, the person has to have a compelling vision of what is positive enough in the long run to justify enduring the short-term distress it takes to get there. Unless Carol has a clear sense that the benefits will eventually outweigh the costs, the costs alone can seem huge and become paralyzing. Second, the person has to have positive coping mechanisms, such as the ability to manage inconsistent feelings as well as the feedback from others, which will invariably be mixed. Carol will inevitably have moments of doubt about the correctness of her decision, and she will probably also encounter others who question what she's doing and why she's doing it. She'll need to be able to follow through on the decision even when in doubt if she wants to avoid the paralysis of indecision. Third, the person needs to have some sense of progress as time unfolds. There must be benchmarks indicating that he or she is indeed moving forward in a progressive manner. Carol must be able to notice signs along the way that she's doing all right with her chosen path if she is to build confidence in herself and in her ability to make sensible decisions that she can trust without suffering later regret.

As I listened to Carol, it seemed to me that she was skilled at analyzing her emotions and was generally quite insightful. These valuable resources that she possessed were ones I could acknowledge and utilize. Yet she also might have been giving her feelings too much attention in some ways. Focusing on, and thereby amplifying, feelings of dissatisfaction with one's circumstances can inadvertently also amplify associated feelings of fear and doubt about changing them. In other words, when Carol uses her feelings as the reference point for making decisions, her mixed feelings can actually delay or even prevent her from making a difficult decision.

Can someone be in Carol's situation and not have mixed feelings? It seems highly unlikely. She was taking a risk and gambling with her sense of well-being regardless of which path she chose. As she acknowledged, she had both fear and excitement, but neither feeling alone. Yet, instead of accepting the inevitability of mixed feelings in such circumstances, Carol wanted the clarity of a single emotion. She said, "I've decided to let it [the decision] unfold and to realize that I'm going to know when I'm ready to do this and when it's right. . . . I believe that knowing more of myself and feeling more strong internally and bringing that outside is going to take me where I really need to go. . . . I think it would be helpful to just know that what is the right thing for me to do will become clearer and clearer. . . . I'm going to know it and I'm going to feel ready to do what I need to do." If Carol's decision-making criterion was to no longer have mixed feelings, her criterion was unrealistic. It is much more realistic to be able to make a progressive decision in spite of having mixed feelings.

Carol was hoping that somehow she would instinctively know what "the right thing" was to do and that her decision would then be a comfortable one. In my judgment, she was wrong on both counts. First of all, knowing what the right thing to do is presupposes that there is the one right thing to do. In fact, a decision such as this one is not about *the* right thing to do; it's about *a* right thing to do. Either decision that Carol makes, whether to stay in her unhappy marriage or to leave it, will be viable. Either decision will have both costs and benefits. The problem, therefore, is that neither decision is going to be comfortable, either now or in the future. Learning to adjust herself to an unhappy relationship is not a comfortable option. Likewise, adjusting herself to the demands of being single and facing new challenges alone is also an uncomfortable choice. Thus, to expect either decision to feel right or to be clearly the better choice is not realistic. This perspective is tied in to the present, when the focus most needs to be on the future: What does each decision path allow, and at what cost? Answering those questions prepares Carol to decide what is worth paying a price in order to have. Then Carol can decide whether she personally can pay that price with a goal in mind and with an awareness of the benefit outweighing the cost.

CAROL'S RESOURCES

Carol is a thoughtful, sensitive, insightful woman. She has a successful career, she has successfully raised children, and she has tenaciously persisted for 40 years in a marriage that has been challenging, to put it mildly. She is clearly able to keep her eyes on the goal, even when the path to the goal is difficult to follow. That demonstrates an ability to set her feelings aside at times and respond to a sense of duty over a sense of desire, one of the most mature and sophisticated skill sets anyone can hope to develop.

Carol also believes in the validity and importance of her emotions. She believes that with enough exploration and consideration, her feelings can be an accurate indicator of her life experience. People who are emotionally attuned to themselves are often able to use their emotions as catalysts for purposeful behavior. The fact that Carol was aware of her mixed feelings and could sense when her excitement was beginning to overtake her fear indicated to me that she had probably already made her decision to leave her marriage. From my interview, I formed the impression that she was simply trying to find a way to make the decision more acceptable to herself (and perhaps others as well). I believe this is what the resource of "impulse control" is about, and I believe such thoughtfulness and deliberateness help define one's integrity. These, too, are powerful resources Carol possesses.

Carol is also aware of her own physicality. She uses feelings in her body as reference points for evaluating herself and her reactions. She commented a number of times on the changes in bodily sensation that she experienced during and after our session, specifically broader shoulders and increased upper-body strength. Thus, her emotional and physical awareness, as well as her intellectual gifts, combined with her insights about the processes of human change to provide valuable resources to utilize in her session.

As a psychotherapist herself, Carol obviously believes that people can grow, that people can change. She surely knows that as they do so old attachments are broken while new ones develop. This belief system was functionally separated, to her detriment, from the decision that she needed to make in her own life. It became a primary goal of my session with Carol, therefore, to remind her in the context of her own decision-making that if she was going to move forward with her life, it would inevitably mean leaving some things behind.

HYPNOSIS AND DELIVERING THE METAPHOR TO CAROL

Following the interview and the delineation of the goals given earlier, the induction of hypnosis began. Hypnotic induction is a process of securing the attention of the client and slowly building his or her focus and receptivity. Hypnosis typically, but not necessarily, involves suggestions for relaxation, reducing the client's anxiety and its potential for interference. Hypnosis also involves building a momentum in the client's thinking, a sense that there is a purposefulness to the suggestions given. This helps establish an expectation that a meaningful learning can take place while the client is absorbed in the process. Hypnosis in and of itself cures nothing—rather, it's the new associations the client forms during the process that have therapeutic potential, and metaphor, within the context of hypnosis, can be a vehicle to assist the formation of such new associations (Yapko, 2003).

Once Carol was focused, her eyes closed and her attentiveness to my words building, I began to describe to her the normalcy of having mixed feelings in some situations and some of the positive personal resources I had found in her. I spoke in a general way about the fact that life inevitably involves changes, whether they be changes in social environments, geographical environments, work environments, friendships, or personal interests. I suggested that what defines mental health is the ability to adapt to these changes. I went on to observe that there are many different ways of making decisions and pointed out that some decision-making processes are efficient in some situations but not others. I next described how much of life is inherently ambiguous, in the sense that there is no apparent clear meaning or best decision. Some of the most important decisions that we all have to make in life are decisions that must be made on the basis of inadequate information. Yet what most determine our quality of life are the consequences of the decisions that we make. So I drew Carol's attention to the concept of ambiguity and helped normalize (depathologize) her feelings of uncertainty, so that she could accept fear or doubt as inevitable while still moving forward with intelligent decision-making.

Once the concept of ambiguity was introduced and developed, I could reinforce the point that uncertainty means risk. This was a natural lead-in to talking about how any decision of importance will have both associated benefits and liabilities. This point allowed me to talk about how even transitions that are clearly progressive will have at least some negative consequences associated with them. It was at this point in the hypnotic process that I introduced the principal metaphor, a segment of the play *Inherit the Wind* (Lawrence & Lee, 1951/2003).

I chose to tell Carol this story due to my impression that she was avoiding making a key life decision because she instinctively knew that whatever decision she made would probably be painful. By spending years exploring possible decisions, she was avoiding having to actually make one. Carol wanted to avoid the pain of either staying married or divorcing, yet continuing her life of ongoing indecision and stagnation was also painful to her. Thus, I wanted to focus Carol on the more realistic and empowering notion that if she was going to progress—in whatever direction—her progress would come at a price. I especially wanted to convey the message that *anything* of value will have a cost associated with it, and the wisdom is in knowing that *the cost is justified by the outcome.* For example, a good education takes years of study and the frequent sacrifice of personal leisure time.

The metaphor taken from *Inherit the Wind,* one I paraphrased from memory, makes the similar point that as we advance our scientific and social knowledge, there is a price to be paid for doing so. The character Henry Drummond, played by Spencer Tracy in the 1960 film adaptation, is the attorney defending a schoolteacher who dared to teach the theory of evolution in a deeply religious town whose citizens are quite literal in their interpretation of the Bible. Drummond offers the observation that growth in our knowledge can mean we have to revise or even give up previously held ideas. Though that may be uncomfortable at times, he advises, we should not let our discomfort lead us to choose a more comfortable ignorance. Drummond's speech, summarized in the metaphor I told to Carol, highlights the importance of having the foresight and the courage to pay the price of progress. The metaphor as it was told to Carol, and the verbal introduction leading up to it, are included in the next section.

Inherit the Wind: A Metaphor about the Price of Progress

"There's one thing that makes hard work easier, isn't there? The sense of purpose . . . the sense of what's beyond it . . . and there is no one, no one more powerful than someone on a mission. . . . And what's been unfolding over these years . . . is what happens when you make your self-awareness . . . your self-development . . . a mission . . . and you've been do-ing that. And it's really no coincidence . . . the things you're able to do now . . . that years ago . . . you would have predicted just weren't in your future . . . and so that curiosity that you have . . . as you notice your own evolution . . . and it's interesting that I should use the word *evolution* . . . because, to me, it's a very deliberate word choice . . . I remember years ago being deeply affected by reading the book . . . and then seeing the movie . . . *Inherit the Wind* . . . the story of the Scopes Monkey Trial in Tennessee early in the last century . . . and Spencer Tracy brought it to life . . . when he turned to the jury . . . which was considering the fate of a man who dared to teach evolution . . . and he said, 'Ladies and gentlemen of the jury . . . knowledge, progress, has a price. . . .' And then he went into a sort of reverie . . . talking at the jury . . . but not to them . . . so self-absorbed . . . as he was saying, 'It's as if there's a little man who sits behind a table and dishes out the price of progress . . . who says, "Yes ma'am, you can have the vote . . . and you can participate as an equal in politics . . . but then you won't be able to hide behind your apron any more." And "Yes sir, you can have an airplane . . . and travel great distances quickly . . . but the clouds will smell of gasoline . . . and the birds will lose their wonder." And "Yes ma'am, you can have a telephone . . . and you can share information instantly with others . . . but . . . you'll give up some of your privacy . . .

and distance will lose its charm.'"... And what your Dad was talking about [when he said "Do the right thing even if it's hard"] ... and what Dear Abby was talking about [when she said "Opportunities are often missed because they come disguised as hard work"] ... and what can last ... well, after this session is over ... is what it means to evolve ... every step forward ... means leaving something behind ... whether you step forward into a future of this relationship continuing ... something's going to change.... And if you step forward into the future of this relationship not continuing ... something's going to change ... and those broad shoulders and that upper-body strength ... and that deeper ... much deeper ... sense ... that you don't have to know ... exactly what's going to happen.... You can just know ... that whatever the price of progress is ... you can pay it gladly ... comfortably ... knowingly ... with the power that comes ... from a sense of deliberateness ... and so, Carol, take a moment ... to absorb and integrate in a very deep way ... and when you think about the vote ... and see airplanes ... and you use a telephone ... constant cues ... powerful reminders ... about your own evolution ... your own evolution...."

Carol was then reoriented. As she opened her eyes, her very first words were, "I can afford it!" When I asked for further comments, she said, "I wanted to say, 'I can afford it! I can afford it!' as you were finishing." These comments, spontaneous and forceful, indicated to me that she understood from the metaphor that progress, any progress, has a price. Her decision-making strategy could change from the need to be comfortable to the recognition that she could afford the price of change.

Carol and I then responded to a number of questions from the audience members, and the demonstration session ended with our thanking each other for our respective contributions to the experience. I asked for and received permission from Carol to contact her in order to check on her progress. I had several communications from Carol, the most recent of which was 17 months after our session. Her follow-up comments are included in the next section.

SESSION FOLLOW-UP

First follow-up (by e-mail), 10 weeks later:

> ...I have rented an apartment for myself, and am moving over the next week or so. I also went to an accountant re: financial issues ... to fund the continuing EVOLUTION OF MY PSYCHE AND SPIRIT. ... [I'll have an] open house wine tasting to toast the continuing UN-FOLDING of my life.... Thank you for your interest and help in my EVOLUTION AS A PERSON AND A THERAPIST.
> Regards,
> Carol

Second follow-up (by e-mail), seven months later:

> ...I have indeed separated from him; I may have told you this news (in my last e-mail) when I actually moved out. The theme of our work was evolution of things, namely me. I have used the tape and the video on numerous occasions, including taking it to a very old and huge tree where I go to remember my father. I felt the broadness in my upper-body which I had

noted during our session, and then I continued to listen to the remainder of the tape on my way out of the deep woods where the tree is located. As I continued to follow the themes and underlying meanings in that tape (I tend to hear and experience additional meanings and associations the times I have reheard it), I was aware of the possibility of my husband benefiting from the themes as well.... He is a man who has great difficulty in accessing his feelings and memories, and I wondered whether a more multi-level approach like hypnosis could help him.... I am not involved in his treatment and did not discuss our tape with him, other than to answer his questions re: my feelings about the experience, so I tried to allow some clarity in the boundary. Thought that you might want to hear of this event.... Thanks for all your help, and by the way, I have listened to the tape and video only a handful of times, though it has certainly positively affected my life and work significantly.

Regards,
Carol

Third follow-up (by e-mail), 17 months later:

...That experience was quite profound for me, and I have watched the tape many times during the past year as a reminder and reexperience of the feeling of strength in my upper body, and the inspiration of my father's words.... The posthypnotic references to planes, women's voting, phones, and evolution have cued me to feel the upper-body strength, especially the planes when I either hear or see them. I also feel that the use of the Inherit the Wind story subtly underlined and validated my father's adage to do the right thing, even if it's hard, in that the attorney and the teacher were indeed modeling that behavior in their portrayals.... My personal life is unfolding slowly, but surely, as we predicted it would. I am in the process of divorce mediation after 44 years of marriage, and am discovering that I can afford it; in fact I have discovered that I can't afford not to do it. My decision to participate in that demonstration was pivotal...."

Regards,
Carol

FINAL COMMENTS

Sometimes people get stuck because they don't know what their options are, and sometimes they get stuck when they know what their options are and just don't like any of them. Hard decisions are hard because they have undesirable, perhaps even painful, consequences associated with them. What justifies suffering through something as painful as a divorce, if not the belief that you will eventually be better off as a result? But what happens when the short-term distress looms larger than the long-term benefits in one's perceptions? If one either thinks too much, especially about the negative (a pattern called "rumination," which increases anxiety), or is avoidant (trying to avoid, delay, or circumvent the inevitable distress), then one makes either poor decisions or no decisions at all, thereby staying in a holding pattern that is itself a very frustrating and uncomfortable place to be (Nolen-Hoeksema, 2000, 2003).

Hypnosis is especially valuable as a means of shifting people's focal points, and metaphor can be an exceptionally powerful means of catalyzing experiential shifts. I think Carol's progress underscores this point. In this case, Carol discovered that ambiguity was more the problem due to the mixed feelings it generates than any sort of personal inadequacy. And she learned that any action she took would have at least some negative consequences, despite her wish to avoid them. It was great to hear her first words coming out of hypnosis: "I can afford it." She's right—she can. Carol has a great many wonderful personal resources, and it was my privilege to be able to work with her in this session.

REFERENCES

American Psychological Association, Division of Psychological Hypnosis (1999). *Policy and procedures manual.* Washington, DC: Author.

Burns, G. W. (2001). *101 healing stories: Using metaphors in therapy.* New York: Wiley.

Burns, G. W. (2005). *101 healing stories for kids and teens: Using metaphors in therapy.* Hoboken, NJ: Wiley.

Erickson, B. (2001). Storytelling. In B. Geary & J. Zeig (Eds.), *The handbook of Ericksonian psychotherapy* (pp. 112–121). Phoenix, AZ: Milton H. Erickson Foundation Press.

Erickson, M. (1958). Naturalistic techniques of hypnosis. *American Journal of Clinical Hypnosis, 1,* 3–8.

Erickson, M., & Rossi, E. (1976). *Hypnotic realities: The induction of clinical hypnosis and forms of indirect suggestion.* New York: Irvington.

Haley, J. (1973). *Uncommon therapy: The psychiatric techniques of Milton H. Erickson, M.D.* New York: Norton.

Lankton, C., & Lankton, S. (1989). *Tales of enchantment: Goal-oriented metaphors for adults and children in therapy.* New York: Brunner/Mazel.

Lawrence, J., & Lee, R. (2003). *Inherit the wind.* New York: Ballantine. (Originally published 1951)

Lynn, S., Neufeld, V., & Mare, C. (1993). Direct versus indirect suggestions: A conceptual and methodological review. *International Journal of Clinical and Experimental Hypnosis, 41,* 125–152.

Lynn, S., Kirsch, I., Barabasz, A., Cardeña, E., & Patterson, D. (2000). Hypnosis as an empirically supported clinical intervention: The state of the evidence and a look to the future. *International Journal of Clinical and Experimental Hypnosis, 48,* 239–259.

Nolen-Hoeksema, S. (2000). The role of rumination in depressive disorder and mixed anxiety/depressive symptoms. *Journal of Abnormal Psychology, 109,* 504–511.

Nolen-Hoeksema, S. (2003). *Women who think too much: How to break free of overthinking and reclaim your life.* New York: Henry Holt.

Schoenberger, N. (2000). Research on hypnosis as an adjunct to cognitive-behavioral psychotherapy. *International Journal of Clinical and Experimental Hypnosis, 48,* 154–169.

Yapko, M. (1983). A comparative analysis of direct and indirect hypnotic communication styles. *American Journal of Clinical Hypnosis, 25,* 270–276.

Yapko, M. (1992). *Hypnosis and the treatment of depressions: Strategies for change.* New York: Brunner/Mazel.

Yapko, M. (2001). *Treating depression with hypnosis: Integrating cognitive-behavioral and strategic approaches.* New York: Brunner/Routledge.

Yapko, M. (2003). *Trancework: An introduction to the practice of clinical hypnosis* (3rd ed.). New York: Brunner/Routledge.

Yapko, M. D. (Ed.). (2006). *Hypnosis and treating depression: Applications in clinical practice.* New York: Routledge.

Zeig, J. (Ed.). (1980). *A teaching seminar with Milton H. Erickson, M.D.* New York: Brunner/Mazel.

CHAPTER 7

The Woman Who Wanted to Lie on the Floor

A Social Constructionist Use of Metaphor in a Tale of Two Clients

Valerie E. Lewis

CONTRIBUTOR'S STORY: A PROFESSIONAL AND PERSONAL PERSPECTIVE

Valerie Lewis, PhD, received her doctorate at the University of Houston and subsequently established Australia's first graduate diploma in counseling psychology at the West Australian Institute of Technology (now Curtin University). She entered private practice in 1981, continuing to teach part time at the University of Western Australia, James Cook University, Edith Cowan University, and the Milton H. Erickson Institute of Western Australia, until her recent retirement.

She has been a member of the Australian Psychological Society, the American Psychological Association, and the International Society of Hypnosis, and still tutors with Massey University, New Zealand. In the last years of her career she made a major philosophical turn to postmodern therapy, and is now aligned with the social constructionist point of view.

Valerie resides at Coolum Beach, Queensland, Australia, where she is an active volunteer with the environmentalist movement, and is the grandmother of Gillian, 12, and Tatiana, 7. She has an interest in health, fitness, and antiaging medicine.

PREVIEW THE CHAPTER

From time immemorial, stories have taught us how we can learn from other people's challenges, experiences, and discoveries. Here Valerie shows how this principle can be applied clinically, using the story of one client's learning to facilitate the therapeutic growth of a second client. It is a story within a story of two clients who have very different presenting problems (anger and depression) but who are going through very similar processes regarding high demands, family relationships, and lack of self-nurturing. Taking a social constructionist and postmodern perspective that avoids prescriptive protocols, the chapter demonstrates the use of questioning and collaboration in the therapeutic process. Crucial to this approach is the therapist's willingness to join the client's metaphoric world, moving out of her chair and continuing the conversation while lying with the client on the floor. We see how such actions can facilitate the client's search for, discovery of, and application of her own personal insights, action, and meaning.

Therapeutic Characteristics

Problems Addressed

- Feelings of anger
- Depression
- Ruminative thinking
- Feelings of guilt
- Feelings of confusion regarding personal change
- Lack of self-caring

Resources Developed

- Accepting new feelings as having positive meaning
- Accentuating coping mechanisms
- Following through on new decisions
- Having feelings of progress and fulfillment
- Building confidence
- Building skills in self-caring

Outcomes Offered

- Recognition of new meanings in self-understanding
- Enhanced sense of worth
- Self-development and evolution
- Progress in relationships
- Acceptance of self-caring as okay

A SOCIAL CONSTRUCTIONIST USE OF METAPHOR

The following case story is an embedded tale of two women who were struggling with very similar issues for very different presenting problems. The main story is of the principle client, Reina, who was provided with a story about another, second client (Margrit) as part of therapy. It was customary for me to ask clients who had particularly instructive stories for permission to retell their story, disguised of course, to benefit others. So it was in these two cases.

By way of background, let me offer some information on how I have come to view therapy after a professional lifetime in the career and exposure to most of the major schools of thought. Social constructionists conceive the mind as being socially constructed and largely the product of a discursive set of stories, involving the creative use of language that necessarily reflects cultural practices and social interactions. Mind, therefore, does not appear in a vacuum, but becomes an expression of social interchange via the medium of languaging. For the social constructionist, language does not provide a picture or a map of what is the case. Rather, meanings are found from within the use of language in social intercourse, of which therapy forms one part.

Therapy may be seen as an example of discursive practice between two or more people. Current narratives are discussed and other narratives are collaboratively constructed that might assist clients to re-story their lives and who they are in a manner that is consistent with a sense of well-being for them. There are no fixed rules about how this may be done, and different therapeutic approaches may be utilized along the way, often guided by the clients' expressed wishes or suggested by spontaneous events that happen both in and out of the therapy room. For example, the client might express the wish to try hypnosis, or the therapist might suggest hypnosis if it appears to be potentially helpful as an adjunct to therapy, such as when the client expresses a need to let go of physical and mental tension.

There is a tradition in social constructionist therapies to use witnesses and reflective teams in hearing and sharing in the stories of clients. This reflects a trend largely emerging from the context of family therapy but which philosophically has taken hold in individual therapy. The term *witness* simply means anyone who is brought into the therapy process who can retell the client's story or who might tell a story of his or her own that is very similar and is thus instructive. In this way, then, the telling of another's story by the therapist symbolically brings in that person as a witness. The many exponents of narrative and other discursive therapies often utilize witnesses and report in the literature that this approach of sharing stories is beneficial to the clients. It can bring clients a sense of not feeling so alone in their story, but of being part of a larger story that is repeated in many places as part of the human condition. Many cultures embrace the notion of the passing down of stories as part of the living memory.

The postmodern turn, as it is often called, refers to a turning away from the modernist models of the singular self and the notion of mind as an object of analysis. Postmodernism in therapy is largely a skepticism of all-encompassing theories, and therefore this approach does not view the therapist as approaching the therapeutic encounter as an expert who prescribes a particular technique, but rather as one who adopts a questioning and collaborative stance. Along the way, the client and therapist together find stories and conversations that are useful and therapeutic to the client. The postmodernist would not consider that his or her construction or narrative is somehow superior to that of his client, but instead provides a space for alternative stories to emerge.

So we come to the case being presented here. As I listened to Reina's story I found that gradually I kept remembering the words of Margrit, a previous client. It was almost as if the two lived in parallel universes, so that I felt that Margrit could be a witness for Reina, and that retelling Margrit's story would be like inviting Margrit into the room with us to share her journey with Reina. I had known Margrit many years earlier and in a different place, and although I could not bring the two clients together on a person-to-person basis, there was a way that evolved for this to happen, for Margrit to be a witness to Reina's story.

REINA'S TALE

Reina was a small, wiry woman of 40, with dark hair worn wrapped around the top of her head. Born in South America, she had spent the past 25 years in Australia. Her English was very expressive as she told me that she was married and had two children, twin girls. "I was always a cheerful, happy person," she said, "always singing and working very hard, very hard. My daughters are going to high school and I have to do lots for them—always running around. My husband is a good man, but he is very quiet and lets me run the show." He worked as a commercial cleaner while she had been working as an assistant in a hospital kitchen.

All was well until she was involved in a near-miss car accident. "The person driving in front of me did something very stupid," explained Reina. "She stopped her car suddenly and I ran off the road and crashed my car so I wouldn't run into her. But I was okay. I wasn't hurt bad and after a while I got out to look at the other person. I saw that there was a small child standing up in the back of her car." This would prove to be a significant factor in her experience.

Since the accident, she reported, she had undergone a personality change. "Now I am always moody, I don't want to do things for my family, and the worst thing is that now I feel angry with them." She had withdrawn from them. "Who is this person I am now?" she asked.

By asking this question, Reina appeared to be acknowledging that she felt perplexed by the changes to her behavior since the accident. I, too, had wondered about this, and was curious about how these changes seemed to make her a different person. Therefore, I inquired, "What do you think about this person?"

"I don't know if I like this new person," she answered, "but you know what? I don't feel like I can go back now. I don't feel like I want to go back there."

Reina was very outspoken, and seemed to be someone who could take charge and always knew what to do. Her demeanor was not that of a depressed person.

Observing a Pattern of Responsibility

I wanted to hear Reina's personal story and so asked her to tell me about her life history. She told me that she had been born to poor parents, and her mother had died when she was very young. "My father was a wonderful man," she said. "He worked very hard all his life, but he was a very demanding father. He expected me to help him with raising my three younger brothers and running the house, and I always did. I mean, you don't question your father, and who else was going to do it? I was the mother."

The family migrated to Australia, and Reina continued to be very involved with her family until she married in her early twenties. At the time of our first session, her own children were in their last year of high school. As I listened to her relate her story, I got the picture of a woman who had always been responsible for others, whose sense of self seemed to hang on those particular responsibilities, with little or no thought of herself.

Something important had happened with her near-miss car accident, or "near-death experience," as she described it, in particular seeing the child in the other car, who might have been killed if she had not swerved away. "Something about seeing that child there in that car has changed me," she explained. "I don't know why."

While she talked about this, she added, "You know what? When I think about all this stuff I just feel more and more angry with my own family. I don't understand it."

"Tell me more about this," I requested. "What it is that makes you feel angry now that didn't make you angry before the accident?"

She said, "Well, you know all of them are expecting me to be cheerful and to do everything for everyone. I always make my girls' and husband's meals, including their lunches. I do all the shopping, washing, and cleaning and still go to work as well."

Reflecting on Reina's history, I wondered if this represented a pattern in her life story. One component of narrative coconstruction that contributes significantly to my work with clients is to be aware of the patterns or structures that form around or within what the clients tell me, and to reflect these to the client as we go along. Any story forms a pattern or multiple patterns, or themes, and often it is of interest to the client to be shown how these emerge in the various stories about their life that are revealed in therapy. It must be acknowledged that the patterns as perceived by a particular therapist may be informed by the therapist's own life experiences and point of view. Thus, the patterns reflected by the therapist should not be considered to be the last word but are offered as part of the ongoing conversation, for consideration.

"Is this how it was in your own family, with your dad and brothers?" I inquired.

"Yes," she replied. As we continued to explore this she added, "You know, I don't just feel angry. I also feel real tired all the time. What happened to my energy?"

While she had had some minor bruising in the accident, she did not feel the fatigue was so much physical as mental. She described it as "feeling like suddenly I no longer have the 'go' to do all the things I used to . . . what I normally did. You know, my family think I've lost the plot. They're running a bit scared. They were real happy that I was coming here."

Redirecting Resources

Despite all this, Reina still was able to show a sense of humor. When she returned for her next session she described how she had deliberately made dreadful sandwiches for her family, and was able to laugh about this. She said, "I don't know. It's mean, but at the same time it feels real good . . . like I'm getting some kind of revenge or something. And I felt a bit better this week. Like, I came here and you didn't tell me I was crazy. Tell me, what's wrong with me?"

I asked her why she thought it was wrong to have bad feelings. She replied, "Well, it is wrong to not want to do all that stuff for your family, I reckon, but you know what, I think that maybe it's not so wrong. I had more energy this week. Not a lot, but some."

I then wondered if that energy meant she was once more doing things for the family or if she might have done something different. So I asked what she had done with the little bit of energy.

She told me that she had gone to visit a friend. "My friend had a good idea," she said. "Something I've always wanted to do. You guys do hypnosis here, don't you? Well, I'd like to try it. I don't know why, maybe because in the old country there were lots of spiritual folks, and my mother used to tell me stories that made me feel good. My friend went to a hypnotist, and she was told this amazing story that helped her so I want to see what it does for me. Maybe you've got a story that would help me the same as her."

"What sort of story do you think you might like?" I asked.

"I don't know, maybe a story that will help me understand what I am going through better."

If Reina had not specifically asked to use hypnosis, I might have simply told the story I used in our therapeutic conversation. In other words, while the hypnosis may have enhanced the learning process, it is not a necessary ingredient to working with metaphors. As it was near the end of the session, I explained that all we could do that day was to begin learning about hypnosis and that I would think about a good story to include next time. So for the remainder of the session I taught her autogenic relaxation, which I often use as a means to a hypnotic induction. When I did this, it was very collaborative, as I prefer to work in a collaborative manner no matter what we are doing, and hypnosis is no exception. I see hypnosis as a skill that is within the client, not the therapist. The therapist simply provides a space via almost any ritual behavior that is set within the language and discourse of "hypnosis." Clients will use that ritual, in this case autogenic relaxation training, to put themselves into hypnosis.

I asked Reina what kinds of feelings she had when she totally relaxed her hand, and she said that it felt deeply heavy. She was then invited to create a feeling such that it would be almost impossible to move her hand, and once she accomplished this, she was asked to allow that feeling to flow up her arm and throughout her body and to tell me what the feeling was doing as it went. As I continued with this approach, she was able to achieve a very deep relaxation.

Finding a Place for Stories

When I asked her to tell me about a peaceful place that she might like to visit while in this relaxed state, she recalled her little bed in South America when her mother was still alive and told her bedtime stories. So I asked her to describe the room for me if she could still visit it in her mind's eye. She described a place that had a view of greenery from a small window and whose walls were decorated in cheerful colors. She liked to lie on the bed and stare out the window. "I could make myself feel just like this even then," she said, "but it's been a long time." I suggested that at the next therapy session she might find it very easy to return to this lovely place for a story. "My mother told me stories about little girls like me," she volunteered.

When Reina returned the following week, her energy was slowly returning, and she was not thinking as much about the child in the car. She said, "I am still frustrated with my family and they still make me mad, though. But they are trying and they are all tiptoeing around me. It's pretty funny in a way."

Reina was very keen to get started with her hypnosis session and quickly achieved relaxation with very little instruction from me. When she told me she was imagining herself lying on her little bed in her childhood room she asked for a story.

During my sessions with Reina, I kept being visited in my mind by an old client from years before, Margrit, whose story reminded me a great deal of Reina and whose story I felt might be instructive to Reina. This is the story I told.

The Woman Who Wanted to Lie on the Floor

"A few years ago, I saw a client who I will call Margrit. Like you, Margrit came from another country—in her case, from Russia. She and her husband and two young children migrated to Australia after first establishing residence in another Eastern European country. They had to sell their wonderful furniture and had nothing when they arrived here. They could speak little English, and her husband managed to find work as a builder's laborer. Margrit took a job in a fish-packing factory, where the factory floor boss befriended her and persuaded her that she must buy a home to ensure her future. To do this, she and her husband had to borrow almost the whole amount, putting themselves deeply in debt.

"Margrit worked very hard for many years and established a home for her family. She did everything for them: cooking, cleaning, shopping, sewing. The family became accustomed to her looking after them well, and she took pride in this. About a year or two before coming to see me, Margrit suffered a severe depression and took medication for this. Her husband, who was present at our first session, said that at that time she had transformed into this different person but had eventually returned to being her normal self. Now here she was again, severely depressed, and this time they were looking for psychological help. The family felt Margrit was sick and needed help.

"When I saw Margrit alone, she told me that she felt like a different person when she was like this. She did not want to do anything for her family. She spoke slowly and with little expression, as very depressed people do. I asked her to tell me about her own family. She said that she had a stern father whom she could never please, and that she had run away into an early marriage to escape this, but that her husband was similar to her father. She was expected to do everything for them, and generally she was happy to do that.

"I asked Margrit if there was one thing that she would like to do for herself. She said that she just wanted to lie on the floor. I invited her to do that, but when she said she felt embarrassed, I suggested that we both lie on the floor. So we did.

"Margrit told me when she was lying down on the floor that she could feel she had left all her old life and demands behind and could relax entirely. I suggested that we both relax for a while and see what it felt like. After a while, Margrit began telling me that her daughter had to do everything when she was like this. I asked her how she felt about this. She thought about it and said, 'Well, I feel very guilty, but perhaps it isn't bad because it helps her to learn.' As we continued to lie on the floor and converse, I asked if she thought the lying down had any special meaning for her, how she felt while there. She said, 'I feel, well, free. I am not doing what I am supposed to do. I am not supposed to be lying down.'

"As it was near to the time for our session to end, I mentioned this, and we returned to our chairs. I asked Margrit if she would think about something until I saw her again: whether she felt that doing things for herself could only happen when she was 'sick' or whether it was possible for her to still do things that pleased her, just for her, without being 'sick.' I also asked her to do something. Her homework was to lie on the floor at least once a day.

"Well, Margrit did both of those tasks. In answer to my question, she said, 'No, you do not need to be sick to do things for yourself.' In the weeks that followed, as well as lying on the floor, she began to do other things just for herself. When her husband initiated work in the garden, she allowed herself to sit in the sun and relax. Instead of spending the budget solely on family needs, she put aside a little for herself and bought some jewelry. She no longer did everything for everyone any more, and found it interesting that, as she loosened the reins, others began to take more responsibility, like her daughter doing more around the house. Over time, her depression lifted . . . and she always remembered to lie on the floor when she felt like it.

"Now I know that this is a story about another person, but I think Margrit's story has provided a message to you and me, Reina, and I don't know what that message is, but perhaps you will be able to tell me when we return from hypnosis and you have had some time to think about it during the week. I will think about it too, and we can talk about it when we next meet."

SHARING CLIENT STORIES

The sharing of client stories can be a most powerful means to bring in a sense of witnessing, as discussed earlier. Clients can take from the story whatever they feel is useful to them in their own re-storying and recreating, both in therapy and in their lives. When you are listening to a particular client relate his or her own stories, you are often reminded of the stories of past clients who have trodden a similar path or who have found solutions that might be valuable to share. As I listened to Reina, I was reminded of Margrit. Both of these women had similar backgrounds, coming from working-class, non-Australian families, and both had been the stalwarts of their families. I felt that they could have much to say to one another, and while I was not entirely sure what that might be, I felt it would be worthwhile to let Margrit tell Reina her story, using me as the mouthpiece. I also felt it would satisfy Reina's wish to hear a story about someone like her.

With Reina, the use of stories was important in her own history, and she specifically asked for the use of hypnosis with a story as a means to helping her in her therapeutic journey. It is important to note that using such methods can be (or can sound) prescriptive, and so the therapist might wish to remain collaborative and explore the use of metaphors, stories, hypnosis, cognitive behavioral analysis, psychodrama, or other approaches with the client.

If the therapist and client arrive at the decision together that storytelling would be useful, the therapist has to choose from a panoply of stories. They could, of course, be therapist-generated metaphors, as described elsewhere in this book, or they could be client stories, as used in this case study. I doubt there are any rules to follow in making such a choice, but in general I try to be alert to cues from the client's own personal tales and expressed wishes. Sometimes the similarity between one client's process and another's makes it an obvious choice, as was the case with Margrit and Reina. At other times, it might be that a previous client had a unique solution to a similar problem, or it could be there was an embedded lesson that you feel, from what this client has told you thus far, he or she might find useful.

In the retelling, I prefer to keep it simple and pare off unnecessary details, retaining the ones that pertain to this client. Again, there are no rules or set formulas to follow here, and the therapist needs to be guided by the personality, needs, and goals of the client. For example, if you are in conversation with someone who likes to get to the point, it may not be a good idea to tell a story that goes on for most of the hour.

It is my belief that telling stories to clients is a facilitative process rather than an intervention. "Intervention" sounds like a medical practitioner intervening in the progress of the infection by applying an antibiotic, or the expert therapist employing some sort of clever technique. That is not what is happening with this style of therapy. The Ericksonian, narrative, solution-focused, and other discursive therapies tend to lead us away from an "expert" stance to the use of stories and metaphors derived and/or adapted from the client's own words. Because such stories may be constructed collaboratively in some instances, and appear to set off a creative healing process, I prefer the word *facilitation* to *intervention,* or even some other word that captures the essence of what is happening.

Another example of facilitation might be when I chose to lie down on the floor with Margrit. Having experienced Margrit as somewhat hesitant about taking initiative, it was apparent to me that she would not willingly do something so unusual as lying on the floor without encouragement. What better encouragement than to do it with her? I had a sense that if I joined her she would feel more comfortable about the whole process of doing things that were self-nurturing. Also, it added a sense of fun, which was important to bring into our relationship, as there was little fun in Margrit's life.

Storytelling is similarly facilitative. It forms a fundamental basis for all human communication, and our very language is based on, and laced with, metaphor. Clients can use the story or ignore it, draw particular aspects from it or build on it. It is not up to the therapist to suggest what clients do with the story, but to put the story out there so as to provide a conversational or discursive space from which clients may journey forth, and report back about, in the continuing conversation that is therapy.

MARGRIT'S MESSAGE FOR REINA

Reina phoned to cancel her next appointment and returned to see me several weeks later. She was very upbeat and looked a bit like the cat that ate the canary. She told me, "Wow, that was such a great story about Margrit. I thought about it a lot and it really meant a lot to me. Lots has happened. Wait till you hear! You know I understood exactly what that woman wanted when she said she wanted to lie on the floor. I realized that I wanted it, too. When I almost got killed and I saw that little kid who almost got killed, it was like, 'How come other people can just take stuff from you?' But when I felt Margrit's desire to lie down, I knew what that was. It wasn't her family at all, it was her. *She* needed to do the lying down and not feel bad about doing it. And it wasn't *my* family either. They didn't make me do everything. I did that to myself. I've been doing it all my life. It was me I was angry with, and I was taking it out on them, like it's their fault that this had happened and I was almost killed or something."

She told me that, like Margrit, she had made a life's work out of creating a rod for her own back. "I always shoved down my own feelings about it. I wasn't allowed to feel resentment or to feel pissed off." She said she felt that it took the accident to strip away her own facade from her eyes. "I had been kind of pretending that parts of me didn't exist, all my life. But I couldn't look at myself, could I? I have the need to do things, too, but I never allowed myself to do it. I needed to lie on the floor, too."

"What is your 'lying on the floor'?" I asked.

"Well," she replied, "that's just what I've been thinking about and doing since I saw you. Mine is different. I want to learn how to dance and to paint." She went on to explain that she had not been allowed to do creative things, as a young girl, after her mother died. Later, as a parent, she felt restricted from doing so because of her responsibilities. She said, "I felt that something more was cut off from me when my mother died. She was a creative woman, you know. She used to do this incredible embroidery. When we were doing the hypnosis I could sort of see some of her embroidered pictures. I need to do something like that too. I could draw really well in school. But I always thought it was sort of silly, not what grown-ups do, you know. And I love to move to music, too." Acting from a deep conviction that she must do this for herself, she enrolled herself and her husband in dance classes, and herself in a drawing class.

"Hey," she said suddenly, "you haven't told me what it was you thought about Margrit's story."

"I had come to much the same conclusion as you have," I said, acknowledging that I hadn't known about Reina's mother's embroidery and her frustrated artistic side, although it didn't surprise me. I added, "I thought you didn't have to be 'angry' just like Margrit didn't have to be 'sick' in order to do things for herself."

Over the ensuing weeks, Reina and I talked about positive ways to tell her family about her own needs and engage them in doing more to help her. To Reina's surprise, they did so readily, as they truly wanted to see her return to being happy. Her anger slowly dissolved, her energy returned, and family communication opened up. She loved the dance and drawing classes and, through them, met some new friends.

REINA AND MARGRIT'S MESSAGE FOR US

When I first met Reina and heard her story, I was struck with the parallel with Margrit's story. While they had quite different presenting problems, their backgrounds and their having made a life's work of being responsible for everyone had amazing similarities. I had a sense that lying on the floor symbolized for Margrit the ultimate in self-indulgence that she had never permitted herself. Instead of becoming angry as Reina had, she became depressed, but by giving herself permission to be open to her own needs Margrit found a way through the depression. I felt that as Margrit could not be there to tell her own story, I stood in her place, becoming a part of the creative process that is re-storying. Reina heard Margrit's tale of wanting to lie on the floor, and understood the metaphor entirely. For Reina, being free to look at her own needs awakened her long-unfulfilled and unconsidered creativity, and in this way Margrit helped Reina to find her own path.

As therapists, we too are often expected to behave in certain ways by our particular cultural subsets, and have much to learn from such metaphorical tales. Our clients bring us the inspirations to continue linking to, and with, them in an ongoing chain of stories and understandings. Like Margrit, Reina has given permission to tell her story, and so now both of these remarkable women, and the therapist who shared their journey, are telling it to you, the reader, who may in turn take something from these stories, or the process of working with them, and share the experience with future clients and therapists. In such a way, we all may pass down the shared experiences and metaphors of life in traditional human fashion: by telling each other stories.

CHAPTER 8

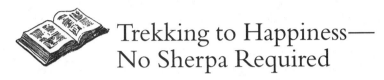

Trekking to Happiness— No Sherpa Required

A Utilization Approach to Transcending an Abusive Relationship

Gregory Smit

CONTRIBUTOR'S STORY: A PROFESSIONAL AND PERSONAL PERSPECTIVE

Gregory Smit, MA, is a marriage and family therapist intern in Sacramento, California. He graduated from the University of San Francisco with a master's in counseling psychology and is a professional member of the Association of Family Therapists of Northern California and a prelicensed member of the California Association of Marriage and Family Therapists. His first exposure to storytelling occurred when he saw Stephen Lankton's presentation on metaphor at a brief therapy conference in 2003, which encouraged him to become a more effective storyteller with his own clients.

Gregory lives in Ripon, California, with his wife, Sharon, and son, Ethan, and believes that the indirect style of communication inherent in stories can be used to foster positive relationships with children and engender a more generous parenting style. When he is not working with his clients, you will find Gregory at the beach, playing volleyball, reading at Starbucks, or at the zoo with his wife and son.

PREVIEW THE CHAPTER

In this chapter Gregory presents us with a challenging therapeutic situation: What do you do when faced with a client who is being physically and emotionally abused, who has not acquired the skills to cope with such experiences, and who does not have the supportive network of a caring family? Having set the challenge, he walks us through his thinking and the interactions with his client as he sought to specifically define her goals, discover her resources, utilize those resources in therapy, and assist her toward her desired outcome of happiness. He describes the choices he weighed in considering what interventions would be most helpful for this client. His rationale for selecting a therapist-generated metaphor is clearly explained, as well as the ways he saw the story matching his client, modeling appropriate coping mechanisms for her, and reaching a point that would enable her to achieve a different perspective. In a useful, self-reflective conclusion, he examines what working with Mariah offered him in validation and discoveries that could be beneficial for other such cases.

Therapeutic Characteristics

Problems Addressed

- Lack of self-esteem
- Lack of happiness
- Unhappy marriage
- Lack of family support
- Physical abuse
- Mental abuse
- One-down position

Resources Developed

- Perseverance
- Hope
- Openness to change
- Positive belief system
- Expanding view of happiness
- More flexible relationships
- Ability to face new challenges
- Development of new perspectives
- Ability to navigate around obstacles and problems
- Responsibility for solving own problems

Outcomes Offered

- Expanded perspective
- New possibilities
- Responsibility for own happiness
- One-up position

The tall stature and large frame of the 28-year-old African American woman were masked by her slouching shoulders and unassuming smile as she walked through the door of my office in San Diego. Mariah's demeanor, I observed, was friendly but reserved. Her verbal utterances were soft, with long pauses in between. In stark contrast, her nonverbal expressions exuded a raw and intense energy that surfaced through rapid foot tapping and hand gestures.

To pay for college, Mariah said, she worked as a waitress, where she had met Darnell, a regular customer. She never intended to develop a serious relationship with him, but at the age of 19 she became pregnant and decided to ensure a secure future for her baby by marrying him. However, things did not turn out as she had planned. Darnell spent a considerable time at the local bars, often coming home drunk in the wee hours of the morning. He caroused with female friends from the bar, which made Mariah feel insecure. As a last-ditch effort to save the marriage, she got pregnant a second time, hoping that the new baby would solidify the couple's relationship. In reality, the added pressure drove them further apart and provided Darnell with another excuse to drink.

In spite of all these setbacks, Mariah completed a degree in art history and later became a successful mortgage broker in San Diego. However, she told me, her potential had been marred by a series of crises Darnell created that caused her to lose several key accounts. The stress of constantly having to smooth things over with her bosses took an enormous emotional toll on her over the years, diminishing her self-esteem, and robbing her of the one outlet where she had a sense of competency.

Mariah said she entered therapy because she was no longer experiencing happiness in her life. Before her marriage, she thought of herself as a happy-go-lucky person. In the intervening years, a lack of interest in the marriage, coupled with her husband's drinking problem, forced Mariah to spend a considerable amount of time pondering whether she was on the right course and what type of action would be necessary to bring back the happiness that occurred so naturally in the past.

Four months prior to entering therapy, she and the children left her husband, then subsequently moved back. The separation, however, did not change the couple's underlying problems. Mariah said that according to her husband's logic, men and women were inherently different and were therefore subject to different rules. When she tried to point out the inconsistencies in his logic, he told her that women were too weak to be trusted and that men have a biological need to roam with other wolves in a pack rather than staying at home all of the time.

Darnell was also physically abusive. During the first session, Mariah downplayed the fact that he had broken her nose during a recent argument, presenting it as a one-time event. However, as therapy continued, the extent of his violence became more evident with stories of multiple assaults. Mariah even recounted an incident several years back when Darnell came at her with a knife because she had been out late one evening with friends.

SEARCHING FOR RESOURCES

I used the assessment time with Mariah to begin to utilize and amplify her resources and strengths, while buffering her deficits (Lankton & Lankton, 1983). The process of utilization can be thought of as a therapeutic position where the therapist explores "a patient's individuality to ascertain what life learnings, experiences, and mental skills are available to deal with the problem . . . [and] then [utilizes] these uniquely personal internal responses to achieve therapeutic goals" (Erickson & Rossi, 1979,

p. 1). I embarked upon this tack because I have found the concept of utilization to be highly effective in inducing change on the client's terms. Practically, I wanted to use her narrative to develop a better understanding of how she viewed her problems and what changes she thought would help her reach her goals so that I could utilize this information to construct future therapeutic interventions. I also wanted to expand my understanding of her beliefs, role definition, communication patterns, and family structure so that these factors could be cultivated as fertile opportunities for utilization in subsequent sessions (Lankton & Lankton, 1986).

One of the most important factors that I wanted to understand, and subsequently utilize, was whether Mariah was ready to change significant aspects of her life and what she thought would be the most straightforward way to initiate the desired change. As I began to query her, she formulated two statements that led me to believe that the seeds of change had been sown, at least partially. Mariah articulated that she could no longer deal with her husband's controlling nature or his alcohol binges. She also thought that her children were suffering from the couple's constant arguing. According to Mariah, the major impediment to change was her fear that she would fail if she was forced to be the sole breadwinner, as her mother had been after her father abandoned the family when Mariah was a child. To overcome this fear, Mariah believed that she simply had to revert back to her own happy personality that was present before she married—a common belief among victims of abuse, who often compare dire present circumstances to fuzzy and less menacing memories.

Wanting to dig deeper, I inquired how Mariah perceived the concept of happiness. Before marriage, she said, she enjoyed the small things in life and would not spend a great deal of time pondering the future. This contrasted sharply with Mariah's current situation, in which she spent an inordinate amount of time ruminating about all of the bad things that could happen.

Mariah's communication patterns and family structure were key considerations in my assessment of her situation. During the assessment period, it became clear that she would often become involved in rigid complementary relationships with significant individuals in her life (Watzlawick, Beavin Bavelas, & Jackson, 1967). For instance, she almost exclusively ended up in the "one-down" position with her husband, as evidenced by his verbal and physical abuse. From a family structure perspective, Mariah's position in the hierarchy of her family of origin was much lower than her age, accomplishments, and abilities warranted. Her mother ensured that the hierarchy would remain unchanged by constantly berating Mariah and undermining her confidence. Even Mariah's younger sister would scold her and mock her decisions. Only her older brother, T'Shaun, acted as an ally, suggesting that, as a grown woman, she had a right to make her own decisions and follow her own heart.

One of my most important functions in the assessment process is to become more aware of my client's resources. Mariah was able to retrieve several key intrinsic resources that could be used therapeutically, including perseverance, hope, a positive belief system, and openness to change. Her perseverance was underscored in therapy during our discussion of the numerous challenges and obstacles that she overcame in her work as a mortgage broker. Her ability to envision a pathway to happiness suggested that she retained hope about the future. Maybe she displayed a Pollyanna-ish view of her past level of happiness, but the very fact that she was able to anticipate a positive outcome, unlike many sad individuals, suggested to me that this feeling could be used in therapy. Mariah's hope, coupled with her firm belief in happiness, could be used as a catalyst to help her retrieve additional resources that would be useful in the process of change.

Mariah was mindful that her present behaviors, beliefs, and relationships were keeping her stuck in unpleasant circumstances and that she needed an openness to change. This solution-focused mentality is often initially difficult for clients to accept because, although they wish that their lives were better, they ultimately believe that their fate is already sealed. Mariah was cognizant of the fact that she was a major part of the solution and was not looking to other individuals to solve her problems.

As a family therapist, I believed it was necessary to unearth Mariah's extrinsic resources. This was difficult given the many stories she told about her unsupportive family. However, it became apparent that she could enlist her brother, T'Shaun, and several of her friends as resources to help her make changes in her life.

PLANNING THE DIRECTION OF TREATMENT

While developing my treatment plan, I utilized the resources that Mariah had already embraced. I believed that it would accelerate the process of change by reducing resistance to the plan. Therefore, Mariah's beliefs in happiness and herself as a source of solutions were used as the focal point of all therapeutic interventions and were constantly amplified in therapy. Her openness to change and her perseverance served as the foundation of subsequent interventions. Specifically, these concepts were used to enrich the process of metaphor development, and, in turn, the metaphor became the vehicle that was used to elicit change-oriented behavior.

In defining and discussing the therapeutic goals with Mariah, my first objective was to utilize and expand her view of happiness to engender specific changes in behaviors and self-image. I also wanted to help Mariah move from a strictly complementary one-down position to a more flexible relationship with her husband. These two goals were inextricably linked because my client's long-term happiness would be extremely difficult to maintain if she continued her pattern as the one-down player in the relationship with her husband. Finally, I wanted to use her brother and social network to strengthen, support, and amplify these changes. In short, I hoped that they would serve as a bulwark to reinforce any nascent changes.

I decided to use metaphor as the centerpiece of my therapeutic intervention. Several factors that coalesced during the assessment process influenced my decision. One of the major factors was that, like many victims of domestic violence, my client did not respond well to direct discussion of the dangers associated with enduring physical abuse. When I discussed creating a safety plan or explained that physical violence is never acceptable, she downplayed the seriousness of the issue by saying that the abuse happened only rarely. In contrast, the psychological distance created by indirectly participating in the metaphorical process allowed her to become more engaged and ready to accept change. Another benefit of the metaphor was that she became much more relaxed while listening to the story, deviating from her usual anxious behavior. Mariah also found that listening to the metaphor reduced her confusion to a more manageable level. At the beginning of therapy, she was not sure if it was really wrong for her husband to abuse her, but as our sessions continued she accepted the fact that she deserved safety. As the confusion waned, Mariah was able to focus on potential solutions rather than continuing to focus on her problems. Metaphor played a key role in this forward-thinking process. Most important, she began to make significant changes once the metaphor was introduced into therapy, so I wanted to continue to use what was working.

DEFINING THE THERAPEUTIC AND METAPHORIC OBJECTIVES

One of my main objectives in creating the metaphor was to encourage Mariah to creatively utilize her available resources as a foundation that could support new resources as they were uncovered, strengthened, and developed through the process of affiliating with the protagonist in the unfolding story. The protagonist, like Mariah, is on a journey. He uses her currently available resources of hope, perseverance, openness to change, and a positive belief system to help him overcome obstacles along the way. He employs these resources in a myriad of new ways and combines them with other valuable resources to face new challenges, develop new perspectives, and reach his ultimate goal. My expectation was that as Mariah experienced the protagonist's success in completing his journey, she would be more willing to integrate this new learning, which would engender changes in her own beliefs, behaviors, and roles.

At the beginning of therapy, Mariah's hopeful attitude had been unmistakable, although apparently fragile. The metaphor was designed to strengthen this hope as she reflected upon the protagonist's unique ability to look beyond obstacles and ignore the people who try to dampen his spirit as he focuses upon his final destination. I believed that helping Mariah to develop the ability to ignore negative comments was critical because the majority of her family members would probably begin to attack her character once she began to make changes that altered the family's dynamics. I believed that this could easily stifle any further progress in therapy. By remaining hopeful, my client could re-frame these attacks as a mere nuisance rather than a massive roadblock to her progress.

Woven into the metaphor was my conviction that Mariah's innate resource of perseverance was a perfect foundational structure, able to support the development of additional resource building blocks, including the ability to learn to navigate around obstacles and problems while continuing to journey toward a goal (Burns, 2001). The protagonist personifies this conviction through his dogged determination to not let bad weather, impassable paths, or detractors' criticism keep him from reaching his destination, thus foreshadowing Mariah's ability to use the perseverance she had developed in her professional life to solve problems that dogged her in her personal life.

Mariah's belief that she was an integral part of the solution to her problems had already laid the foundation to help her learn to take care of herself, to stand on her own two feet, and to develop more effective self-assertion skills (Burns, 2001). The metaphor encouraged my client to layer these new roles and behaviors into her personal experience. In the story, the protagonist does not expect someone else, such as a Sherpa, to solve his problems or to carry him to his destination. Rather, he actively sets his own agenda, overcomes his own obstacles, and reaches his desired objective on his own. Learning to utilize these behaviors would increase the probability that Mariah could stop being victimized by her husband and take a proactive assessment of her self-image.

The metaphor was designed to be a fish-eye lens, utilizing Mariah's openness to change as the tool that would alter the way she perceived things (Burns, 2001). At the top of a mountain, the protagonist develops a different perspective as he surveys his environment from a 360-degree perspective rather than the myopic view that is normal at the base of the mountain. Mariah's base-camp view of herself, perpetuated by husband and family, was as a one-dimensional failure. The metaphor encouraged her to expand upon this perception with new frames and possibilities, including an assessment of which behaviors would increase her happiness and consummate a functional relationship with her husband.

At the highest level, my goal was to illustrate that the path to a more functional life winds through unexplored territory. The protagonist is not afraid to traverse new territory if it enables him to reach his goal. Similarly, Mariah would benefit from trying out new beliefs, roles, and behaviors, both in and out of the therapy sessions. Significant progress toward her destination would be made as she learned to integrate these new learnings.

Another goal for the metaphor was to seed the idea that Mariah was responsible for cultivating her own happiness and should adjust her beliefs, behaviors, and roles to promote this feeling. Zeig defines seeding as "activating an intended target by presenting an earlier hint" (Zeig & Gilligan, 1990, p. 222). The protagonist presented Mariah with the ultimate hint regarding the path to happiness by pursuing a style of living, extreme as it is, that creates this feeling in his life. He is not willing to placate the masses of detractors at the expense of an opportunity to truly enjoy his journey, a potentially poignant lesson for Mariah to learn.

Woven into the fabric of the metaphor was the message that Mariah did not have to always assume the one-down position in her relationships but could become more constructively assertive with the individuals in her life. The story point in which the protagonist stands on top of the mountain, looking down upon his detractors, was designed to provide a cue that the one-up position is an attractive destination and that the decision to capitulate on a specific issue can be a choice rather than a constant relationship pattern.

PLANNING THE STEPS FOR A METAPHOR INTERVENTION

I start the process of metaphor creation by listening intently to the client's language and then using the material from our discussions to create an analogy that will link the client's desired outcome—in this case, happiness—to the metaphor that follows. I said to Mariah, "When you say that you are looking for happiness, it is as if you are looking for a peak mountain experience, an experience that many mountain climbers have when they finally reach the pinnacle of the mountain." By sequencing the intervention in this way, I attempted to ensure that Mariah would not resist the subsequent metaphor because she would already be comfortable with the creative bridge between the ideas of happiness and a peak mountain experience. Of course, if Mariah resisted the analogy, I would have the opportunity to develop a more suitable metaphor. However, Mariah's nonverbal communication indicated that the analogy fitted her worldview, so I proceeded with the metaphor development.

I see the second step in the metaphor creation process as an opportunity to develop a character who personifies the new resources that are useful for my client to cultivate. With Mariah, I wanted to use a bona fide mountain climber who had overcome significant obstacles so that she could identify with a real person who had defined his own version of success and happiness. Ideally, I would have been able to find a female mountain climber who embodied all of these characteristics. However, after significant research, I believed that Reinhold Messner came closest to epitomizing the characteristics that would be useful for Mariah on her new journey. He is a unique individual who is "probably the only person who truly climbed [Mount] Everest alone" (Jerberyd, 2002). He was the first to climb Mount Everest without supplementary oxygen (Jerberyd, 2002). He was not interested in being defined on other people's terms, such as world record recognition, but in defining his own happiness and success (*Reinhold Messner,* 2003). Throughout his life, Messner overcame criticism about

his unique style of climbing. He learned to conquer obstacles, develop unique solutions while journeying toward his goal, stand on his own two feet, and build the perseverance to both reach his goal
and enjoy the journey along the way. My hope was that by reflecting upon Messner's characteristics,
Mariah would start an internal search process that would clarify which of these resources would be
useful for her own journey.

The final step in the process of metaphor creation is to develop, expand, and enrich the story, in
this case linking the end goal of happiness to the interim step of a journey. As I developed the story, I
wanted to focus as much on Messner's experiences as he journeyed up the mountain toward his goal
as I did on the feelings he had when he reached his final destination. I wanted to embed the aspects
of Messner's life experiences, character, and personal resources that would be useful to Mariah's own
search for happiness into the main plot of the story. With each step of story development, I wanted
to encourage Mariah to take a risk by beginning her journey.

BEGINNING THE TREK

This is how I used those different aspects of Messner's life in the final version of the metaphor.

I remember hearing the story of Reinhold Messner from my favorite college professor. Now,
Reinhold is a very successful and unconventional mountain climber. He was the first person
to climb Mount Everest by himself without using the traditional method of employing a
Sherpa and without the use of oxygen bottles. He was also the first person to climb all of
the Earth's fourteen tallest peaks. His ability to reach so many difficult destinations has given
him the reputation of being the greatest mountain climber of all time.

Reinhold was able to set himself apart from so many other climbers because of the
strong internal compass that guided him along the journey. While other climbers were looking to Sherpas to guide them along the path, Reinhold focused on his own resources to help
him reach his destination. He used his clever mind to quickly assess all of the possibilities and
then made his decision. He had a knack for finding the best route, for knowing when the
weather was turning bad, and for finding the best place to set up camp. He didn't want to
waste time trying to build consensus with a large group of other climbers on the mountain
because he was confident of his path and didn't want to be taken off course.

While he was at base camp, many of his detractors would try to talk him out of moving toward his new destination. They were quick to call him a lunatic and criticized him
for the way he did things. They would often say, "Reinhold, stay with us at base camp and
have a drink, live a normal life, stop being so crazy." Reinhold overcame their criticism by
focusing on the vision of what he wanted his life to look like. He persevered and remained
hopeful that he would reach his goal.

Once on the mountain, he had to be flexible because things were not always easy. Sometimes the normal passageway was too dangerous to use, so he would have to try a new one.
Other times, bad weather forced him to set up camp for the night early and he would have
to make up time after the storm passed. On one occasion, he had to climb up one side of
the mountain and descend on the other side, a side he had never seen. All of these experi-

ences provided new resources that Reinhold could use when he faced a difficult situation. He might not have known the exact path to the top at that moment, but he recognized that he had succeeded in the past and would find a way to succeed now.

At the summit, Reinhold saw views that could not help but change his perspective. The criticism from people at base camp faded as he realized that he was far above them now. As he slowly turned in a 360 degree circle, he was excited that he could see for miles and miles. Happiness flooded his body. The kind of happiness that comes from recognizing that he was in the perfect place at the perfect time . . . that no one had carried him up the mountain . . . that he had used so many unique gifts along the way . . . and that no one could take away his accomplishments because this journey was his own unique journey.

OFFERING MORE THAN A METAPHOR

It is important to put the metaphor in the proper context of the therapeutic plan because it was not the sole intervention that I used with Mariah. The metaphor was used early in the therapeutic process as a catalyst for change. After Mariah had the opportunity to retrieve internal resources based on her personal connection to the story, we began to discuss her issues within the context of the metaphor. For instance, at one point in therapy, she suggested that her desire to set up camp for the winter, due to exhaustion, meant she was a failure. I normalized this desire as an internal self-protection mechanism meant to ensure that she would not become sick and be forced to return to base camp and miss out on her journey to happiness.

Once the story had been presented, I asked Mariah to pretend that her future self entered the room to provide her with support in initiating and developing new behaviors. She reacted positively, detailing the panoply of characteristics embodied in this vision of her future self. Then I suggested that Mariah's future self might have some useful advice for her because she was older and more experienced. As she told me the advice her future self wanted to share with her, she became noticeably more relaxed, letting out a big sigh and developing a slight smile on her face. "Lighten up on yourself and take one step at a time," was what her future self wanted her to remember.

Prior to listening to the metaphor, Mariah would shrug off suggestions to develop a safety plan. Once she retrieved the necessary resources from the metaphor, she was more willing to make positive changes in her life. This openness provided the opportunity to offer a psychoeducation intervention, encouraging an increase in personal safety within her abusive relationship. First, I suggested that she might want to have a safety plan in place. Second, I provided her with the patterns of the early warning signs that suggested violence might be imminent. While Mariah was learning these patterns of violence, I attempted to help her develop her own resources among family and friends, suggesting she call her brother, T'Shaun, or one of her friends every time she noticed one of Darnell's destructive patterns. The contact with her support system was designed to reinforce her recent learning and break Darnell's pattern of attempting to isolate her through manipulative behavior.

As Mariah's confidence and creativity increased, she began to change her beliefs about the role she should play within her family and altered her communications with them in previously unexplored ways. I encouraged these explorations through the use of weekly homework, which included learning to discriminate between aggression and assertion, monitoring her responses to her family, and determining which communication styles she liked and which ones left her feeling dissatisfied. One significant outcome of this role development was that she was more willing to stand up for herself during conflicts with her mother.

Once Mariah changed her role definition to include the belief that she was worthy of respect, she was no longer willing to accept Darnell's demeaning and abusive behavior. She left, telling him she would be willing to work on the marriage if he attended an anger management group and individual counseling. He did not. If he belittled her during visitations with the children, she would tell him she did not like the way he was treating her and would ask him to leave, without losing control or screaming at him. Mostly he complied. This transformation in her ability to be assertive was a major therapeutic accomplishment.

Mariah became much more relaxed, was not as concerned about what others thought of her, and learned to again enjoy being in the moment, thus handling problems as they arose rather than constantly catastrophizing about the future as she had done in the past. From this new perspective, she developed more satisfying relationships and rekindled a love of her job. These factors, she considered, were critical to ensuring that her happiness would continue over time.

LEARNING FROM AN EXPERIENCE

Working with Mariah certainly validated some of my thoughts about the therapeutic process. First, the case reminded me of the power of utilization. Aligning with Mariah and utilizing her need for happiness was a major contributor to the success of this case. Second, it strengthened my conviction in the importance of using metaphor to create an expectancy set with a client who appears to be confused about how to proceed in making changes in his or her life. I noticed a significant improvement in Mariah's ability to analyze possible solutions once the story was introduced into therapy. Third, the case also deepened my appreciation of how metaphors play an important role in developing resources that are useful to the client. This story appeared to help Mariah access courage, creativity, and confidence as she began her journey. Finally, the case reminded me that telling stories builds rapport with the client by accessing a familiar bonding ritual, one that the client may have experienced while hearing bedtime stories in childhood. This rapport is strengthened every time the storyteller and the client immerse themselves in the common experience of a new storytelling encounter.

It may be trite to make the point that effective storytelling is at least as important as creating an appropriate story: The rate of utterance, attention to detail, inflection, and intonation of speech are critical factors. However, I also realize that any intervention will never be perfect and that client outcome is a better indicator of success than a perfectly presented story. As a therapist, I amplify or de-emphasize an idea during a story, but I never really know if the intervention will be successful until change occurs in the client. This ambiguity is simply inherent in a major swath of the therapeutic territory and needs to be embraced.

The story of Messner helped Mariah envision that change was possible. Seeing Messner reach his destination allowed Mariah to retrieve her own internal resources. Yet the most important outcome from therapy was that Mariah saw her situation from a different perspective, overcame difficult obstacles, and regained a sense of happiness by climbing a metaphoric mountain—no Sherpa required.

REFERENCES

Burns, G. W. (2001). *101 healing stories: Using metaphors in therapy.* New York: Wiley.

Erickson, M. H., & Rossi, E. L. (1979). *Hypnotherapy: An exploratory casebook.* New York: Irvington.

Jerberyd, P. (2002). *Reinhold Messner.* Retrieved November 15, 2006, from http://www.jerberyd.com/climbing/climbers/messner/

Lankton, S. R., & Lankton, C. (1983). *The answer within: A clinical framework of Ericksonian hypnotherapy.* New York: Brunner/Mazel.

Lankton, S. R., & Lankton, C. (1986). *Enchantment and intervention in family therapy: Training in Ericksonian approaches.* New York: Brunner/Mazel.

Reinhold Messner. (2003). Retrieved November 15, 2006, from http://www.everesthistory.com/climbers/messner.htm

Watzlawick, P., Beavin Bavelas, J., & Jackson, D. D. (1967). *Pragmatics of human communication: A study of interactional patterns, pathologies, and paradoxes.* New York: Norton.

Zeig, J. K., & Gilligan, S. G. (Eds.). (1990). *Brief therapy: Myths, methods, and metaphors.* New York: Brunner/Mazel.

CHAPTER 9

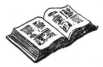

And the Two Snakes Fought

Storybook Therapy to Help Deal with the Divorce Monster

Joy Nel

CONTRIBUTOR'S STORY: A PROFESSIONAL AND PERSONAL PERSPECTIVE

Joy Nel, MEd, is an educational psychologist from Johannesburg, South Africa. Specializing in narrative therapy and Ericksonian psychotherapy, she trains educators and fellow psychologists in narrative ideas, focusing on the utilization of stories of hope. This work she has presented at international congresses in Germany and South Africa.

Working at a primary school, she became involved in the stories that young people told about themselves and their families, and grew interested in finding ways of collaboratively conversing with them to open up hopeful possibilities in their lives.

Her parents, true to the Afrikaans culture and tradition, shared stories around the dinner table of heroes who lived, loved, and fought with hope. When she was a young child, the family's African gardener filled her mind with fascinating stories of the Zulu-speaking people and the ways they witness and live hope in their lives. Now, as a therapist, Joy teaches stories of hope and peace to others.

PREVIEW THE CHAPTER

Parents can be embarrassing enough for a child even without a "not real" divorce. Joy tells us of a 10-year-old girl who self-presented to the school psychologist because of distress, unhappiness, and altered behaviors related to her divorced parents' continuing to live together in an ambivalent relationship. With a narrative therapy orientation, Joy collaboratively engages her young client in creating a storybook that draws on the child's interests and past experiences to build a metaphor of two snakes fighting. We are guided through the processes of "storybook therapy" from listening to the client's problem-saturated story, externalizing the problem, and deconstructing her "bad ideas" to coconstructing a healthier counterplot to the story. In a cooperative interaction between client and therapist, the preferred story is written up, edited, and formatted into a storybook that is then shared and celebrated with significant others in the client's life. This playful, educational approach teaches essential life skills and builds hope.

Therapeutic Characteristics

Problems Addressed

- Divorce
- Parental conflict
- Unhappiness
- Loss of hope
- Aggression
- Withdrawal
- Deterioration in schoolwork
- Worry

Resources Developed

- Learning to externalize problems
- Learning to deconstruct problem-saturated stories
- Learning to create preferred stories
- Standing up to old problems
- Being honest
- Feeling nice
- Learning to celebrate

Outcomes Offered

- Effective problem-solving skills
- Empowerment
- Improved relationship skills
- Management of "bad ideas"
- Enjoyment
- Strength
- Hope

Jamé, a 10-year-old girl in fourth grade, referred herself for therapy using the mailbox system by which children at the school could write a note telling about the problem that was invading their life and then post it in a mailbox. We, the school psychologists, would collect them and invite the child for a conversation. Jamé's note said that her parents had divorced the previous year and that she was extremely upset by this. Stating that she couldn't get rid of her unhappiness, she said, "My brain keeps on saying it over and over again."

The story was that her parents divorced when Jamé's father suspected her mother of having an affair with another man. Although the divorce case was settled, her father never moved out of the house, as he felt that her mother would not be able to look after the children by herself. Her parents' continuing to live together resulted in a lot of tension and fighting in the house, which left Jamé feeling scared and confused. She described the divorce as "not real because it is not the same as the other children in my school." Although Jamé's father was building a new house, this too was surrounded with uncertainty. Would they all reside there together, or would he move to the new house alone? In addition, both her parents were not sure whether they really wanted to be divorced or whether they would try to work things out.

It seemed that Jamé was what Kathy Weingarten referred to as "bereft of hope" (2000, p. 401). She had lost her sparkle and enthusiasm for living and seemed to be lost in the sad and confusing world of a "not real" divorce. She displayed and was living with a number of the wide-ranging effects that divorce leaves at one's doorstep. Jamé's mother said with concern, "She was a fun-loving and confident young lady prior to the divorce but is now overtly quiet or overtly aggressive. At times she becomes violent and throws things around, or sometimes hits me or her sister. She snaps very easily at anyone but especially at me."

Her schoolwork was also starting to suffer. Her mother said Jamé was withdrawing from her friends at school and was either "constantly fighting with them or telling stories about them." She thought Jamé found the divorce "embarrassing" as it "made her sister take drugs." Additionally, she felt Jamé's father was influencing her negatively against her mother and sister. Jamé had shared a very special bond with her father, but even this relationship became uncertain as the divorce continued to cause havoc in her family. Consequently, she experienced confusion and loneliness as the bonds between her sister and parents deteriorated.

NARRATIVE AS "STORYBOOK THERAPY"

Thinking about the continuing direction of my work with Jamé, I leaned toward narrative therapy because it is concerned with the tales and stories we tell about ourselves and about our lives (Epston & White, 1992; Morgan, 2000; White, 1989, 1995; White & Epston, 1990). As I often invite children to put the therapeutic tellings and retellings of these stories in writing, I refer to this approach (consistently with Linda van Duuren, 2002) as *storybook therapy:* the writing, editing, and publicizing of the child's own storybook. Jamé's storybook displays her "life-world" of hope and tenacity in dealing with divorce. It became the proof and ratification of the steps she took in challenging divorce along with its other problem monsters. It also voices her hope-filled "life-story" and calls all readers into believing and following hope with her (Kotzé & Morkel, 2002; Weingarten, 2000). The child's own

story is a personal representation of her world, has greater value and meaning than an externally offered story, and allows the therapist to readily enter the child's life.

Jamé was very excited about the prospect of being reminded of her therapeutic learnings by
writing up her story. In doing this, we utilized her snake metaphor (which is described later), writing a story about a snake family plagued by divorce. The creative time used in the writing up and
publicizing of this story gave us an opportunity to extend our conversations and to revisit and retell
her knowledge.

THE PROCESSES OF STORYBOOK THERAPY

"Storybook therapy" provides the opportunity for our clients to unearth problem-saturated stories
and negative perceptions about themselves. This leads to the reclaiming of knowledge, skills, and, of
course, the self.

Assisting my clients in writing their stories steers me as therapist down the avenue of respectfully
and gently entering a client's life-world, wherein I can guide them into rediscovering and celebrating their self-empowerment. The therapist, during this process, works from a not-knowing position
(Epston & White, 1992). Only from this position, where we accept that we are knowledgeable about
the therapeutic guidance and space we provide but not about the client's world, are we able to give
justice to our clients' stories (Epston, 2002). Therefore, children are the owners of their stories and
lives, and the therapist is only the scribe.

The process of storybook therapy with children is not a fixed process, but rather a creative and
flexible process wherein we discover and enjoy our strengths. During this process I am mostly guided
by my client and therefore provide only the practical structure of each therapeutic conversation and
the storybook. A brief outline of the basic process I used with Jamé follows.

LISTENING TO THE PROBLEM-SATURATED STORY

Hearing Jamé's Story

During our first conversation, Jamé sat with her head bowed, fidgeting nervously with her fingers.
Her body language spoke of all the emotions she had bottled up inside her. I asked, "Will you tell
me more about the divorce that is staying with your family at the moment?"

She shook her head and replied, "I don't know, it's not nice."

Being alert to the risk of exposure and embarrassment for my young clients, I wanted to respect
her private space in the lack of verbal responsiveness, and so sought to move to another realm of communication. Mindful of Freedman and Combs's comment that "just listening and asking facilitating
and clarifying questions from a position of curiosity can be very therapeutic" (1996, p. 45), I asked,
"Would you like to build a story in the sand tray that could tell me something about you?"

Jamé proceeded to build a "game reserve for all the animals on the shelf," telling me as she did
about the times she went hunting with her father and all the things that she enjoyed in life. Speak-

ing about her dad, she added, "I don't always understand what he says. He always changes his story. It makes me worry. When they are not fighting he says, 'We are all going to stay together,' but when the fighting is bad, he says, 'I am going to stay on my own, where nobody can shout at me.'" While Jamé took her time to build a fence around her "game reserve," to make sure that "they never run away" or "feel sad" like her, I made use of the opportunity to ask her clarifying questions regarding the sadness she was feeling and whether that was what she wanted to talk to me about.

During our second session, Jamé played with the snakes in the sand tray again, telling me about a pet snake she had called Mrs. Brown. Mrs. Brown was a boa constrictor, and Jamé said, "I love watching her and feeding her mice." She explained that they had put another snake in the cage with Mrs. Brown, but Mrs. Brown had killed it. I commented on the loss of her snake, whereupon Jamé replied, "I'm okay with it now, I knew it was going to happen."

"How did you know that?" I asked, and she explained that she had spent "hours" observing the two snakes and she could see that Mrs. Brown wanted to kill the other snake, because she was always hissing at the small one. I wondered out loud, "Have you spent time observing the work of divorce at home, like you have the snakes?" With a smile she produced her notebook and aptly explained, "Divorce is like two snakes fighting or like two snakes running away from each other." She added thoughtfully, "I was watching Mrs. Brown and the other snake closely. They were always hissing at each other, sometimes wanting to bite each other." Relating it to how things were at home, she said, "We are always fighting—especially my mom and dad." Feeling scared and worried, she explained, "When divorce makes fighting so bad, I just want to run away and never come back." Then she added, "At times I feel like doing what Mrs. Brown did and just chomp up everyone around me."

Aware of Jamé's earlier reluctance to talk about the divorce directly, I recognized that her use of the metaphor of "the two snakes fighting" afforded us the opportunity to externalize the problem and explore her relationship with divorce from a distance. In order to stay with Jamé and her metaphor in our conversations, I made sure that the plastic snakes, shrubs, and the picture she later drew of "Divorce" were always available for her to utilize in the sessions.

Externalizing the Problem(s)

Jamé and I both agreed that it was imperative for us to understand all we could about the divorce in her life in order for her to deal better with it. I asked her to imagine the two of us as detectives, who needed to gather information about the mean problem that was trying to steal her happiness so that we would know how to outsmart the problem. This caught her attention and a little smile started. "So, detective Jamé, what should we call this problem that we are trying to outsmart?" I asked. Her answer was definitive: "Let's just call him Divorce!" From there we used language that helped us personify this problem, naming it Divorce as if it were something visible and tangible—something that could be destroyed. Personifying a problem with children instantly creates empowerment for the child, as it opens up a new reality wherein she and the therapist stand in opposition to the problem and its tricks. I asked her to draw me a picture of Divorce, saying, "I would like to see what this thing is that has been invading your happy life." As she put it up on the wall she said, "This is what has been causing all the fighting at my home."

"Divorce changed everything and everybody in the house," she explained. "There are so many things that Divorce did to them. Too much to talk about in one day." Jamé decided it was best if she wrote all these things down in a book and brought it to our next conversation, as we didn't have much time left in the session and she still wanted to "dig a hole for the snakes in the sand tray, make a river, and go find some sticks outside to use as trees." Respecting her wishes and trusting that she would take time at home to think about Divorce, I agreed and handed her a small notebook that she could use.

Deconstructing the Discourses

The "broader stories" or "dominant narratives" that exist in our culture influence the ways in which we give understanding and meaning to our lives (Freedman & Combs, 1996; Morgan, 2000). The power that discourses have over people's lives—such as discourses about what should happen in a "real" divorce—was evident in Jamé's life. Consequently, I considered it a prime responsibility for me to deconstruct with Jamé the dominant discourses surrounding the problem. A further opportunity to do so arose during one of our conversations when Jamé gave me an informative lesson regarding various venomous snakes. "The venom of some snakes can either kill you, let you lose an arm or leg, or blind you or leave you paralyzed," she stated with authority. "I saw a film where a huge anaconda spat a man full of poison, covering him in poison slime so he was stuck to the floor and could not run away."

"Have you ever been stuck to the floor by poison slime that other snakes or people have spat at you?" I asked.

"Lots," Jamé revealed. "Mom and Dad often spit me with poison slime. It makes me want to cry or hit them." She explained that it usually occurred when she asked what was happening with them and the divorce. Jamé had many questions about the divorce that she wanted her parents to clarify for her but were not being addressed: Who is going to move? Do they still love each other? Why did they have to divorce? Is Dad still cross with me and Mom? Can they stop their fighting? What is going to happen?

When she asked such questions, she said, "They spit poison slime, telling me to stop moaning. Mom says I must not ask her things that are too difficult for me to understand. Dad, he told me I shouldn't worry about what is happening, because it is big-people problems." This upset Jamé tremendously, leaving her to conclude that "nobody cares about me anymore." She explained, "If they don't tell me and they don't listen, but just fight, fight, fight, it makes the Worry monster appear and grow bigger."

A strong theme that reoccurred within this discourse was the idea that children can and must cope with any adversity from the adult world. This idea was so strongly imbedded within Jamé that she refused to tell her father that she was conversing with me, a psychologist. During our deconstruction of this discourse, Jamé stated that her dad told her, "It is not so bad. You will get over all your crying one of these days. A lot of kids come from divorced homes and are okay." Consequently, she explained, "If I tell him, I'm scared he will get mad at me or stop taking me hunting with him."

During our fifth conversation, I said, "Well, Jamé, perhaps there is one thing that you can do during this week to boot the monsters out of your life and to prove to yourself you can do it. Do you have any ideas of what you can do?"

"I will stop the Worry monster, by telling my dad I talk to you," she decided. When I questioned her on this decision she had made, she explained, "It is not good to keep secrets. It makes people worry, and I do not want my father to worry anymore." She added, "I don't want Worry in my life anymore, and I don't want it in my house!"

Coconstructing the Counterplot

Jamé was also influenced by the discourse of the perfect family. This discourse implies that a family can only be happy and loving if the parents are married. It had an overwhelming voice in Jamé's life, leading her to accept and believe that her life would never again be happy. The voice of this discourse was so powerful that Jamé refused to inform any of her friends about her parents' divorce, concealing it by "telling them nice stories about Mom and Dad that are not real." She stopped inviting her friends to sleep over at her house in case they thought it "weird" that her dad slept in the living room. The comments and jokes her friends made about other kids whose parents were divorced fueled her beliefs, raised her anger, and resulted in both physical and verbal hostility toward them. As a result she lost most of her friends.

Toward the end of this conversation, Jamé exclaimed, "I might be able to stop the fighting with my friends and get them back."

"How do you see you could do this?" I asked.

"Perhaps I need to tell them all the truth," she replied.

When I passed Jamé in the corridor at school a few days later, she happily pointed to her friends and said, "They are friends again and are very nice now that they know the truth." The deconstruction of this powerful discourse gave Jamé an opportunity to reach out to her friends and rebuild her relationship with them. It also facilitated her deconstruction of other discourses, enabling her to acknowledge and honor other personal knowledges such as "My mom cares about me. She is just different than my dad." "My dad was worried that he might lose me." "Moms and dads do things that they don't always mean to."

REAUTHORING AND STRENGTHENING THE PREFERRED STORY

Writing and Designing the Storybook

In the second session I introduced the option of writing a story about how she had triumphed over problems in her life, reflecting, "I have listened to your story of what is happening in your life with the snakes fighting. If you and I were able to change this story into a better story for you to live your life by, what would you call that story?" She answered, "And the two snakes fought."

Knowing we were going to write a story, we kept thorough process notes of every conversation. At times, as in Jamé's case, clients want to make their own therapeutic notes either during the session or afterward. These notes were incorporated into the writing up of the story. All artworks created by Jamé were kept in our therapy room. It is a good idea to take photos of certain artworks during the session if the client prefers to take some of the work home.

The actual writing of the storybook starts as soon as I realize that a rich counterplot is emerging in our therapeutic conversations. With Jamé this happened in our eighth session. It is important to use your own discretion and check with your clients whether they are ready to start the writing process during the therapeutic conversations. I have found it useful to have a "writer's table." The clients know that when we work there we spend time writing, editing, and designing.

First, Jamé chose the title of her book. Second, she selected the appropriate format of her book after looking at stories written and designed by previous clients. She was shown pop-up books, matchbox books, poster books, pocket books, talking books, and computer books, before choosing to make a poster book. It is wise for you as a therapist to copy your client's storybook, if you have received permission to do so, as this can help establish a library of hope-filled stories to share with future clients. Third, we took some time choosing the characters, setting, and message of her story, as well as designing the front page. Finally, it was time to write up the story. We compared notes. I worked collaboratively with Jamé, suggesting some ideas and helping with the formulation of sentences and paragraphs.

Editing the Story

The editing of the story happened throughout our therapeutic conversations. When Jamé was satisfied with the draft I typed it out for her. I then gave her the draft to take home. This allows clients to do further editing of their own, and, if they want, they can check it with their parents or loved ones.

In our following session we made a few changes before printing the final copy of *And the Two Snakes Fought*. Hereafter, we took great care in painting, cutting, crafting, and pasting Jamé's book. Before putting it all together Jamé chose her own ISBN number and we designed our title page, selecting "Pandora's Press" as the name for our "printing company," after the story of hope as told in the legend of Pandora's box (Kershaw, 1990).

This is Jamé's story, which I have translated from her native Afrikaans. It was created in a book that folded out to take the shape of a snake (see Figures 9.1 and 9.2).

And the Two Snakes Fought

Once upon a time, long, long ago, there were two snakes. The one snake's name was Mr. Brown. He was the biggest and strongest snake that was ever seen on earth. He had a beautiful smooth skin, with the most beautiful yellowish golden brown spots. The spots always glistened in the sun. The other snake, his wife, Heidi, was just as beautiful as he was. Her skin was even smoother and it had beautiful large scales with golden-yellow stripes. The two snakes had two daughters. The older daughter's name was Trudy, and the younger daughter's name was Jamé. They were just as beautiful as their mother and father.

One day something very sad happened. For some reason or other the snakes started to fight. They made loud hissing sounds and bit each other's tails with their sharp teeth. When they first started fighting they couldn't stop. They fought over silly things. The man snake, Mr. Brown, fought because he thought the wife snake liked somebody else.

One evening when mother snake and her daughters went to visit granny snake, father snake turned up there as well. Another man snake was also there. He was a friend of granny

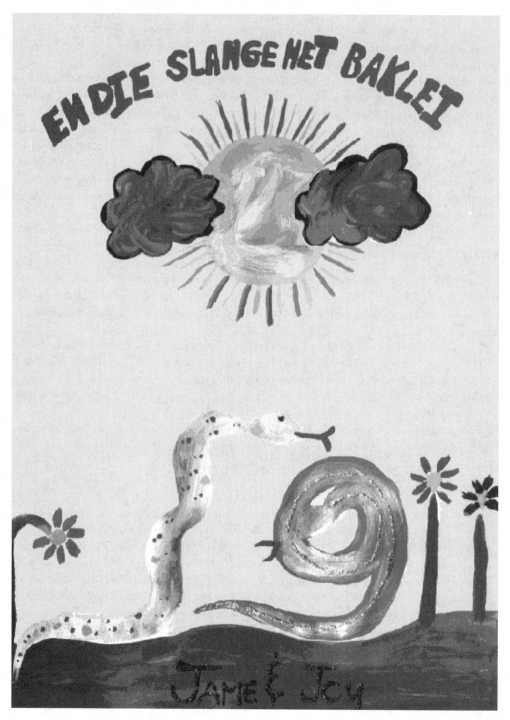

Figure 9.1　Cover of Jamé's story, *And the Two Snakes Fought*.

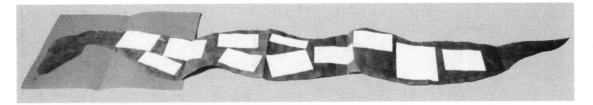

Figure 9.2   Jamé's story unfolds along the snake's body.

and also lived there. His name was Jack. He was very friendly. Mr. Brown was jealous of Jack and was angry with him. He thought that Jack and Heidi liked each other too much. That was not true!

That evening Mr. Brown became furious when he saw Heidi and Jack sitting beside each other on the sofa. He was so angry that he twirled his strong body around Jack and spat poison at him.

Mr. Brown decided to divorce his wife Heidi. They got divorced, but everybody still stayed in the same house. Divorce turned many things upside down in the house. The snake family had lots of fights. They hissed very loudly and spat poison all the time. Mom and dad snake bit each other with their poisonous teeth. Divorce made sister snake Trudy very angry at everybody, especially at father snake. Divorce was so bad for her that she started using drugs. Everybody was so scared of Divorce that it made them feel so confused.

Jamé was also very upset by Divorce. Divorce started telling Jamé some lies. Divorce said to her that:

It was her fault that Mom and Dad were getting divorced.
The snake family would never love each other again.
Mom and Dad didn't love each other anymore.

All these lies that Divorce told made Jamé feel very bad about herself. Divorce was so sneaky and wanted to hurt Jamé so badly that he brought along other problem monsters too.

Divorce and the problem monsters were like a bad gang that just wanted to hurt Jamé. In the gang there were the Fighting monster, the Sad monster, and the Worry monster. These problem monsters did many things and told Jamé many lies.

Fighting monster told her to fight with Mom, Dad, and sister snake all the time. He told her that if she did that she would feel better about herself. He said she would become stronger than the fighting in the house. He said that if she fought the most Mom and Dad would stop striking and spitting at each other. The monster told her that if she fought all the time and was miserable to everyone in the house, they would never forget her.

Divorce was so big that everybody in the house started forgetting about one another and about love.

The monster lied and told her that her friends did not like her anymore because Divorce was living with her. He told her to strike at them and spit poison to get them back.

Sad monster was also very sneaky and teased her a lot. He said that nobody in her family loved her anymore. He also told her that her teachers and friends at school were laughing at her and that they thought she was stupid. The monster said that she should not sleep at night, but should cry all the time. He said that if she cried all the time Mom and Dad would no longer divorce because they would feel sorry for her. She believed him when he told her that that was the only way to keep them together.

Actually the Worry monster was there all the time but grew in size when Divorce came to the Brown family. This monster always had a good laugh when he got Jamé to worry all the time. He let her worry over where she was going to stay when dad snake moved out one day. He told her that mom snake would be sad and lonely if she went to stay with Dad. Then he said that dad snake would be cross and sad if she stayed with Mom. He whispered in her ear that maybe she would have to go to another school and that she would never have friends again. He made her believe that if she worried all the time Divorce would go away.

What the stupid problem monsters did not know was that Jamé was much stronger than all of them. Jamé decided that the monsters were not going to hurt her anymore. She decided to fight back. While she fought back she learned many things about herself. She used these things to say to the monsters: "GO AWAY and LEAVE ME ALONE!!!"

These are the things that Jamé learned about herself:

She is special.
She is important to many people, also to Mom and Dad, even though they are getting divorced.
She has lots of guts.
She is a good friend.
She is a good sister.
She is a good daughter.
She is friendly.
She is helpful.
She cares about other people.
She can feel good about the things that she is good at, like athletics and mathematics.
She is honest.
She chooses to be happy.
She always shares with others.
She is clever.

Jamé learned many things about Divorce. She decided that she would use these things to help her snake friends should their moms and dads ever get divorced. She would show them that Divorce is not that big!

She could teach them the following things:

Divorce is not the end of the world.
One's life goes on and you can still do all the nice things you used to do before.

You are not going to see so much of your mom or dad if you decide to live with
one of them but you can speak to them on the phone every day or you can
make cards for Mom and Dad.

When you go and visit over weekends you can enjoy a movie or a meal together or
you can just talk.

Nobody is going to forget about you!

Jamé also got two more friends that helped her to remember how strong she is and
how she killed all the monsters. The names of her special friends are Blackie, the cat, and
Redspot, the rabbit. They are different from her other friends because they speak to her
alone. Other people do not know that they can talk.

These friends are very special and Jamé takes them with her wherever she goes. Sometimes they stay in her pencil box and sometimes she puts them in her shirt pocket. They
are always close to her heart.

Every time the problem monsters try to worry Jamé, she just strokes her special friends
and they remind her of how strong she is and that she shouldn't listen to the stories the
monsters tell.

These two friends help Jamé to remember that:

Monsters tell lies, and she must not listen to their stories, no matter what.
She is always special.
She is never alone.
She is strong.
She has a good life even though Mom and Dad are divorced.
She must be happy for each day.
She can always believe in herself.

Publicizing the Story

The sharing of preferred stories and preferred ways of being can support people in reclaiming their
lives from the effects of a dominant story and dominant discourses (Freedman & Combs, 1996).
Writing up the story with Jamé helped her tell her preferred story, but publicizing it gave her a voice
that spoke of courage, hope, and strength. I invited Jamé to consider sharing her story, celebrating
her new ideas, and rejoicing with friends and family about her choice. This invitation had a twofold
purpose, described in the following subsections.

To Share and Celebrate

First, my therapeutic aim was for her to share and celebrate her new, coconstructed story of preferred
ways to handle divorce. The purpose was to have her acknowledge her reclaimed and newfound
knowledge.

Jamé made invitations to her celebration and delivered them to five of her close friends. She
decided that she wanted to read her story, *And the Two Snakes Fought,* to her friends because she was
so proud of her beautiful book and of how she had conquered the problems in her life. This gesture

from Jamé was, to me, a defining moment and proof of immense change in her. I knew now that Jamé's voice was much stronger than divorce.

To further validate her new ways of processing, I presented Jamé with a certificate of excellence for reclaiming her life from divorce and invited her friends to share any special messages or insights they had regarding Jamé and her story.

"Jamé is a good friend," responded the first. "She must always remember that she is special. It is good that she can teach other children about divorce." Another said, "She writes very good stories and I feel happy that I heard it. I am glad we are not fighting anymore." Others followed: "I am glad that Jamé is my friend, and that she always helps me with math." "I am happy that she told us that her mom and dad are divorced because I know that I must help her and not fight with her." "Jamé, I think you are a very good person and I am glad that I am your friend." "Jamé's story is very nice." "I like her very much, and I think she is strong."

To Build Better Understandings

These special messages from her friends ratified all the personal knowledge that Jamé discovered and reclaimed during our conversations and the writing of her storybook. This matched with my second aim of our celebration: to affirm that wrong ideas can be turned into better understandings, through discussion with her friends. I see this stage of including peers as so important that I wonder whether any challenge to old, unhelpful discourses can be sustained without an audience. If other people's beliefs and ideas can help maintain a problem, then surely they have the potential to help bring about and maintain more helpful perceptions of ourselves and our abilities (McKenzie & Monk, 1997). When I asked Jamé's friends, "What better understandings have you gained from this discussion?" the responses were affirming.

"It is not a child's fault when a mom and dad do not want to stay married, and it is not nice to tease children because they are sad about it," said one of her friends. "Children are not bad because their mom and dad do not want to stay together anymore," said another. "You are still happy and a good child when your parents are divorced." "You will still have lots of friends to play with if your parents are divorced." "When parents divorce your mom, dad, and friends still care about you." Jamé added, "Divorce is not the end of the world."

FINDING HOPE IN A CHEESEBURGER

Toward the end of my 11 enlightening conversations with Jamé I wanted to ascertain whether, and in what manner, she had experienced them as helpful. I also wanted to determine whether she felt her therapeutic aims had been met. With this in mind, I asked, "Can we have our own little celebration wherein we could also take the time to reflect our learnings to each other?"

Jamé replied, "That will be a good idea, if we could tell each other about these things in McDonald's!"

So, sitting at a table in McDonald's, she said, "Our conversations have helped me enjoy life again. They have stopped the voice in my brain telling me that because of my parents' divorce I will have a bad life." She explained, "Our work together has helped me to know that I am very strong and can tell problems to leave me alone. I feel in my heart that life is good, and I always want to feel this way. I keep hope safe in my heart and believe in myself again."

"And how are things with your friends and family now?" I asked.

"Mom and Dad have stopped fighting in the house. I think this is a good thing that they learned from me." She reflected further, "I have learned to never listen to the wrong ideas of other people, but to rather listen to myself. And I know my friends have learned that it is not nice to be ugly and joke about children whose parents are divorced. They now understand divorce better. I think I have helped teach them to be stronger than problems."

Then, contemplatively looking at the Quarter Pounder with cheese in her hands, she summed things up aptly: "You know, my life is almost just as good as this cheeseburger."

REFERENCES

Epston, D., & White, M. (1992). *Experience, contradiction, narrative and imagination: Selected papers of David Epston and Michael White 1989–1991.* Adelaide, Australia: Dulwich Centre.

Epston, D. (2002). Putting the narrative back into narrative therapy workshop. Pretoria, South Africa: Institute for Therapeutic Development. In L. Els (2000), *The co-construction of a preferred therapist self of the educational psychology student.* Unpublished doctoral dissertation, Rand Afrikaans University, Johannesburg, South Africa.

Freedman, J., & Combs, G. (1996). *Narrative therapy: The social construction of preferred realities.* New York: Guilford Press.

Kershaw, S. (1990). *A concise dictionary of classical mythology.* London: Basil Blackwell.

Kotzé, E., & Morkel, E. (2002). *Matchboxes, butterflies and angry foots.* Pretoria, South Africa: Ethics Alive.

McKenzie, W., & Monk, G. (1997). Learning and teaching narrative ideas. In G. Monk, J. Windslade, K. Crocket, & D. Epston (Eds.), *Narrative therapy in practice: The archeology of hope* (pp. 82–116). San Francisco: Jossey-Bass.

Morgan, A. (2000). *What is narrative therapy? An easy-to-read introduction.* Adelaide, Australia: Dulwich Centre.

van Duuren, L. A. (2002). *Children's voices on bereavement and loss.* Unpublished master's thesis, University of South Africa, Pretoria, South Africa.

Weingarten, K. (2000). Witnessing, wonder and hope. *Family Process, 39*(4), 389–402.

White, M. (1989). The externalizing of the problem and the reauthoring of lives and relationships. In M. White (Ed.), *Selected papers* (pp. 37–45). Adelaide, Australia: Dulwich Centre.

White, M. (1995). *Reauthoring lives: Interviews and essays.* Adelaide, Australia: Dulwich Centre.

White, M., & Epston, D. (1990). *Narrative means to therapeutic ends.* New York: Norton.

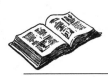

PART THREE

Changing Patterns of Behavior

CHAPTER 10

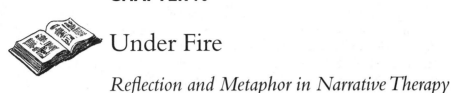

Under Fire

Reflection and Metaphor in Narrative Therapy

Christine Perry

CONTRIBUTOR'S STORY:
A PROFESSIONAL AND PERSONAL PERSPECTIVE

Christine Perry, M. Counseling, is in private practice as a family counselor, working extensively with couples, children, and individuals facing a variety of life challenges. With many years' background in primary teaching, pastoral care, and family counseling, she is currently facilitating a diploma of community welfare through Community Training Australia. She is a member of the Queensland Counsellors Association, a clinical member of the Australian Counselling Association, and on the national register of the Psychotherapy and Counselling Federation of Australia. As part of her master's studies she explored the ways in which clients "story" their lives, with specific focus on the use of metaphor in helping understand how they see themselves and their problems.

On a personal note, Christine is happily married to Hugh. Together, they love spending time with friends and family, including their young grandson, as well as traveling to new places and enjoying the tranquility of their property in sunny Queensland, Australia.

PREVIEW THE CHAPTER

Narrative therapy proposes that stories both explain and shape our lives, that we live by the stories we have of ourselves, and that those stories are changeable. Christine explores how this therapeutic approach can be applied clinically with a male client in a situation of work-related stress that has resulted in uncharacteristically aggressive behavior. Listening carefully for client-generated metaphors, she selects two of these with which to work in different ways. In the first, she asks her client to draw his problem story on a whiteboard. Then, using carefully crafted questions, she engages the illustration to examine the story of the client's resources, before requesting that he also represent his new or alternative story visually on the board. In an innovative touch, she uses a "reflecting team" whose role is to join with the client, provide feedback, and open possibilities for change. The second metaphor is explored, and shaped, by both questions and team reflections, permitting us to see opportunities beyond the single-therapist, oral-story approach to metaphor work. The chapter elaborates and builds on an article originally published in *Psychotherapy in Australia* (Perry, 2004).

Therapeutic Characteristics

Problems Addressed

- Work-related issues
- Aggression
- Verbal abuse
- Stress
- Managerial pressure

Resources Developed

- Humor
- Life skills
- Decision-making ability
- Adaptability
- Acceptance

Outcomes Offered

- Acceptance
- Discrimination
- Responsibility
- Awareness of triggers

Only the eyes moved as he surveyed the mountain ahead, the eyes and the racing heart. He remained weighed down with indecision and helplessness. His eyes desperately searched for a way forward. Fear gripped his guts as the shots sounded. Where had they come from? Where to hide? Eyes frantically scanned the dark places on the mountain. No flash. No movement. Awareness. The shots had come from behind. He was the target for what those trapped in the surreal depravity of a war zone call friendly fire. Survive this situation and know that you truly are a warrior.

This quotation comes from an unpublished story that was written as a personal response from my supervisor, David Axten, after we discussed and reflected upon the case of Paul. Paul worked in security as a doorman at a men's hostel, and came to counseling seeking assistance for a "work-related" issue. He struck me as an imposing figure: tall, well-groomed, efficient in manner and imperative in speech. He described his main roles at work as "peacekeeping, administering first aid, and observing people." Approximately four weeks before, he had had a "blowup at work" and became verbally abusive toward one of the hostel inmates—something he described as being "out of character." As he spoke he did so with a rich use of metaphors. He perceived his stress as reflecting organizational problems at the hostel. In discussing his therapeutic goals, Paul said that he needed "ideas, avenues on stress management." Currently, he was off work, "taking time out to deal with stress."

My question became "What therapeutic approaches might best help him achieve these goals?" To describe the processes I followed in developing those interventions, I will first provide a background to my work and therapeutic thinking before discussing the applications in this particular case.

THE "NARRATIVE" METAPHOR OF THE COUNSELING PROCESS

The use of stories and metaphor enriches counseling and psychotherapy regardless of the theoretical approach a practitioner may hold. Metaphor is recognized as a pervasive aspect of ordinary language. Not only do we use metaphor to construct our talking, but our thought processes, our construction of reality, and our actions are all structured by metaphor (Wickman, Daniels, White, & Fesmire, 1999). If human beings regularly use metaphor to communicate with each other and to structure their conceptual world, then it behooves us as counselors to be aware of, and engage with, the conceptual metaphors that clients bring to the counseling context. Indeed, one study found an average of three metaphors per 100 words in a single hour of therapy (Ferrara, 1994). Such frequent use of figurative language in therapy indicates that metaphor can play a powerfully significant role in the therapeutic process.

Metaphors as a way of viewing the mind have a tendency to drive psychological theory, research, and practice. For example, a researcher who holds a metaphor of the mind as a computer may ask about the information-processing systems underlying intelligent thought. A theorist with a subconscious metaphor may hypothesize about hidden aspects of childhood, or a clinician with a cognitive metaphor of mind may employ therapeutic techniques to modify thought processes. In fact, as therapists, we should bear in mind that a person's dominant worldview or metaphor of life has a positive relationship to his or her preference for counseling approaches (Lyddon & Adamson, 1992). It may even be that all theories or methods of therapy are themselves metaphoric structures of reality (Kopp, 1995). Thus, we would expect that the way therapists use metaphor will depend on their own individual metaphors of counseling.

The narrative metaphor of therapy maintains that people make sense of their lives through "storying" their experiences, and the more they retell and act out those stories, the more those stories actively shape their lives and relationships (White & Epston, 1990). In other words, we create our own life stories, and our stories, in turn, help to create who we are.

In narrative therapy, externalizing or personifying the client's problem story and attributing oppressive intentions to it enables clients to separate from their problem-saturated identity and the cultural discourses that are subjugating their lives. Externalizing the problem, or seeing it as outside of themselves as a person, helps clients to think about issues such as self-hate or anger as hostile, outside forces in their life, not at all intrinsic to their nature and personality. As the history of the problem is explored and placed in a context over time, the client is more likely to perceive it as changing and less fixed or permanent. This then opens up space for the consideration of other stories about the problem (Morgan, 2000; Sykes Wylie, 1994; White & Epston, 1990).

In assisting the client to consider other stories, the therapist can play an important role (1) in the discovery of moments when the client has not been dominated by the problem, and (2) in the examination of evidence to bolster a new view of the person as competent enough to stand up to the problem (O'Hanlon, 1994). To help the exploration of these unique outcomes, and throughout the re-storying process, therapists may ask questions like "Have you done this before?" and "What did it take for you to do that?" (Epston & White, 1992; Morgan, 2000).

As clients respond to such questions and ascribe meaning to their unique outcomes, they can revise their relationship with the problem. They can be assisted in this process with questions that help build awareness of the resources and skills they employed to attain those unique outcomes, questions like "How did you manage to resist the problem on that occasion?" They may also be asked to speculate about an alternative story that might accompany those unique outcomes. Thus, both client and therapist are involved, collaboratively, in the process of coauthoring a new, more helpful, more healing story to replace the old metaphor of despair.

The narrative metaphor of counseling describes the problems that people bring to therapy as a dominant, oppressive story, while the solution is seen in creating an open space for rewriting an alternative, more helpful story. It is believed that people seek counseling when their dominant narratives represent only a selected portion of their experience. Most therapists will know that a depressed person is selectively aware of the things that fit his or her dominant story of despair and overlooks those things that have or may provide a different experience. Those aspects of lived experience that fall outside of the dominant story provide a rich source for the generation of more helpful and satisfying alternative stories. As people retell their stories in therapy and begin to look for alternative narratives, they commonly become aware that they have already started to experience them.

REFLECTING TEAMS, METAPHOR, AND NARRATIVE THERAPY

Some therapists have incorporated a "reflecting team" approach to create a virtual therapeutic community whereby clients have access to a smorgasbord of ideas and are able to select those ideas that best fit with their experience (Andersen, 1987). The reflecting-team format begins when the client meets with the therapist in front of a one-way mirror, with the team observing from behind the mirror. The reflecting team composition is quite flexible, but frequently comprises consulting, guest, or student therapists, and usually includes from three to six people. At some point the therapist and client swap places with the team. While the team members discuss their ideas in response to the client-therapist conversation, client and therapist become observers behind the mirror. When the team members finish their "reflections," they again swap places, and the client comments on what she or he heard from the team.

Reflecting team members' comments are usually based on curiosity and speculation, are grounded in their own experience, and are intended to "open up possibilities rather than arrive at a consensus" (Lowe & Guy, 1999, p. 38). The use of a reflecting team in narrative therapy puts the postmodern concepts of collaboration, multiple perspectives, and transparency into action. The three tasks of team members are, first, to join with the client, clients, or family; second, to support the development of a new narrative; and, third, to facilitate a deconstruction of problem-saturated descriptions (Freedman & Combs, 1996).

The discussions emerging from reflecting teams are often metaphorical in both their language and nature. One example relates to a couple in therapy who spoke of feeling "lost" with each other. The team observing the session pondered aloud what it would be like to be "found." The members discussed journeys in which people and ideas can be both lost and found. If the couple ventured on a trip into unknown territory, what signs or guidance might they find along the way? wondered the team. Following these reflections, the couple began to talk differently about their journey together. They discussed what signs they might find, and in the process their feelings changed from desperation to hopefulness. They began to explore new directions for themselves and their relationship. As a couple they found a new narrative "that was neither one's story nor the other's" (Lax, 1994, pp. 71–72).

The following case study is another, more detailed example of how a narrative therapist and reflecting team can work together with client-generated metaphors: (1) to externalize the problem, (2) to map and deconstruct the problem story, (3) to explore unique outcomes, and (4) to build an alternative story. This represents a summary only, with particular focus on the interventions pertaining to the collaborative use of metaphor.

THE CASE OF PAUL

Paul was the client I mentioned at the beginning of this chapter who was experiencing a work-related issue and sought assistance on stress management. As I attended to his "problem story" about stress in the work situation, I was aware that I also needed to be listening for any times when the problem had less influence over Paul (unique outcomes), so I asked, "What sort of strategies do you currently use to deal with stress?"

He told me, "I read a lot. I enjoy movies, and participate in Masters Super League football." In the work situation, "taking a breather" (such as having a cup of tea) and "having a laugh" helped to reduce his stress level.

When I asked him, "How do you manage in this difficult role?" Paul described a tendency to rely on his own resourcefulness and to make correct decisions at the right time while simultaneously remaining calm. Discussing his increasing skills in finding resolutions to situations of conflict, he said, "Instead of seeing in black and white I'm making up my own grey."

This initial exploration into Paul's stress-coping strategies and strengths was done intentionally to lay the foundation for a new perception of himself: not as a person deficient because of succumbing to stress, but as one having the ability to remain standing strong in an extremely stressful situation.

The reflecting team who had been observing this first session swapped places with Paul and me, and we observed their discussion. They commented on Paul's "confidence and trust in his own ability" to deal with situations and his "high expectations of himself." The team wondered, "How does he manage himself in that environment so he doesn't constantly blow up?"

One team member remarked, "Paul is a big person. Even if he got a little bit angry, he would seem more threatening." The team considered how "the body we're born with can affect how others perceive us," and they asked, "What can Paul do about that?" They also wondered whether he could "advocate for some sort of group process" to deal with the stress at work.

Paul described the team comments as "all constructive," and he identified with the observation that his size might affect the way people at work perceive him. With regard to an organizational approach to reducing stress at work, he said, "I've explained to management about the way things are, but they do nothing about it. If they sat down and talked to us [the security staff] they might understand. I've tried to initiate this, but it didn't happen." I acknowledged his attempt to be proactive in the system by trying to initiate change.

"Maybe the sounding board of coming here might be helpful," he commented. "I think my high standards cause me to get frustrated by them not acting." With regard to options for the future, he added, "I don't want to keep fighting the system. The easy way would be to walk away, but I want to stay."

I asked, "What are the reasons that you want to stay in your job?"

Paul answered, "I do the job because I enjoy it, I help people, and because of the pay, but I feel like I'm getting shot at."

After that first session, I reflected on Paul's comments about "fighting the system" and "getting shot at" as representing a metaphor of the problem story. I considered that the externalization of stress in the case of Paul might be less useful therapeutically than an externalization of the problems between people at work (e.g., "getting shot at") since the problem story seemed to be partly systemic in nature. As I thought further about the metaphor of Paul "getting shot at," some questions began to form in my mind: "Who is shooting at him?" "What is he defending?" "Is he armed with anything?" "Does he engage the shooter?" "How does he remain standing?" "What skills or strategies could he be using in this situation?"

Identifying, Exploring, and Transforming the Client's Metaphor

By the second session, Paul had returned to work at the hostel and had the prospect of a new part time job doing "security parking." Reflecting on his role at the hostel, he commented, "I had a cause. I wanted to help these guys."

I affirmed the strengths that Paul exhibited in this role: "You were helping and standing up for people." I was intending to further explore the personal attributes and strategies that enabled him to remain standing in that difficult situation; however, Paul reiterated his comment from the previous session: "I feel like I'm getting shot at." I observed much emotional energy (anger) and bodily stress attached to this statement, so I decided to pursue the metaphor. I reflected back to Paul my mental picture, "You're standing up and helping people, but being shot at while standing there." Paul acknowledged this verbal description of his metaphor.

The Problem Story

At this point in the session, I considered that further exploration of Paul's metaphor of the problem (stress at work) might help to capture the whole meaning of the story and enable him to help build a new version of the story. A collaborative style in metaphor generation can assist a mutually shared understanding of the meaning of a metaphor and increases the perception that the therapist is deeply connected with the client. Furthermore, I was mindful of Barker's comments (1985) that therapeutic metaphor can take a variety of forms, including blackboard diagrams, artistic metaphors (e.g., painting), metaphorical objects (e.g., toy blocks), tasks with metaphorical meaning (e.g., "couples choreography"), and nonverbal language (e.g., facial expressions, body postures, movements, dance).

Due to the availability of a whiteboard, and my desire to collaboratively represent and explore Paul's metaphor, I asked, "Would you mind if we try an experiment in drawing?" Initially, he told me what to draw, and I attempted to represent his verbal description of the metaphor with a very basic level of drawing skill. Paul then helped to modify the drawing and add in further detail as we discussed what he described as "being in a battle."

As we conversed, Paul and I worked collaboratively to create a visual representation on the whiteboard of the battle metaphor: his problem story about the work situation. Paul's resultant drawing was a figure representing a soldier making a stand, with bullets being fired at him from one direction.

I asked Paul a number of questions to further elaborate his battle metaphor: "Who is shooting at the soldier? Is it the enemy or is it friendly fire? Is he armed with anything to shoot back? What is the soldier defending?"

In response, Paul said that he was being "shot at by friendly fire" and that he was not carrying, or wanting to use, any weapons against those shooting at him. He told me that he was defending the hostel inmates, whom he believed were not being treated fairly by other workers, especially management.

Commenting that the drawing was incomplete, he added a group of inmates standing behind the soldier, to illustrate his attempt to defend the hostel inmates from the bullets of the other workers and management. He also changed the picture to include bullets from both sides—from the other workers (criticism) and the inmates (verbal abuse). He saw himself as being caught in the middle between a barrage of bullets from each direction. He had the role of having to be the mediator between both sides. Using this pictorial metaphor, we discussed several incidents (unique outcomes) in which Paul had been able to mediate without losing his cool.

A Story of Resources

Attempting to further explore the metaphor with Paul, I asked, "How is the soldier able to remain standing while being shot at? What would the soldier need to be carrying (strengths, skills) to enable him to keep standing and mediate between both sides?"

Paul responded by drawing a backpack on the soldier, and described a list of supplies that the soldier was carrying. I wrote these on the whiteboard as he told me: "Humor, life skills, decision-making ability, bullshit detector." These skills or attributes were the ones he considered most significant, so we discussed each of these as we listed them (e.g., "How have you used humor to help you stand in that place?"). Through further discussion of his ability to work with and coordinate others, he added another figure, which represented his work partner. I acknowledged that he was not standing alone.

Paul discussed the intuitive way in which he and his partner worked together during a crisis. For instance, Paul told me how his partner and he coordinated their efforts when an inmate became violent (one protected the other inmates while the other attempted to defuse the situation).

AN ALTERNATIVE STORY

I then encouraged Paul, "Now, draw a different picture. A picture of how you would like it to be at your new job."

Paul engaged enthusiastically in this new task, drawing two figures. The one on the left represented himself, and the one on the right represented the customer. Paul drew a double-headed arrow between the two figures, indicating communication going in both directions.

I wondered aloud, "Where does management fit into this picture?"

He described other staff members as making up a supportive network, and he drew some other figures around him to illustrate this support.

Again Paul drew the backpack on the figure, and listed the qualities the figure would need in his new job, discussing each of these in detail: "humor, life skills, adaptiveness," and so on. We explored the scope of adaptiveness as involving his ability to adapt his interaction style to different types of people and to readily deal with novel situations in his new job. For example, he had told me of the immense variety of people with whom he interacts at work in the capacity of a "listening ear" (e.g., "people with a drug habit"). I acknowledged his versatility and empathy in being able to relate to such a variety of people. He seemed confident in his ability to adapt in the new job and, additionally, seemed pleased that it might place him in a less stressful environment ("no bullets being fired"). He began to recognize and acknowledge the strengths that he was able to bring to the work arena, but with regard to the situation at the hostel, he commented, "I can't move the mountain."

Having observed the session through the one-way screen thus far, the reflecting team began by working with the visual metaphor already on the whiteboard —the drawing reflecting Paul's new job situation. The team brainstormed and wrote on the whiteboard some more skills to add to Paul's backpack, which reflected qualities they had observed in Paul: *handles the rough stuff, plain-talking man, handles crisis calmly, acts, is proactive.*

One team member described Paul as a "mountain mover" but noted that "something enabled him to make a decision that he can't move this mountain." Other team members wondered, "Is that a new learning for him?" "Have there been other mountains in his life that he has moved?" "He has a strong sense of social justice and integrity." "He is passionate about injustice." "But he is going into a situation where there might not be any mountains to move." "Is he a mountain seeker?" "If there's not a mountain at his new job, is that okay for him?"

With reference to the additions to the whiteboard metaphor ("acts, is proactive"), Paul remarked: "I've been known for the fact that I'm not scared to get my hands dirty. The ones shooting ammo at me, they call me a control freak. I don't want to be that, but I need to sequentially order the things to do in a crisis."

After these comments, Paul and I talked more around the metaphor of "moving mountains." He said, "There have been a couple of hills in my life that I've moved." We spoke about what the "mountain moving" represented for him.

I asked, "Is it about fighting injustice, or does it represent something else? Are you a mountain seeker?"

"It's more about having new experiences. I love a challenge," he responded.

I asked him, "Will your new job be enough of a challenge for you?"

Paul replied, "Yes, it will be a challenge. It might not be a mountain. I don't want to see another mountain for 10 years. The mountain where I was, was bigger than I thought. I bit off more than I could chew, and I ended up with a mouthful of rock. . . . I'm happy to see a Nullabor Plain (a flat Australian desert) for a while."

Affirming and Extending the Alternative Metaphor into the Future

In the third and final session, Paul told me, "I feel good about the last sessions. What I've learned is that talking can de-stress and I can change."

He was still doing some shifts at the hostel, but he had commenced working part time at his new parking job, and scheduled a date to leave his old job completely. He discussed the ways in which his new job was matching the new story we created on the whiteboard the previous week.

I attempted to extend the mountain metaphor relevant to Paul's new position. "You mentioned that you didn't want to see any mountains for a while—you wanted to remain on the Nullabor Plain. Have you encountered any mountains in your new job?"

"No. I'm still on the Nullabor Plain," he replied. "However, I have encountered some cool rock pools and streams." He described the appreciation that his ongoing customers showed toward him, including tips.

"That must be *refreshing* for you," I reflected.

Paul affirmed that he was enjoying his new job and went on to say, "My wife has noticed that I'm still smiling when I come home from work. I'm having a laugh. The new job is a big contrast from the old one at the hostel, where I was beating my head onto the mountain." And, realistically, he acknowledged that he "might come against a few mountains" in his new job.

I asked, "What will you do if you encounter mountains in your new job?"

He replied, "I'll put the mountain into the landscape. I'll stand back and check out the mountain, as part of the bigger picture. I'll look at the easiest way of scaling it and decide whether I want to climb to the top or not. I might ask others who have already climbed it. I don't want to be like a goat and butt my head on it." Later he added, contemplatively, "Sometimes I can climb the mountain and sometimes walk away from it."

When I asked what he would like the reflecting team to comment on, he said that he would like them to notice "how I may have changed over the last three sessions."

"How do you think you have changed?" I asked.

"I can step back and look at myself as a hill—with my own strengths and weaknesses. I can be responsible and not blame others." Paul then described his learning experiences in terms of the serenity prayer that he recently read. "I can accept the things that I cannot change."

The reflecting team observed how the landscape seemed to have become much clearer. "There's been a huge leap where Paul's got a sense of what is appropriate to tackle and what's not," they said. The team speculated about Paul not letting a problem go as far this time, by checking out the mountains that come along. They observed that Paul is "able to see the mountain emerging, rather than suddenly finding himself facing one."

There were further questions related to extending the mountain metaphor: If Paul decides to climb the mountain, how does he plan the route? What will he use to keep himself safe—a rope, boots to grip? Is Paul a skilled climber, or would it be a hard slog?

Paul described the mountains in his old job as being more like a "cliff face—you can't go over it." He remarked, "It's about being responsible—seeing the triggers. I won't get into that situation again."

I asked, "How will you manage not to get into that situation again?"

"By recognizing the triggers. By taking a step back, sniffing the flowers, and recognizing the whole landscape," he said.

We thanked each other and finished the final counseling session at this point.

IMPLICATIONS FOR PROFESSIONAL PRACTICE

The most important contribution of the battle metaphor seemed to be in expanding Paul's sense of the personal meaning and interpretation of the battle, as expressed through his appreciation of the personal qualities that enabled him to stand strong in the battle. The role of the reflecting team in discussing and elaborating the mountain metaphor was crucial because team members introduced questions, such as "If there's not a mountain at your new job, is that okay for you?" enabling Paul to connect his actions with his sense of identity. The team also reinforced and affirmed Paul's growing sense of what is appropriate to tackle and what is not. Paul and I were then able to build upon his new story about how he might deal with mountains in the future.

Overall, both the battle and the mountain metaphors were used collaboratively by the counselor and the reflecting team to externalize and explore the dominant story, as well as to create an alternative story that would impact Paul's future landscape of action. Each metaphor was used in a different way, yet both metaphors proved valuable in evoking change for Paul. Combs and Freedman (1990) claim that the more metaphors clients have to choose from for a given situation, the more choice and flexibility they have in how to handle it.

It is well recognized that the collaborative utilization of client-generated metaphors enables therapists to more accurately reflect feelings, clarify underlying meanings, and enhance rapport building (Wickman et al., 1999). However, the therapeutic efficacy of metaphor seems to depend on the therapist's ability to *identify* and reflect the client's metaphoric language, to collaboratively *explore* and *transform* the client's metaphor, and to *affirm* the changed metaphor by extending it into the client's preferred future. The role of the reflecting team is to elaborate the client's metaphor by offering different perspectives and to become a participating audience for affirming the client's emerging new story.

Following our discussions of Paul's case, my supervisor David Axten completed his unpublished story:

> *The warrior moved cautiously through the landscape, silently placing the weight on the soles of his feet. Soon he was in dead ground, out of line of sight and fire. He quickened his pace, surefooted, traversing the rough scree slope. Again he studied the mountain, and his face visibly relaxed as he saw the change. From here he could see the sheer rock was broken with chimneys and ledges. He could find a route and take the high ground. The eyes smiled.*

REFERENCES

Andersen, T. (1987). The reflecting team: Dialogue and meta-dialogue in clinical work. *Family Process, 26*, 415–428.

Barker, P. (1985). *Using metaphors in psychotherapy.* New York: Brunner/Mazel.

Combs, G., & Freedman, J. (1990). *Symbol, story, and ceremony: Using metaphor in individual and family therapy.* New York: Norton.

Epston, D., & White, M. (1992). *Experience, contradiction, narrative and imagination: Selected papers of David Epston and Michael White, 1989–1991.* Adelaide, Australia: Dulwich Centre.

Ferrara, K.W. (1994). *Therapeutic ways with words.* New York: Oxford University Press.

Freedman, J., & Combs, G. (1996). *Narrative therapy: The social construction of preferred realities.* New York: Norton.

Kopp, R. (1995). *Metaphor therapy: Using client-generated metaphors in psychotherapy.* New York: Brunner/Mazel.

Lax, W. (1994). Postmodern thinking in a clinical practice. In S. McNamee & K. Gergen (Eds.), *Therapy as social construction* (pp. 69–85). London: Sage.

Lowe, R., & Guy, G. (1999). From group to peer supervision: A reflecting team process. *Psychotherapy in Australia, 6*(1), 36–41.

Lyddon, W., & Adamson, L. (1992). Worldview and counseling preference: An analogue study. *Journal of Counseling and Development, 71*(1), 41–47.

Morgan, A. (2000). *What is narrative therapy? An easy-to-read introduction.* Adelaide, Australia: Dulwich Centre.

O'Hanlon, B. (1994). The third wave. *Psychotherapy Networker, 18*(6), 19–29.

Perry, C. (2004). Reflecting on narrative: Metaphorically speaking. *Psychotherapy in Australia, 11*(1), 54–59.

Sykes Wylie, M. (1994). Panning for gold. *Psychotherapy Networker, 18*(6), 40–48.

White, M., & Epston, D. (1990). *Narrative means to therapeutic ends.* New York: Norton.

Wickman, S., Daniels, M. H., White, L., & Fesmire, S. (1999). A "primer" in conceptual metaphor for counselors. *Journal of Counseling and Development, 77*(4), 389–394.

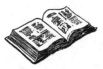

CHAPTER II

The Door Is Open, the Bird Can Fly

Merging Therapist and Client Metaphors in Child Therapy

Joyce C. Mills

CONTRIBUTOR'S STORY:
A PROFESSIONAL AND PERSONAL PERSPECTIVE

Joyce Mills, PhD, has inspired audiences internationally with her heart-centered, playful, and creative approaches to communication, problem solving, and healing. She uses her expertise as a masterful storyteller, along with principles of Ericksonian hypnotherapy and her experiences with transcultural teachings, to communicate with severely troubled children, youths, and families.

Awarded the 1997 Annual Play Therapy International Award for outstanding career contribution to the field, Joyce is executive director of the StoryPlay® Center, codirector of the Phoenix Institute for Ericksonian Therapy, a licensed marriage and family therapist, on the board of a nonprofit organization, and the acclaimed author of seven books (see Resource Section).

Joyce and her husband Eddie enjoy living in Phoenix, Arizona, where she provides workshops, consults internationally, and is in private practice. Joyce is a grandmother of two, Tyler and Parker, who hold a special place in her heart. Her interest in indigenous cultures, stories, creativity, and nature enriches her personal life and nourishes the soul of her work.

PREVIEW THE CHAPTER

Just as our clients have metaphors that describe their problems and open up possibilities for change, therapists also have their metaphors that shape and inform their work. In this chapter, Joyce describes the formation and evolution of her metaphor of "butterfly magic" as a means of healing and transformation. It is a metaphor that closely parallels the processes commonly followed by clients in their healing and, consequently, the processes therapists need to follow to facilitate that healing. Just as the evolution of a butterfly occurs in four stages, we are guided through four passages: from creating a safe environment to crawling before flying, cocooning for greatest change, and finally emerging in a new, transformed state. How this metaphor can shape therapy is illustrated in the case of Joey, an 11-year-old boy in residential care with autistic characteristics and an "obsession" with keys. Joyce models how a problem can be transformed into new possibilities by being sensitive to a child's metaphor, acknowledging that metaphor, and utilizing it for effective change. Based on a chapter in *Reconnecting to the Magic of Life* (Mills, 1999), Joey's story emerges like a butterfly from its cocoon.

Therapeutic Characteristics

Problems Addressed

- Residential treatment
- Serious school problems
- Violence
- Delusions
- Dissociation
- Abuse
- Neglect
- Emotional challenges

Resources Developed

- Seeing possibilities rather than problems
- Acknowledging client metaphors
- Utilizing client metaphors

Outcomes Offered

- Enthusiasm
- Calmness
- Smiling
- New possibilities

A long, long time ago there were two Caterpillar People who were very much in love. One day a sad thing happened and the Caterpillar Man died. The heart of the Caterpillar Woman was broken. She didn't want to see anyone or talk to anyone, and so she wrapped her sorrow around her like a shawl. Then she began walking and walking . . . and while she walked, she cried.

Caterpillar Woman walked for a whole year, and because the Earth is a circle, she returned to the very place from which she had begun walking. The Creator took great pity on her, saying, "You have suffered too long. Now it is the time to step into a new world of color . . . a new world of great beauty." Then the Creator clapped hands twice . . . and the Woman burst forth from the shawl as a beautiful butterfly. And it is said that this is why the butterfly is a symbol of renewal for many communities: It tells us that at the end of all suffering, there is the gift of relief.

This is how I remember the story of the Caterpillar Woman as originally told to me by a traditional storyteller from the Warm Springs Tribe. Spiritually, the ancient story provides us with an important teaching about healing and renewal, while scientifically there is another story that can help us to see how each stage of the butterfly's transformation parallels our own.

With Diana Linden, a neurophysiological biologist at Occidental College in Southern California, I was discussing the use of metaphors to explain science. Diana enjoyed using stories to teach biology to her classes, and I enjoyed listening to Diana talk about her amazing research into muscular dystrophy. During this visit, Diana asked me how I viewed healing. While I pondered my response for a moment, an image of a butterfly came to mind. "When I think of healing, I think about the butterfly. You know, we are like a caterpillar crawling around, until at one point or another, we go inside our cocoon and transform into a butterfly."

Chuckling a bit, Diana said, "Oh, Joyce, that's not exactly what happens. You're leaving out a big part of the process of transformation." She went on to tell me the story. "As most of us know, there are four stages to the butterfly's transformation: the egg, the caterpillar, the chrysalis, and the emerging butterfly. What most of us don't know is what makes the metamorphosis possible, what changes the caterpillar into a butterfly. This is the part you are *really* going to like. Caterpillars have special cells in their bodies called 'imaginal discs,' which contain all the seeds of change."

Imaginal discs, I echoed within myself. Diana was right: I loved it! As a matter of fact, even though I really didn't know what they were, I wanted to run right out and buy some imaginal discs for myself. "Where can I get some?" I humorously quipped.

Diana laughed along with me and then continued. "You see, the caterpillar prepares for this great change by eating and eating. When it is big enough, it shakes its body and sheds its skin, which it has now outgrown . . . shakes and sheds, shakes and sheds. Then, just at the right time, it finds a leaf or a branch and attaches itself by weaving a thin, silken thread and a small pad, becoming what is known as the chrysalis. The chrysalis is a hardened skin that develops and protects the caterpillar as it goes through its changes. Inside of the chrysalis the caterpillar completely breaks down in structure, becoming a souplike substance."

Diana went on to explain that it was only at the point of this breakdown that the imaginal discs release the seeds of change contained within, allowing the caterpillar to transform itself into a beautiful butterfly, as the magic of metamorphosis completes itself.

After hearing Diana's description of this amazing process of biological change, I purchased many books on the metamorphosis of the butterfly in the hope of finding a way to translate this scientific metaphor into my teachings. In *Butterfly and Moth* (Whalley, 1988) I found beautiful illustrations and descriptions of each of the stages, combined with the knowledge Diana had shared with me. As this model of transformational healing and change began to unfold, I realized that so often in life we go through times of fear, uncertainty, darkness, feeling like we "can't take one more thing." Then somehow, after what could be called a moment of miracle, we find the inner strength to go on . . . our own imaginal discs . . . and eventually experience a breakthrough in our personal and spiritual growth.

And so it is with the greatest awe and respect for this winged teacher of change that I share the following stories as they relate to each stage of the butterfly's growth, and to our human ability to embrace and achieve the magic of change.

PASSAGE ONE: A SAFE ENVIRONMENT

In the world of the butterfly, after an elaborate courtship dance with the sole (or "soul") purpose of attracting the opposite sex and mating, the female selects just the right plant on which to lay her eggs. She does this so that her eggs have a safe home on which to hatch. In a parallel of this first stage, we as therapists—and as human beings—also need to discover the importance of creating a safe environment in which all new ideas, relationships, and personal awarenesses have the opportunity of developing. Without this safe environment, nothing positive develops. We all need support and encouragement to go on—both therapists and clients.

I remember a time when I was in the fourth grade and was given an assignment to make a map of the world. Loving art, I did this assignment with great enthusiasm. However, I did not have blue paint to use for the water. I only had red paint, and I didn't have the money to go out and buy blue paint. I worked for hours detailing the map in the best way that I knew how, and when it was done I proudly brought it into my classroom. We were each asked to show our work, and when I stood before the class, holding the large poster-size map I had painted, the teacher commented, "What is all that red? We all know that the water is blue." At that moment the class laughed, and I began to shake with embarrassment. I never raised my hand to volunteer for anything in that class again. My teacher's classroom was not a safe "leaf" for my "eggs" of childhood creativity.

As I look back on that experience today, I can see its positive influence on my life. I know that when I teach a workshop or see a new client, the most important thing for me to focus on is creating a supportive environment so that each person can feel safe exploring and discovering new ideas and choices. Let me illustrate how I go about applying this in my work with the story of Joey. I have broken his tale into four parts and placed it at the end of my description of each of the four passages to best show how they shape and guide my therapy in a practical way.

JOEY'S STORY: CREATING A SAFE ENVIRONMENT

I met Joey on a visit to a residential treatment center for abused, neglected, and seriously troubled children and adolescents in Oregon, where I had the opportunity of working in one of the cottages that housed 24 children who were described as having the most serious problems in the school. I decided to work with these children, who ranged in age from 8 years old to 17 years old, in a large group. The staff wondered how this would work, since many of the children were identified as being violent, delusional, dissociated from reality, and unable to sit still for a long period of time. I wondered as well, since I had never worked with such a group before.

I noticed a large round handheld drum hanging on the wall as I entered the cottage and asked if we could use it. "Sure," was the enthusiastic response of the cottage manager. My thought was to first tell the children about the drum and how it is a connection to their heartbeat—an important teaching I learned from the many Native American people I have worked with for close to two decades of my life. Since most of these children are often disconnected from their own heart songs, I felt this would be a good way to reintroduce them to their own rhythms. My second intention was to pass the drum in the circle and have each of the children hit it once with the drumstick, thereby putting their "voice" into it.

I then went into the gymnasium and asked the children and staff to sit in a circle on the wood floor. The circle was the first step in forming an environment of safety (the first passage in the process of transformation), as no one is above or below another, no one in front or in back of anyone. Instead it allows us to sit beside one another in the quest for healing and connection.

I began to spread out many of the things I had brought, such as sweetgrass, sage, a shell, feathers, my grandmother's shawl, salt from Hawaii, and my two endearing turtle puppets, BT (Big Turtle) and LT (Little Turtle)—my medicine. I explained that in many cultures medicine is not just something that comes in bottles but instead can be found in all aspects of life, such as in stories, rocks, plants, many things of nature, as well as in those special objects given to us by special people. I shared stories about each of the things I brought. For example, I picked up the braid of sweetgrass and said I learned to use it for bringing sweetness into life. I demonstrated by picking it up and bringing it close to my nose and inhaling its sweetness, and touching my heart. I did the same for sage and told the group how I learned that it is a sacred herb that can be burned for purification and for creating a sacred space in which healing can occur. I said that sometimes when I am having a hard day I burn some sage and the heaviness of the day seems to lighten. I use the abalone shell in which to burn the sage and sweetgrass. I told them about the Hawaiian salt and how it is used by the Hawaiian people in much the same way as the sweetgrass and sage: It is for prayer, purification, and healing. There are many stories that go with the salt, but one such story, told to me by a Navajo man I call my uncle, is that of Salt Woman and how she brought the first laugh to a little child by just the salty touch of her finger to the child's mouth. My grandmother's shawl always goes with me to remind me of the wisdom she shared with me throughout her life. I then picked up my puppets BT and LT and introduced them to the group. With BT in hand, I moved his head inside of the shell and said that turtles are very wise. When they are scared they go inside and seek comfort from within. When they feel ready, they stick their heads out and move forward.

A young boy sitting next to me proudly told me that he had a drum, some feathers, and a medicine bag that his grandfather, a respected Lakota tribal elder, had given to him some years ago. Knowing how important it is for children to be connected to that which brings cultural and family pride, I leaned over and whispered, "Well, what are you waiting for? Go and get your special things." He was clearly delighted and went to his room, accompanied by a staff member, and came back in a few moments with his very sacred treasures . . . his medicine.

I continued to lay out the special things I had brought to share with the group. Somehow the veil of mental and emotional illness that seemed to separate us slowly began to lift, and I was simply sitting in a circle of children in which we could all feel safe to journey into the following passages.

PASSAGE TWO: YOU GOTTA CRAWL BEFORE YOU FLY

Do you hear clients making the following statements? "I am not happy in this relationship; I am outgrowing my partner, job, or lifestyle." "I know that I need to make some changes in my life." "I need to shed my skin and become a new person." "I'm not happy living in this body." Well, if they are pondering any of these thoughts, it is a good indicator that they have entered the second passage. Like the caterpillar, they know it is time for a change in their lives. I welcome this news with gleeful anticipation.

Often there just seems to be an overall sense of discontentment with life as it is in this second passage, but discontentment is not necessarily always negative. It can be used as a positive indicator pointing to the need for change in our lives or letting us know that change is on the way, whether we have asked for it or not. This is particularly true of adolescents. They don't like their bodies, hair, or selves in general. It is as if teenagers are in a psychic search for another form. However, although they want something different, they don't seem to know yet what that form is. Just how do they, or we as therapists, know when it is time to change?

"You watch the sail, and feel the wind, and you just know inside when it is time to change." These are the words that were shared with me by Leonard, a young man whose innate ability to sail the challenging oceans of Kaua'i matched the grace and vision possessed by the soaring eagles of the skies. Leonard and I set out for an afternoon sail on his two-person catamaran. At one point I glanced up and noticed that his deeply set brown eyes were focused upward toward the mast, while he skillfully maneuvered the sails with his long sun-browned fingers and manipulated the rudder with the toes of his bare foot. We were heeling sharply to one side while the powerful winds carried us across the azure blue ocean with swift grace.

At another time the waves were increasing their height and intensity. Leonard motioned for me to change positions and move to the other side of the catamaran. After carefully wobbling across the small boat and regaining my balance, I asked him, "How do you know when it is time to change?" I thought that I was referring to the situation on the catamaran, but as I thought about it later, I realized that my question was far more about life in general than about an ocean adventure. And so was his answer: "You watch the sail, and feel the wind, and you just know inside when it is time to change."

At this point you may be asking, "So what is going to help my client transform from a caterpillar to a butterfly?" In the metaphor of the butterfly, the answer is imaginal discs. Like the butterfly, each of us has imaginal discs that contain all seeds of change. These imaginal discs are our inner resources, interests, skills, and past learnings that may be lying dormant and, in a sense, are just waiting to be awakened . . . to be released. As the little caterpillar carries these cells within its fuzzy body, we too carry these cells within our own caterpillar stage, not consciously knowing that we even have them or what they can do for us when their time comes. I like to think of imaginal discs as our winged assets of change, enabling us to renew a sense of hope, recognizing that unseen possibilities are truly present to help us move forward, no matter what challenge or obstacle is placed in our paths. Again Joey's story helps illustrate this passage.

JOEY'S STORY: THE IMPORTANCE OF KEYS

As I began to talk about how each of us has special things that make us feel good, Joey, the 11-year-old boy sitting to my left, with cinnamon-colored hair and smiling blue eyes, began to talk rapidly and told me he wanted to share something that was important to him in the group too. It was his "medicine." I excused him also, and he went to his room to get his special gift. When he came back he had many pieces of paper on which keys were drawn. All kinds of keys. Car keys, door keys, storage-box keys, and pictures of keys he had drawn on multiple pieces of paper. In a rapid-fire fashion, he began telling me all about his keys.

As he talked, it became apparent that the other children in the group were becoming increasingly annoyed with his monologue. One girl huffed and said, "We heard this before. That's all he ever talks about." Apparently she and the others saw this preoccupation as an obstacle or problem for Joey, but maybe the keys also offered unseen possibilities. I knew Joey was providing me with a valuable "key" to his inner world, a world filled with obsessional thoughts and fear. In order to open the door to Joey's world, I needed to recognize his obsession as an imaginal disc, a seed for change that could possibly release Joey's positive potentials and possibilities. I acknowledged the young critic's statement with a nod, turned to Joey, and said, "You know, keys are so very important. Without keys I couldn't start my car, I couldn't open the door to my house, or for that matter, I wouldn't be able to lock it in order to keep everything safe inside. Yes, keys are *very* important." In talking to Joey about keys, I was also using them as a metaphor for the whole group. All of these children and adolescents needed to find their own keys for unlocking their unseen potentials. I continued by saying, "Sometimes we need to lock things away in order to keep them safe, and sometimes we need to open those boxes at just the right time in order to find what we need."

As I spoke of keys, Joey quieted his chattering and moved closer to me. The other children in the group nodded their heads slightly in agreement. Yes, keys are very important. For this boy, they were his medicine . . . the keys to his inner life.

PASSAGE THREE: A TIME OF GREATEST CHANGE

This third passage draws attention to the greatest mystery of change. With the chrysalis completely formed, the caterpillar is now ready to break down and have its special cells, the imaginal discs, release the seeds of change. While the chrysalis appears inactive and quiet on the outside, the most amazing and dramatic changes take place on the inside. *It is during this stage that the magic of transformation takes place.* As with the butterfly, it is in this stage that our greatest change occurs as well.

Our chrysalis stage is often distinguished by being a peak time of "not knowing." It is a period of withdrawal, not wanting to socialize, often wanting to hide and not deal with the outside world, with a given struggle, or with a certain situation. I often hear clients say, "I just want to pull the covers over my head and not face anyone." "I want to wake up and have this problem gone." "I can't see a way out of this situation." "My life feels hopeless." Life often feels dark and isolated with little space for movement. Although some people view these feelings as symptoms of depression or anxiety, I choose to view these symptoms as indicators of being in this third stage—the chrysalis—the place where the greatest change can occur.

Like the caterpillar, which must break down into a soupy, gel-like substance before undergoing its transformation, so too do we need to learn how to break down our old limiting belief systems about ourselves in order to transform from our caterpillar-like selves into empowered human beings capable of reaching our full-winged potential.

How often do we all try to hold on to our old caterpillar selves only to find that if we continue to do so, we never discover our fly-away-butterfly selves? I think of all the different survivor groups, with more coming into existence every day. As an alternative, I dream about *thriver* groups. Although surviving is an important stage in the quest for healing from trauma, it is not the *only* stage. Thriving is the next stage.

In the meantime, staying within a quiet space and a time of not-knowing—not having clear-cut answers or quick solutions to our problems, withdrawing from the outside world—is not often honored in our society. We are supposed to have the answers and be able to come up with solutions at the drop of a hat. Yet nature tells us that this is a critical time in the cycle of change. It is important to remember that all creatures in nature have a time of withdrawal, dormancy, or hibernation. There is a life-cycle pattern that allows for a time of cocooning. Think about the cycles of the seasons. There is fall, when the leaves change from green to vibrant colors, only to become brittle and then fall off the trees. This is followed by the coldness and bareness of winter. And through the cold there is an absence of color and vibrancy, as all is asleep. The season of winter is most like this chrysalis stage. All the changes are taking place on an inner level.

The regeneration reveals itself during the next season, spring. It is a reawakening of life and nature. It is a time of emergence. Spring is playful, youthful passion, and fluttering. And then it slowly changes into summer. There is often intense heat, a dramatic change from the seasons that come before, a time when the youthful growth of spring turns into the mature passion of summer. The four cycles of the butterfly are very much like the four seasons of nature. There must be the season of the chrysalis before the season of the emerging butterfly.

JOEY'S STORY: THE PROCESS OF CHANGE

I then picked up the drum and told the group that a drum can also be a *key*—a connection to their *heart songs*—and that I would be passing it around for each of them to hit the drum with the drumstick as loudly or softly as they liked, at the same time saying their name or making a sound. I demonstrated by hitting the drum and yelling, "Joyce." They all laughed and followed suit. Some tapped quietly, while others struck the drum with great fervor. One girl with a cast on her arm stood up and hit the drum hard as she yelled as loudly as she could. Her therapist, who was sitting next to her, commented, "I'm glad Lindy could get her anger out." At that moment, Lindy shot back, "I am not angry, I feel *powerful*." It was a spontaneous moment that allowed me to say to the whole staff how important it is to not analyze someone's intentions but instead to let them tell you what their interpretation is. Allowing the process of transformation to take place is what is important, not trying to make it happen. I linked analyzing and forcing change to picking apart a cocoon, which is the private place where the caterpillar transforms into the beautiful butterfly it is destined to become.

Joey gleefully took the drum when it was passed to him, struck it with great enthusiasm, and shouted his name. As it came full circle, Joey was calm, with a beaming smile on his face.

PASSAGE FOUR: FINDING YOUR WINGS

A long time ago I heard a story about a man who found a large cocoon and decided to take it home to watch the butterfly inside emerge. As I remember it, the man watched and watched until one day he noticed a tiny opening in the cocoon. He thought the butterfly was struggling to make its way out of the cocoon and that something must be wrong. So he decided to help the butterfly along by making a larger slit for it to emerge with greater ease. When the butterfly finally came out, its wings were shriveled and small, and its body misshapen. The man thought that the wings would spread out in a few hours, but they did not. Instead the butterfly was unable to fly; it was crippled for life. Although the man meant well, he did not know that there was a purpose for the struggle: It was nature's way of propelling the body's fluid into the wings of the butterfly so that it could emerge and ultimately fly with strength and beauty.

This story shows us that even though the butterfly is completely formed, it has to use all of its pulsating strength to push itself through its protective chrysalis into the light. It then hangs upside down, gently fluttering its still-wet wings. You see, even though the butterfly is fully developed and born into the world, it is not quite ready for flight. If the wet-winged butterfly is rushed along, it will be crippled for life. The butterfly knows when it is time to fly . . . no one has to tell it or coax it.

In our own lives, the beginning of this fourth passage is often marked by our taking more and more risks—flexing our newly acquired wings, so to speak. On an inner level we experience the first inklings of hopefulness after a dark time of unconscious change. This passage is a time of awakenings, of "aha" insights, of breaking through our cocoon. It is critical to our well-being that we not be pushed during this stage, but supported to move forward at our own pace. Just as the butterfly awaits the right time to fly, at a certain point we will feel ready to assert ourselves in the world.

We begin to feel more secure with our new learnings and abilities. We may take that leap of faith to change jobs, enroll in a class we have thought about for some time, initiate a new friendship or relationship, or take that long-envisioned trip. Whatever outer action is chosen, we are ready to fly with new wings of vision and courage.

This fourth passage is the stage in which we are likely to hear our clients expressing metaphors like the following: "I feel like I'm finally beginning to see the light at the end of the tunnel." "I feel like I could soar." "I can finally hear the music in my life again." "These ideas are finally taking off." If you have experienced any of these feelings, you will know that you are well into the fourth passage of change.

JOEY'S STORY: FLYING FREE

Since that visit when I first met Joey, I have returned to Oregon many times and have had special visits with Joey. On one such occasion Joey drew a picture of himself next to an apple tree, a birdcage with its door open, and a bird flying. In his quick-worded fashion of communication, pointing to the open door of the birdcage, he said, "The door is open, the door is open, the door is open." Joey took a breath and continued, "The bird is out now, the bird is out, he can fly . . . the door is open."

I smiled and replied, "Yes, Joey, the door *is* open and the bird can surely fly."

Later, in a staff meeting, I asked if Joey usually drew or told stories. The staff said no. They hadn't seen him draw in such detail before, nor had they heard him tell such a story. The sensitive and gifted staff continued on a daily basis to help Joey use his obsession with keys to unlock the hidden pathways to his private world. On my last trip I learned that Joey no longer talks about keys but is interested in cameras. He is busy taking pictures of life.

With the butterfly model of healing in mind, I clearly saw Joey's use of keys in his life as his *imaginal discs*—his personal medicine. Keys became the medicine to help him open the doorway to his inner abilities. Instead of looking at his fixation as a problem to be extinguished, I chose to *utilize* it in a positive way, not just for him but as a metaphor for the group as a whole. Since these children and adolescents had multiple problems stemming from abuse, neglect, and emotional challenges, it became apparent that they all needed to find the *keys* to their own wellness and comfort.

REFERENCES

Mills, J. C. (1999). *Reconnecting to the magic of life.* Phoenix, AZ: Imaginal Press.
Whalley, P. (1988). *Butterfly and moth.* New York: Eyewitness Books.

CHAPTER 12

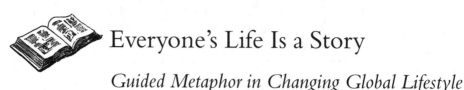

Everyone's Life Is a Story

Guided Metaphor in Changing Global Lifestyle

Rubin Battino

CONTRIBUTOR'S STORY:
A PROFESSIONAL AND PERSONAL PERSPECTIVE

Rubin Battino, MS, holds a master's degree in mental health and is a licensed professional clinical counselor. He is the president of the Milton H. Erickson Society of Dayton, Ohio, and a fellow of the National Council for Hypnotherapy. Trained in Gestalt therapy, neurolinguistic programming, bio-energetic analysis, and Ericksonian methods of hypnosis and psychotherapy, among other disciplines, he has authored or coauthored seven books, and is currently writing another on very brief therapy (see Resource Section). In addition to a small private practice, he offers therapy training and for over 12 years has voluntarily facilitated groups for people with life-challenging diseases. Most of his professional life has been as a professor of chemistry, a profession in which he continues to be active.

On the personal side, he and his wife of 45 years have two sons and seven grandchildren. He likes to travel, is involved in community theater, and has written over 15 plays.

PREVIEW THE CHAPTER

Rubin guides the reader of this chapter through the step-by-step processes for working with guided metaphor, a unique approach to therapeutic storytelling that he has developed for working with client-generated metaphors in a way that does not leave the therapist waiting and hoping for clients to come up with some workable metaphoric description of their situation. He actively elicits the clients' own stories of their lives to date, and then invites them to reframe these stories toward a more desired and desirable future story. As demonstrated in the case example of George, a clinical counselor, Rubin avoids the traditional approaches to diagnosis and assessment, simply working with the client's own story and the changes he or she wishes to make. His work is based in a conviction that stories not only reflect what has been, but can also shape what will be. Though his approach does not actively seek to elicit or define the therapeutic characteristics of the metaphor he works with, the case presented illustrates the following core characteristics.

Therapeutic Characteristics

Problems Addressed

- Relationship issues
- Being stuck
- Lifestyle issues
- Self-doubt
- Self-criticism
- Emotional pain

Resources Developed

- Being present
- Increasing fun
- Building joy and confidence
- Being more assertive
- Finding oneself
- Being more open
- Taking risks

Outcomes Offered

- Confidence
- Realistic hope
- Openness to life and love
- Courage
- Appreciation

Guided *metaphor* is a made-up term. It is an approach that was devised to combine Kopp's term *metaphor therapy* with my work on guided imagery and metaphor, as well as with elements of traditional approaches for the use of metaphor (Kopp, 1995; Battino, 2000). Following Kopp's recommendation of using client-generated metaphors in preference to therapist-generated ones, I believe that the best way to use guided imagery for psychotherapy or healing is to structure the session around the client's own image of what will work for him or her. That image is actually the client's own metaphor.

One could ask, "Is telling a person's actual story—past, present, and desired future—really metaphor? Would terms like *guided narrative* or *guided life storying* be more accurate?" To me, metaphors are stories, and stories are metaphors. The stories that clients have about their lives, whether actual or made up, are the metaphors of their life. The old story, to which a person may hold, is neither actual nor real. It has evolved during the client's life, and, although it may be rooted in real events, it has been modified and transformed by his or her life experiences. Consequently, what clients tell me about their "real" life is the metaphor about their life, as they believe it.

In this chapter I initially present and discuss a six-step process for using guided metaphor for psychotherapeutic purposes. The process is illustrated by a case example of a client I have called George. The case is followed by a discussion about who might benefit from this approach and how it might be applied. Guided imagery for healing and improving health has been treated elsewhere (Achterberg, 1985; Achterberg, Dossey, & Kolkmeier, 1994; Battino, 2000; Naparstek, 1994).

STEP-BY-STEP PROCESSES FOR GUIDED METAPHOR

Step 1: Open the Therapeutic Discussion

During the initial session with a client, the first step I take is to offer an explanation of the importance of all people having their own life story: the story they tell themselves and others about how they got to the present time. These life stories have beginnings, middles, ends, themes, and key episodes. An illustrative example of how this opening to therapy may be phrased is provided in the case of George, which I will discuss later.

Step 2: Elicit the Client's Story

In the second step, I ask the client to relate his or her life story, initially as if it were a one-page summary, then a single sentence, and finally as a word or a phrase. If we, as therapists, are going to use client-generated metaphors, then we need to know the client's life story, or what the client *believes* is his or her life story. Condensing this story to a single sentence forces clients to find and enunciate the central theme of their story, thus describing who they believe they are at this moment in time. The distillation into a word or phrase sharpens their sense of themselves. For example, clients may represent themselves as dreamy, depressed, lovable, unlovable, creative, or ordinary. Usually, clients readily respond to the elicitation of their "old" story. Both the client and the therapist can find this process helpful, as the client can define himself or herself, perhaps in a new way, and the therapist receives much information in a condensed form.

Step 3: Elicit How the Client Would Change This Story for Personal Benefit

Clients are now asked how, from the perspective of the present, they would change their life story for the better. Assuming they could create a miracle, how would they want their present and future lives to be? What would need to be different for them to feel more comfortable and freer of old constraints? The new life story is the clients' magical transformation to their desired self, the person they wish to be, with the past they wished they had. Since memory is malleable, why not create a new past life? This process is part of the therapeutic approaches that involve asking clients to adopt an "as–if" scenario, in which something is "as if" it was desired to be. Talking about a new past makes it seem real (as is discussed more in step 5). Condensing the new life story to a sentence and then distilling it to a word or phrase helps focus the client and reifies the new story. It may seem surprising, but in my experience clients find no difficulties in writing or expressing a new life story.

Step 4: Elicit How the New Life Story Has Already Changed the Client's Future

Having elicited the new life story, I then take the next step, asking, "What is going to be different about your future?" In such a question there is an assumption that the client's future *will be changed* simply by the adoption of a new life story. To make this new future more real, the client is requested to describe in some detail how his or her future will have changed. This is an "as–if" frame and a reframing that changes the client's perspective and beliefs about his or her future. In effect, it helps consolidate all of the previous work.

Step 5: Deliver the Client's Personal Life Metaphor

Using the style of a guided imagery session, I then retell the client his or her life story and new life story, and reiterate how his or her future may be changed. The typical guided imagery session usually lasts about 20 minutes and consists of the following elements:

1. A 5- to 7-minute relaxation period
2. A trip within the client's own mind to a safe, secure, special, individual healing place
3. The delivery of the image for healing or change using the client's own ideas about him- or herself
4. A brief affirmation that the healing/change work will continue
5. A reorientation to the present with a suggestion such as "When you are ready, you may take a deep breath or two, then return to this room, now."

When listening to these stories, the client is typically in a trancelike state because a person's attention commonly shifts internally when listening to stories. (For more information, see Achterberg, 1985; Achterberg et al., 1994; Naparstek, 1994; Battino, 2000; Burns, 2001, 2005.)

Step 6: Ratify and Reorient

The final step, ratifying or validating the process and learning, is achieved by inviting an ideomotor signal (such as a nod of the head) by which the client indicates that he or she has indeed experienced a change of: (1) their story, (2) the effects of the story, and (3) the anticipation of how this will alter the future. At this point, I compliment him or her on the courage to do this work, and invite a reorientation to the present. I invite a reorientation by changing my vocal delivery to an ordinary conversational tone and making suggestions for returning to the here and now via stretching, breathing, blinking, or a combination of these.

THE CASE OF GEORGE

Having thus set out the procedural steps for using guided metaphor, I will now illustrate their application with a case example. The following information was obtained when I asked George to provide me with a brief statement about his concerns and what he wanted out of counseling. Obtaining the client's history and directions for counseling usually takes about five to seven minutes, and I generally find this is all the time that is needed.

George is a 47-year-old who has twice been divorced. At the time of our meeting he was dating, but he was "wary" because he feared getting trapped or lost in relationships. He said that self-doubt was a theme in his issues. Previously, he had been diagnosed with an Obsessive-Compulsive Disorder, although he said that his symptoms fluctuated and were not that troubling. Interestingly, he was a clinical counselor, but one whose conversations expressed considerable self-criticism and uncertainty. As I want to offer my clients maximum gain from our time together, I frequently use the session for both teaching and personal change when that client is also a fellow helping professional. Since George appeared to be stuck in an amorphous place with general issues rather than specific ones for which tailored interventions would be useful, I suggested to him that it might be appropriate to work toward a global lifestyle change. This process is what I call "guided metaphor," and it is designed to provide a client—here, George—with a new life story. He was intrigued both by the possibility of changing his life story and also by the prospect of learning something new. What follows is a reconstruction based on my clinical notes.

The Opening

Because the therapist's opening statement, in some form adapted to your individual client, is the entrée into eliciting the client's story, I began by explaining to George, "Everyone's life is a story, one that you may tell to others, or one that you tell yourself about how you arrived at this point of your life. You are the hero of that story, of all the things that have happened to you, and that you have done. There are many remarkable things you have done, like learning how to walk and talk and read and write.

"There are so many parts to a good story. There is a beginning, middle, and end, and all the transitions from one phase to another. There are so many roles that we try on, and also live. Most lives have a central theme or role that provides us with meaning or purpose. When you look back over your life, you can identify key incidents. Many people have thought that their life story would make a good book simply because our individual lives are so endlessly interesting, and everyone has and is a story."

The Elicitation of the Client's Story

I then asked George, "If you were to write the jacket blurb of your life's story, what would that be in a few short paragraphs?"

He told me that he was born in the Midwest, where he had mixed experiences at school: At some times other kids teased him, and at other times they wanted to play with him as friends. He experimented with drugs but still did well enough academically to obtain a counseling degree and launch into his lifetime career. After graduating he married for the first time; his divorce and the death of his mother occurred around the same time. He moved to the western United States, where he married and divorced again, prior to returning to the Midwest.

"Thank you," I said supportively. "Now, please condense those paragraphs down to just one sentence."

"I have had a lot of pain," responded George, "but also a lot of joy. I have liked life."

"And, now, please distill your old life story into a word or two, or a just a single phrase."

"Being present," came the response.

I encourage therapists to write down what the client tells them in as much detail as possible, being careful to record the client's own words, expressions, and metaphors. Remember that the sentence and the word(s) are *self-diagnoses* and, therefore, more significant than authority-generated diagnoses. In *The Heroic Client,* the authors make a strong case for what they call "client-directed outcome-informed therapy" (Duncan, Miller, & Sparks, 2004). By that they mean that therapists should *follow* the clients' leads since the clients know themselves better than we do or ever will. In addition, it is the clients who also know what outcomes will satisfy them. Their own words carry the structure, significance, and emotions that the therapist can only guess at . . . and, possibly, mis-state. The process I have described here is for eliciting clients' own stories in *their* words. How a person describes himself is actually who he is, since he *acts as if* that story is the norm by which he lives.

The Elicitation of the Client's New, Changed Story

"Imagine," I said to George, "that you had the power of an editor to change your life story. How would you now rewrite the story of your life so that it comes out the way you want? Please briefly tell me your new life story."

George replied that his new life story did not involve any changes in parents or family, though his father would have played a more active role in his life. School would have been better if he had taken more care of himself, and he would have started dating at a younger age but not married his first wife. There would have been more arts and music, more male friends, and less time in therapy. He would not have married his second wife, and would have felt more self-assurance. He would not have done drugs, and would have permitted himself to have much more fun and joy.

"Now, condense that new life story into one sentence," I suggested.

"I will have had a lot more fun and worry less."

"And now distill your new life story into just a word or a phrase."

"Joy, confidence, lighten up," George concluded.

The Elicitation of Future Change

I then inquired of George, "Thinking about your future, how has your new life story changed your future? Please give me some details about your new future. What is different?"

He described being more open with people, being more certain in what he did, taking more risks, and having a lot more fun. He would go through the different phases of his life with less fear of death, change, or women. He would stay more open to learning, to meeting others, and to testing and challenging himself. There would be more of a sense of control and direction in his life.

"So what is the sentence summing up your future story?" I asked.

"I am more realistically hopeful. I am more open to embracing life and love," he answered.

"And in a word or two?"

"I feel both courageous and appreciative."

It is amazing how readily clients like George have generated their new stories and future changes. In the guided metaphor approach the therapist simply facilitates the overt telling of the client's own wishes, dreams, desires, and hopes. As in responses to the miracle question ("If you could wave a magic wand and make life as you want it to be, what would be different?") that is used by solution-focused brief therapists, the client's new story with its life changes is remarkably realistic (Berg & Miller, 1992; de Shazer, 1994; Miller & Berg, 1995). The client knows what changes are possible in the story of his or her life.

The Delivery of the Guided Metaphor

Based on the understanding that the client's story is that person's metaphor about his or her life, a guided metaphor session is similar to a guided imagery session, in that the therapist initially utilizes the client's imagery to basically retell the client's story. Using the client's language, metaphors, and details about change, the therapist then guides the client through his or her new story and into a potential future story. This retelling of the story has the effect of ratifying it and making it more real. Typically, the client's new story is significantly shorter than the old story. Yet it is important in the retelling to reverse this proportion and spend much more time in the telling of the new story and future changes. The more detail I can supply for the new story, based on the client's words and ideas, the more real it becomes. The client's "as-if" becomes the "reality" I talk about, convincingly. In doing so I am, after all, just sharing in the client's dream with him or her.

This is the guided metaphor I retold to George and how I told it.

Relaxation Phase

"And now, George, we can just start with you paying attention to your breathing. Just notice each breath as it comes in and goes out . . . with each inhale, chest and belly softly rising . . . and with each exhale all those muscles relaxing. Softly and easily, naturally, simply . . . just one breath after another. And if a stray thought should wander through, thank it for being there and just go back to your breathing. This breath and the next one. And if your eyes should close, that's fine. Just one breath after the other. . . ."

The Individual Healing Place

"And within your mind, now, you can just drift off to that safe, secure, special healing and learning place that is just yours, uniquely yours. Your special place. Enjoy being there . . . and while you are there I am going to tell you your life stories—the old, the new, and your future."

George's Old Life Story

"You were born in the Midwest. Being in school involved a rough transition since you were teased a lot by other students. There was a bright side for you in playing with friends. High school was a positive experience. You experimented with drugs for about ten years. After getting your counseling degree, you entered your first marriage. You loved her very much, but didn't trust her. You got divorced, and your mother died about the same time. You moved out West, married again, enjoyed that marriage at first, struggled with it, and then divorced for the second time. Then you moved back to the Midwest. In a *sentence,* your old life involved a lot of pain, but also had a lot of joy. You did like life. In a *few words,* that life was 'being present'."

George's New Life Story

"Your new life story involves no changes in your parents or family. However, your father would have played a more active role in your life—being there for you when you needed him for guidance and love. School would have been better because you would have taken better care of yourself by 'bopping' a few kids. You would have started dating at a younger age, and would not have married your first wife. There would have been more arts and music, and more male friends. You would not have spent four to five years in therapy, and you also would not have married your second wife. Somehow, there would have been more assurance in your life and your activities, doing more things that you like to do, particularly physical things. One manifestation of this would have been staying closer to your roots in the Midwest. There just would have been much more fun and joy and living in your life, and worries would have been so minor as to almost not be there. Looking back, and looking forward with this new life, you would not have done drugs—in your new life they are just not needed for you to find yourself and happiness and comfort and joy. And in your new life your parents would have lived longer and been there for you longer. In a *sentence,* you would have had a lot more fun and worried less. In a *few words,* in your new life there would be joy and confidence, and you would lighten up."

George's Future Story

"In your future, the one you will have created for yourself with your new life story, you will be a lot more open with people, and . . . you will know who to do this with. There will just be more certainty in what you do and how you do it. You will just be able to let yourself go naturally and simply through the different phases of your life. You will be taking more risks and having a lot more fun. A lot more fun. And, interestingly, somehow, you will not only be less afraid of death, and change, and women, but more open to learning, and meeting, and testing, and challenging yourself. There will simply be, there *is,* more of a sense of control and direction in your life. Yes? The *sentence* to which you have sentenced yourself is: You will be and are realistically hopeful and open to embracing both life and love. And those wonderful words you have chosen, the words that describe your new life, are *courageous* and *appreciative*—that's wonderful—courageous and appreciative."

Affirmation of the Healing/Change Work

"And you know, George, that your new life has already begun, this moment, with all of your dreams and hopes and reality becoming available. As you experienced the listening to your new life story and your future, these new ideas have already become part of you. Just being realistically hopeful. Yes. Finding and experiencing the courage to be courageous and appreciative. Wondering about your life, and change . . . changing, becoming, being, your new story, your future, what an interesting future. Yours, yes."

Reorientation to the Present

"And I want you to know, George, how much I appreciate your courage in coming here, your sharing so much of yourself, and your trust. Thank you. And whenever you are ready, you can take a deep breath or two, stretch, blink your eyes, and come back to this room. Thank you."

The Ratification

The ratification comes in the retelling of the stories by another person. Typically, the client's old story is longer than the new story he or she tells you. However, in the delivery it is important to spend *more* time retelling the new story and the future changes than going over the old story. The more detail you can add about the new story and the future, the more real it becomes. In reorientation, you wonder about the uniqueness of their stories and how interesting their future has become. The therapist marvels at the client's daring and imagination: "Your new story and its future are just fascinating to me. I don't know about you, but I can hardly wait!" George left with apparent wonderment at what he had done.

There was a second session that occurred some six months later, in which George reported some continuing lack of direction and loss of a "zest for life." As a central theme of this session I decided to use Bill O'Hanlon's idea of *inclusivity,* in the sense of George's being able to be *both* of two opposing qualities: depressed *and* light, sad *and* happy, having some physical ailments *and* being healthy, having bad *and* good memories. The inclusivity idea is a kind of reframing that changes clients' belief that they can exist in only *one* state, showing them that life is so interesting that we can actually enjoy experiencing and living in a particular state *and* its apparent opposite (O'Hanlon, 2003). George appeared to be happily surprised that it was okay to be, for example, depressed *and* light. In essence, this session was one where we had an "amiable chat" in which I was a reassuring and reaffirming older presence (I am a grandfatherly 73). It was almost as if George needed to make contact with a father or grandfather figure, full stop. By the end of the session he had lightened up considerably. I believe the earlier guided metaphor session, in which I heard the stories of his life and helped him plan new stories for the future, set the stage for this consolidating session.

WHO CAN BENEFIT FROM GUIDED METAPHOR?

When are guided metaphors most appropriate to use? Are there particular clients for whom they are relevant or appropriate? Are there particular problems or outcomes that this approach addresses better than others? When can a therapist make the choice to use guided metaphor instead of other approaches like therapist-generated metaphors?

Generally, I use the guided metaphor approach with clients who have global or vague concerns about their lives. They are stuck, and can't seem to find a path or meaning or fulfillment. Rather than working with a specific concern (I prefer working with "concerns" instead of "problems"!), my preference is to go for a more complete change, an all-encompassing one, via the mechanism of having *the clients* change their life story. I am not giving advice or making suggestions, but following their lead on how they have described their life to this point, how they would change it, and how that has impacted their future. This is using *their* metaphors or stories about their lives, and how those metaphors can change. Consequently, this approach probably works better with the more amorphous concerns instead of specific ones.

Having said that, I do not want to rule out the option of using guided metaphor when the client is faced with specific concerns. Rather than working with an isolated symptom, why not have clients change their entire outlook on who they are, and how they got here, and what they can do? This more global approach may incorporate all of the minor concerns and at the same time provide the person with a solid basis from which to be able to manage future specific issues. (In saying that, I acknowledge it may reflect something of my own impatience with what may appear to be petty concerns.) Having this "big picture" leads me to ask myself questions like "Why work with the small change rather than large denominations, when the limited time in a session can be used for a more comprehensive solution?" Since the solutions told back to clients are theirs to begin with, I see my role as simply facilitating their own ideas and change on a global, whole-person scale.

In the classical use of metaphor in therapy, the therapist generates the metaphors based on his interpretation of what the client needs. A sensitive therapist can generate effective metaphors with sufficient ambiguity for clients to pick out what they feel will be effective for them. But, I find myself wondering, why go to the effort of creating (or adapting) metaphors for clients when they can provide you with their own unique story of what has been, *and* how they can change it?

MECHANICS OF DELIVERY

Storytelling is hypnotic in nature. Add to that the fact that I am a therapist trained in Ericksonian methods, and you will find it unsurprising that my retelling of the client's stories is done in a hypnotic style and using hypnotic language forms (see Battino & South, 2005, specifically the chapter on language forms). While some skills in the hypnotic area may be advantageous, they are not necessary to use guided metaphor in the form I have described. As all storytelling has a mesmeric quality, it is often enough just to use your best storytelling skills, for they alone can be sufficient to engage and entrance the client in the listening process. (For guidance on building such storytelling skills and effectively using the storyteller's voice, see Burns, 2001, 2005.)

Generally, I suggest that clients close their eyes to minimize distraction. I tell them that they can do this at any time, and that they can also keep their eyes open, in an unfocused way. When I begin telling the client his or her new story, I typically ask if it would be all right to hold his or her hand. If this is okay, then I hold the client's hand through the telling of the new and future stories. This anchor appears to make the new and future stories more real for the client. There is also an extra level of protection and reassurance that occurs via the contact. Since, when being told a story, many people regress to associations of being told a story as a child, the hand holding may reinforce memories of related comforts of childhood.

In retelling clients' stories, I can only retell the *surface* stories that they have told me. (In transformational grammar, the term *surface structure* refers to the partial linguistic meaning of a communication, whereas the *deep structure* is a sufficiently detailed communication that contains all of the linguistic meaning.) The art of effectively telling guided metaphors is, first, in the precise use of vague language. An example is "As you move into your future, what interesting new things will you discover for yourself and about yourself?" The precise or specific part of the statement is that "you *will* discover," and the vague part is "what interesting new things."

The second aspect of effectively telling guided metaphors is to ensure that it is done with sufficient pauses for the client to engage in the mental processing that will allow him or her to fill in relevant connections and details.

Guided metaphor can be offered verbally to the client in a session of therapy, as I have described in the case of George, or it can be offered as a written homework exercise. In the latter technique, you ask the client to write out his or her brief old story, sentence, and word, then the new story, sentence, and word, followed by the future story, sentence, and word. While the actual writing can be an effective and sufficient process in itself, you can additionally request that clients bring their writings into the next therapy session and process them in your office (L'Abate, 2004).

The idea of guided metaphor, as I have presented it, builds upon Kopp's metaphor therapy (1995) and the field of guided imagery. It is grounded in an understanding that clients' stories *are* the metaphors of what their life has been, is, and can potentially be. Additionally, guided metaphor has roots in narrative therapy, pseudo-orientation in time, timeline therapy, changing personal history, and solution-oriented approaches, as well as the classical uses of metaphor in therapy. I have found it to be a rapid way of helping clients to resolve their concerns through the use of their own metaphors in this structured manner.

REFERENCES

Achterberg, J. (1985). *Imagery in healing.* Boston: Shambala.

Achterberg, J., Dossey, B., & Kolkmeier, L. (1994). *Rituals of healing: Using imagery for health and wellness.* New York: Bantam Books.

Battino, R. (2000). *Guided imagery and other approaches to healing.* Carmarthen, UK: Crown House.

Battino, R., & South, T. L. (2005). *Ericksonian approaches: A comprehensive manual* (2nd ed.). Carmarthen, UK: Crown House.

Berg, I. K., & Miller, S. D. (1992). *Working with the problem drinker: A solution-focused approach.* New York: Norton.

Burns, G. W. (2001). *101 healing stories: Using metaphors in therapy.* New York: Wiley.

Burns, G. W. (2005). *101 healing stories for kids and teens: Using metaphors in therapy.* Hoboken, NJ: Wiley.

de Shazer, S. (1994). *Words were originally magic.* New York: Norton.

Duncan, B. L., Miller, S. D., & Sparks, J. A. (2004). *The heroic client: A revolutionary way to improve effectiveness through client-directed, outcome-informed therapy.* San Francisco, CA: Jossey-Bass.

Kopp, R. R. (1995). *Metaphor therapy: Using client-generated metaphors in psychotherapy.* New York: Brunner/Mazel.

L'Abate, L. (Ed.). (2004). *Using workbooks in mental health: Resources in prevention, psychotherapy, and rehabilitation for clinicians and researchers.* New York: Haworth Press.

Miller, S. D., & Berg, I. K. (1995). *The miracle method: A radically new approach to problem drinking.* New York: Norton.

Naparstek, B. (1994). *Staying well with guided imagery.* New York: Warner Books.

O'Hanlon, B. (2003). *A guide to inclusivity therapy: 26 methods of respectful resistance-dissolving therapy.* New York: Norton.

CHAPTER 13

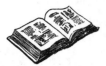

Scared Speechless

Goal-Oriented and Multiple Embedded Metaphors in a Case of Psychogenic Dysphonia

Carol A. Hicks-Lankton

CONTRIBUTOR'S STORY:
A PROFESSIONAL AND PERSONAL PERSPECTIVE

Carol Hicks-Lankton, MA, is a marriage and family therapist in private practice in Pensacola, Florida, where her work explores the individual's generative awareness to confront the challenges of life and embrace the enlarging repertoire of experience that will invariably find expression in therapeutic metaphor. Well known internationally for her workshops on hypnotic metaphor, Carol says, "I have always loved stories and the capacity they have to stimulate thinking, emotion, and direct experience through identification with the protagonist." Central to her work is the permission she offers all of her clients to follow the spark of inspiration that is speaking to them *from within*.

A noted student of Milton Erickson, she was particularly impressed by his use of stories and went on to coauthor two classic books on Ericksonian hypnotherapy and goal-oriented therapeutic stories (see Resource Section). Currently, she is writing a new book, called *Setting the Mind to It,* that is dedicated to facilitating the intentional fulfillment of desire.

PREVIEW THE CHAPTER

Carol takes us into the world of a 51-year-old woman whose abusive and traumatic past has, literally, left her scared speechless. How do you begin to communicate with someone who has difficulty communicating for herself? Here we see how therapeutic stories can open those channels, find client resources—such as this one's ability to express herself through poetry—and build both hope and trust. Each session extends on the former ones, gently offering metaphors and guided imagery to advance the client's progress and culminating in a multiple-embedded metaphor: a story, within a story, within a story. This is presented in columns, allowing us to see both the stories as they were told and the rationale for telling the specific aspects of each tale. The metaphors, which are drawn from a variety of sources, identify with the problems, challenges, or issues faced by the client; offer resources, skills, or reframed concepts; and caringly create the potential for new outcomes that match the client's goals to review and reinterpret her traumatic past, as well as reclaiming her long-overdue power to find her voice and speak freely.

Therapeutic Characteristics

Problems Addressed

- Dysphonia
- Abuse
- Cruelty
- Past trauma
- Past suicide attempts

Resources Developed

- Learning calmness and relaxation
- Building hope
- Developing effective communication skills
- Developing self-expression
- Learning to trust
- Reenvisioning the past
- Learning to say goodbye

Outcomes Offered

- Empowerment
- Resilience
- Strength
- Calmness
- Openness of expression

Judy entered therapy at age 51, desperately seeking healing for an anxiety disorder that manifested as an almost complete inability to speak. Her words seemed to be stuck in her throat. This dysphonia obviously interfered significantly with her talking the necessary talk to tell me about an intensely abusive childhood, the recent onset of this mysterious symptom, speculations by many physicians, and their eventual conclusion that it was psychogenic.

She managed to convey that the dysphonia first developed the previous year following an illness and that it was first believed to be asthma or a throat blockage. She volunteered the possibly relevant historical information that she and her siblings had been frequently choked and tortured by their adoptive parents, who both died in recent years.

Judy wasn't able to say much during our sessions, but she would cry, nod her head, and go into a calm, receptive place while I told stories. At the next session she would bring in poems that captured the essence of what I had talked about the week before and demonstrated how she had integrated that material. She told her stories in writing after hearing mine in our sessions.

THE ASSESSMENT

Through Judy's writing, I learned details of her childhood abuse and how, feeling hopeless, she had attempted suicide twice before graduating high school. She later married an abusive man, had two children, divorced him, and now has good relationships with her adult children. She operated a successful antique business before her illness, and she is currently involved in a healthy relationship with a supportive man. She was severely limited by the speech impediment and hoped that this therapy would be the last time she would have to tell her horror story and that, in telling it, she could re-interpret it, heal the wounds it recounted, forgive herself and others, replace anxiety with relaxation, and speak freely.

Continuing the assessment, I initiated relaxation training to determine if Judy was able to relax. I also wondered how relaxation would impact her ability to speak. I wanted to facilitate her being able to develop and stabilize a calm state from which she could dissociate and review traumatic events from her past that we could reinterpret and pair with relaxation. I invited her to focus attention on her breath and to simply review what she had told me without additional need to speak. I talked to her about these treatment goals and what it was possible to accomplish by setting her intentions on claiming her long-overdue power to find her voice and speak freely. I talked to her about containing the traumatic memories and rethinking them in such a way that she could imagine the happy and safe childhood she had never experienced. I spoke of Milton Erickson's idea that "it's never too late to have a happy childhood." While I talked, she accomplished a calm, relaxed state, and silent tears flowed steadily over her cheeks. Though this relaxation seemed to be beneficial for her, she did not speak any differently upon reorientation. That was the end of our first session.

THE CLIENT'S RESOURCES, STRENGTHS, AND SKILLS

Walking a Guided Path

When Judy returned for our second session, she brought me the following handwritten poem about the hope she had experienced as a result of the first session.

> A little ray of hope, I felt as I spoke to you.
> Even though tears did fall, I felt something good come through.
> Hope's what's kept me going, in hope that I would find a reason to keep living,
>   a little peace of mind.
> A brighter day tomorrow, to shine within my life, to help smooth out the wrinkles,
>   make the wrong somehow seem right.
> I know the things that seem so bad will never go away,
> But I think you can help me find a place for them to stay.
> There's really not a reason for some thoughts to hang around.
> Without them I'd be better, feel more safe and sound.
> I'd like this to be the last time my horror story's shared.
> And then just go on living, each day without a care.
> I like the idea of pretending, changing bad to good,
> Putting wrong things in their place, and leave it as one should.
> And then when it is stormy and cloudy all around,
> I'll just close my eyes, and let the sun shine down.
> I guess this journey makes us friends in some sort of way.
> And I thank God you crossed my path to help me find my way.
> A way to inner peace, a little ray of hope.
> If I find these treasured gifts, then I feel I can cope
> With the things that come within my life each and every day.
> Then maybe I can share a little ray of hope with someone along the way.

Several strengths became evident in this transaction. Her writing and communication skills were excellent. She had the capacity to experience hope and believe in her ultimate healing, not just of her voice but of her defining life trauma. She was willing to trust a stranger although her learning history did not support such a choice. I asked her rather soon to settle into a contemplative state and simply gaze at a painting of a wooded path while I talked to her about pretending that this painting was a dimensional gate through which she could enter to walk in imaginary woods.

It wasn't a formal metaphor but rather guided imagery she could use to go inside and create a context for appreciating her strengths and value. That imagery lent itself to going deep inside herself in the same way that one enters a path that leads deep into the woods. It was a path into a safe and healing place. I directed her to imagine coming upon a river flowing through these woods and to encounter herself sitting beside it. I reminded her about angled mirrors from department stores and how she could see herself in the center panel and also look to the left or right and see an infinite progression of selves in either direction, flowing like a river. I suggested that she look deeply into the eyes of the center panel, her current-age self, and transmit to "her" the validating message "I accept you unconditionally right now." Next, I suggested that when she looked at the infinite selves flowing off to the left that she imagine them stretching back through time getting younger by weeks, months, and years until she could even imagine the innocent baby first emerging into life at the farthest end. Inside this arrangement, I encouraged her to transmit this acceptance message to all the younger selves and to simply review her lifetime in the way people report doing after near-death experiences. They describe their life passing in front of their eyes, in a review in which everything suddenly becomes clear and makes perfect sense. I didn't know all the horrors of Judy's life, but I knew it was important for her healing to be able to remember them differently from when they happened and to accept the traumatized self who had been beaten, blamed, and choked.

I directed her to review this lifetime dispassionately, just as she would objectively observe any life forms, boats, barges, or driftwood that might go floating past her on that river she was imagining sitting beside. I invited her to send the message of acceptance down the lineup of selves as though it were a magical river of hydrogen peroxide that would seek out any particular wounds and bubble up to cleanse and heal them. Particular emphasis was placed on having a communion with her precious baby self and validating her existence, welcoming her to life, holding her with love, and warning her of the rigors ahead that she would experience. But this time she would be supported by this resourceful self who was back from the future to encourage and empower.

A Story of Regrowth

While Judy was pondering these suggestions, I talked about repotting plants and how rewarding it is to free the life force that has been root-bound and choked by constriction in a tight pot without proper nutrients and support. Because I had just been involved in this activity myself, it was on my mind and literally under my nails, and the reality of those imprisoned plants was like what Judy experienced in that the plant manages to tenaciously cling to life, but almost in suspended animation. I illustrated this phenomenon of survival with a digression into the movie *Harold and Maude,* describing how the wise Maude had taken the young and tormented Harold under her wing in order to expose him to the richness of life in all its glory since his mother had fallen down on the job. I described various adventures these two protagonists enjoyed in the process of Harold's coming to life, starting with how they met while recreationally attending the funeral of someone neither knew. I went into particular detail describing the scene where the two of them came upon a horribly root-bound tree clinging to life in a too-small pot, choked by fumes, bereft of sunlight, on a city street where strangers hurried by oblivious to the anguish of the desperate tree. Maude, however, noticed the tree and recognized in an instant that it deserved a better life. She and Harold lifted the potted tree into a pickup truck and spirited it off into the wide-open living, breathing, wooded spaces, where they freed it from the constricting pot; dug a nice, new, moist, and fertile space in the receptive mother earth; and reverently placed the tree inside, blessing it to thrive free and strong, able to breathe freely and give full expression to its life force.

When Judy returned after this second session, she brought a vibrant arrangement of flowers she had grown and collected for me. She also brought her second poem, about traveling down a path and meeting a younger self whom she nurtured. I experienced a deep appreciation for this client's strength. During this session, I asked her to talk about the events of her life that she had viewed in the previous week. She still spoke haltingly as she began to tell me about caring for her father as he was dying, at which time he was still speaking to her abusively. For the first time, however, as she reported his criticism and demands, she suddenly spoke with authority, clarity, and power, telling me how she had spoken back to him for the first time in her life and had told him that she didn't want his money and she was done taking care of his hateful, sarcastic, controlling, and mean-spirited self!

I told Judy I wanted to use her story for this chapter because she inspired me with the tenacity of her strength and tenderness. I asked her if she could share with me the details of the horror story with sufficient thoroughness that she could truly put it behind her. She talked more clearly than she had previously been able to do and shared her pain from a place of safety. She later wrote out an account of her entire life story, beginning with coming to consciousness at five years old in an orphanage and learning that she and her siblings were to get a permanent home with a mom and dad. Their dream life quickly unraveled into their worst nightmare as the adoptive parents unleashed unthinkable cruelty. Judy carefully included every horrible detail as if feeding it to a transformational fire. She also included a poem entitled "The Lost Child," from which I have taken an extract to conclude this chapter. In the poem she expressed gratitude that the wrong done to her had been acknowledged and that "the lost child loves it when you tell her she didn't deserve the pain."

A Mountaintop to Gain

In our next session, I told Judy a story about Milton Erickson's son, Robert, and how as a teenager in Phoenix, Arizona, he would ask his wise and famous father for help whenever he was faced with a problem. In identifying with Robert, Judy could imagine and experience the effect of a loving, accepting father, the likes of which she had never known. I explained to her that the father would always answer every question with the same one-word answer. Pointing his finger at the mountain called Squaw Peak, he would simply say: "Climb." Robert would then have no other option than to climb the mountain with his question weighing on his mind. I described a typical climb up such a mountain and the phases of frustration, pain, fear, isolation, and doubt the climber experiences. I invited Judy to enter that relaxed, receptive state while I described how Robert had been lucky enough to have a father wise enough to recognize that the child was the best expert for solving his own problem and the father's "help" was simply to direct him into that inner space where he could find his own superior answers to what troubled him. I invited Judy quite explicitly to identify with this imagined ideal father as though he had been her real father. After all, the permissions and validation were just as true for her as they had been for Robert Erickson. After this session, Judy brought in a poem entitled "My Mountain Climb." In it she described a child's experience going up a mountain with her father and connecting with her inner child:

> Again I met this lonely child, just waiting for me to arrive.
> I reached out and took her hand, and to the top helped her arrive.
> We knew we each held the answers, to help each other's pain.
> And needed each other's strength the mountain's top to gain.

Judy was now ready to go into the belly of the beast of her past to confess and release her shame and fear. She wrote about a strong feeling of peace at her adoptive mother's death in knowing that her mother would not be back. She wondered whether she should feel bad for having felt this relief. Judy clearly stated her most urgent goals: "I want the lost child on the path to feel the comfort and love and compassion I'm able to give. I want her to feel the worth I feel she deserves. I want her to see the world through happiness and hope and begin to love at its fullest. I want to cover her fear, help her grow strong, and find the power to overcome the chains that haven't completely let her go. I want to help her find a way to move forward and look forward and let the dark tales that haunt her be put away forever, buried to return no more, like at her mother's funeral."

Rarely is a treatment plan as congruently communicated as this was. Her incredible responsiveness to metaphor thus far was my indicator to proceed with an even more detailed metaphoric intervention that would address each of her stated goals.

A MULTIPLE EMBEDDED METAPHOR

I used a multiple embedded metaphor format as a structure to include several goal-oriented stories around this complex business of establishing unquestioned worth, releasing shame, forgiving parents, and opening herself to free expression. This structure is detailed in *The Answer Within* (Lankton & Lankton, 1983) and involves telling not just one but a series of goal-oriented stories designed to challenge limiting beliefs, retrieve and strengthen preferred emotions, and illustrate and allow desired behaviors. In this case, the aim was to give her an opportunity to transform and move through those old traumas, say goodbye to the horrors of that past, clarify her heartfelt desires, and place her mind and intentions firmly in the service of manifesting these desires. I wanted her to discover breathing freely, finding her voice, and giving full emotional expression to all of her experience.

The stories as I told them to Judy are presented in the left-hand column, while in the right-hand column I have sought to describe some of my thinking and rationale for using this language and these concepts, and to illustrate the relevance of those stories.

Story one begins: The man played flute in the symphony orchestra. He was exceptionally talented. One day he uncharacteristically ventured to disagree with the conductor, who severely criticized him, practically slapping him in the face with his biting words to the effect of "give me no lip—how dare you talk back to me?" Almost immediately, the man's lip swelled to such a distorted size that he was completely unable to play his flute. His distraught family took him to many physicians, seeking a medical cure that was not possible for this emotional condition. Finally, the man was referred to Milton Erickson, who carefully listened as the man related the horror story of his abusive past and how the father had forbade any of the children to talk back or make any objection in response to the unreasonable authority he wielded over them in his tyrannical way. The father may have meant well, but his relentless devalu-

I selected this story due to the parallels between the character's and client's lives, the character having developed a symptom (swollen lip) in response to an abusive adult just as the client had done with her throat closing. In both cases, the symptom interfered significantly with the person's giving full emotional expression to those impulses that had been forcefully silenced. Also, the protagonist had been through many physical evaluations without finding a cure for this stress-related symptom.

There is acknowledgment for the client that her survival did depend on her compliance with the demands of her parents. But in both cases contexts had shifted, and now survival and symptom remission required giving that same full expression to what had been necessarily squelched.

ing of his children in favor of his own egotistical control had practically choked the life force from his cowering children, who had held it all inside as if their survival required it. Erickson carefully listened to this sad history and at the end informed the man that his symptom could be cured but that it would require that he give full emotional expression to all the toxic bitterness, resentment, rage, and anguish that had accumulated over this lifetime of pain. The man was desperate and yet still fearful to take this leap into the now prescribed but heretofore forbidden expression. He pitifully wondered whether Erickson couldn't just give him a medication to cure the swelling. Erickson forcefully commanded him to "shut up with your stupid request for medication and get on with the expression you need to give." With that, the man erupted into "a most vituperative" attack on Erickson himself, spewing insult and rage in a powerful flow that had been waiting for a long time. And each person must find the courage to give this kind of thoughtful and thorough and empowered expression of that which has been built up and choked back into her. And you can do that even now from inside this protected place. And you can take all the time you need to give that expression from within yourself even now while I talk about other things.

This is an indirect suggestion designed to give direct permission to the listening client to personally review and give expression to those things she had needed to repress.

Story two begins: The emperor penguins that live in Antarctica make an annual trek of seventy miles to their breeding grounds in the most severe conditions imaginable. It is a love story and a survival story of epic proportions.

    The March of the Penguins is an aptly titled National Geographic documentary that captures the strength, perseverance, and incredible power of the instinct to survive we are all hard-wired to blindly follow. In response to an invisible yet strongly felt signal, the birds suddenly emerge in unison from their life-sustaining waters and begin the incredibly arduous trek, shuffling across the frozen landscape of their extremely harsh and downright abusive home. The ones who survive the challenging trek arrive at the breeding ground and set about the process of selecting their mate for this cycle. Signals are exchanged, vows accomplished, and the dance of love begins and culminates with the miraculous arrival of the egg, which must be

I selected this story as a natural context to reinforce the incredible courage, strength, determination, and will to survive that I see this client as possessing but underrating in herself. I hoped that in admiring the penguins' embodiment of these traits she could identify and begin to appreciate the same strength within herself. Again, the harshness of their context paralleled Judy's abusive home.

I also intended this story as an opportunity to reinforce the precious miracle of Judy's own existence

transferred to the protective custody of the father, while the now famished mother must retrace the same seventy miles to eat and replenish her capacity to nourish her chick. Meanwhile the fathers carefully and precariously hold the precious egg of new life on top of their feet and huddle together against the dark subzero Antarctic winter with its ferocious winds, sometimes of one hundred miles per hour, with nothing to eat for months since they left the life-sustaining sea. There will be nothing to support their survival, only severe challenges and adversity—yet tenaciously they hold on to life and wait for the return of the mothers. The chicks begin to hatch and must be fed soon or they will die. The mothers are making the long trek back. Miraculously, the majority of them return just in the nick of time and recognize their mates and offspring, whom they have never seen outside of the egg. Transfers are accomplished and the life-giving nutrients are transmitted. The fathers, who have now lost more than half their body weight and haven't eaten in months, must trek back to the feeding grounds. On and on this tag-team parenting continues, as the babies come into consciousness knowing nothing other than the harsh reality they were born to—and the inherent strength hard-wired into their very existence to not only survive but thrive as examples of the life force itself and the awesome unquestioned worth and value that you have by virtue of being alive. And each being resonates with an understanding that you can trust this instinct and capacity to trust the power of being who you are. And you feel it deep in your bones and let it bubble up through your heart and in the intake of each miraculous breath—you being breathed by the great life force itself that moves through you, sustaining you through all expression of your unique way of seeing and being and experiencing. . . .

Story three begins: This matter of saying goodbye to a parent is a complicated thing. Getting what we need from a parent is even more complicated. The man had asked for hypnotherapy to control the symptoms of hypertension, which he was afraid would lead to problems of the heart such as the ones that had just killed his father. He could work out or use biofeedback to force this fear to temporarily subside, but as soon as a life pressure arose, back into

and to invite her to "hold that precious egg of new life" that is herself with the same reverence and seriousness with which the father penguins hold their literal eggs.

Here Judy is metaphorically invited to identify with the hatching chicks as they come into consciousness inside this brutal reality. Here I switch pronouns intentionally in the middle of the sentence to transition into an indirect suggestion to again speak directly to Judy's unquestioned worth and value. Additional suggestions further invite her into an experience of feeling this life force as it moves through her.

Judy had directly requested help in putting the deaths of her parents into a better resolution. The man in this story also has a physiological symptom (hypertension) that resulted from the heart limitations of his parents. It is again a parallel metaphor, which I included to stimulate Judy's thinking about the goodbye to her parents that she had not yet completed.

the alarming range his anxiety would soar. I contracted with him to use hypnosis to make friends with his fear and to begin with the fear of emotional vulnerability. He had just buried his father a few weeks earlier, but his goodbyes were far from fully said. He agreed with the goal of experiencing the full catastrophe of emotional vulnerability, and so he followed the suggestion to go in his mind to the grave site, where he could say what needed to be said to finally bury that parent and all the unfinished business waiting to be resolved. When you bury a parent, you start by thanking them for what they were able to give and saying goodbye to the bitterness for all that was unwanted and painful that they also gave. You say goodbye to the hope that the parent will ever be able to make good on the love and acceptance and approval you so desperately wanted from them. It is a terrifying moment when you say goodbye to that dream and let go of any hope of it ever being reality at the hands of that parent. But the more you succeed at releasing hopes for that parent to come through, the more it suddenly becomes possible to become that ideal parent who is able to materialize beside that aching and grieving child self. You are able to respond to those heartfelt yearnings with just what's needed.

So the man sat there at the grave of his parent and released into the fires of transformation all that bitterness and pain. He transmitted to the spirit of the parent that he was going to learn more than the parent had been able to teach, and he issued forth forgiveness that freed not only his own psyche but that of the parent, reassuring the parent that his limitations would not limit the man he had become from realizing and knowing both his fullest worth and the wondrous depths of emotional vulnerability to which we're all entitled. And then he entered into a communion with the child he had been, taking that essence of himself into his heart and arms and soul, tenderly embracing that spirit and receiving questions, assuaging pain, transmitting the deepest acceptance, validation, and permission to be that the child had been hungering for through the eternity of its existence. And the child released the burden of guilt and fear and shame he had been struggling to bear all alone. And that burden was transformed and crystallized into a multifaceted core of unquestioned worth and deep calmness. He was breathing very easily and radiating with

I wanted to encourage Judy to let herself feel the power of fully feeling all of her emotions, including fear and vulnerability.

The second-person pronoun was used to blur boundaries between telling the story of how "he" said goodbye and how Judy can experience this process directly.

This apposition of opposites suggests that a shift can occur when she releases hopes for approval from her parents and in so doing receives nurturing from the unexpected source of herself.

The continuation of the story and what the man told his parents just serves to stimulate her thinking about similar transmissions she might want to make to her parents. And when the man nurtures the child he had been, these details provide an opportunity for Judy to transmit acceptance and love to her inner child as well.

This sentence recapitulates the reassociation in experiential life I want to foster here. She has retrieved and memorized feelings of calm well-being, which I

well-being when he finally finished burying that parent and saying goodbye.

Thereafter, any signal of that previous symptom only served to transport him back into that wellspring of well-being he had memorized that day. And you take all the time you need to bury all that needs to be buried and to memorize the solidness of your connection to this power source at the inner sanctum to which you can always return immediately at the first signal of your anxiety.

Story two concludes: When the penguins return at last to their beloved sea, they instinctively know just where the portal is that promises entry and release into the waters that wait below. They don't pause at the water's edge to behold their reflection on its mirrored surface. If they did, they could see and memorize the indicators of that incredible strength and power and tenacious determination that somehow show up even on a bird's face. Maybe they would see them deep within the soulful eyes. It is a universal experience known to all who have suffered long and prevailed to experience the sweet relief at the journey's transition. And in that moment, it is as if you are giving birth to yourself, fully seeing the unquestioned worth and value, just as you could see it in the infant you once were when you imagined a travel back to that bittersweet beginning when the life force delivered you into the harsh climate you would have to suffer through with those misguided parents who didn't know how to celebrate and nurture the precious life given to them. Perhaps they mourn their missed opportunity, just as those penguins grieved when they inadvertently allowed the precious egg to break and freeze and die. But you are able to immerse yourself in this celebration of witnessing the coming to life you have accomplished. Drink it in. Breathe it in. Feel it in your heart and soul and as if you were sitting beside a mirrored reflecting pool or a deep primordial well; look upon yourself and pronounce it good. I accept you unconditionally right now. And slip even deeper into the daydream you're dreaming and imagine the backgrounds of the various situations in which you are going to want to breathe easy, experience unblocked passages, give full emotional expression, experience the pangs of emotional vulnerability, speak your truth with kindness to anyone

want her to associate with any time she detects an anxiety signal.

I mention the possibility of seeing a reflection in a mirrored surface so that I can encourage Judy to see herself in her mind's eye and notice how she looks as she experiences these resourceful feelings.

I want her to memorize the sweet relief she has earned the right to as she comes into this knowing of her value. I refer to a directive from an earlier session to imagine encountering her infant self. She had been quite moved by her capacity to appreciate the value of that infant self. I suggest that her parents may well have mourned their mistakes and would join in the celebration of her spirit prevailing.

She is encouraged to create a visual self-image that captures this resource state and associates the self-image into and through all the contexts of her life where she wants to have those feelings available. This also allows her to mentally rehearse her preferred interaction in the various situations where she needs to be able to give full emotional expression.

This suggestion is to focus her awareness on identifying what she wants and giving herself permission to adopt that motivation strategy, recognizing that you need to tell how it is for you or what you need or want. Know that wanting to is a good enough reason and you deserve to let your mind's strongest intentions be set to achieve your most heartfelt desires. So just what do you desire, anyway? And what does it look like and sound like when that you who is empowered with all that strength and worth and kindness and compassion goes after what she wants? Notice how it is tempered and balanced with such an exquisite sensitivity and caring for the needs of others. Be very pleased with what you see, and know that this daydream being born now continues forever.

she will inevitably do so with sensitivity to others as well.

Story one concludes: That flute player with the swollen lip vented his rage in an attack on Erickson, following orders to give full emotional expression. One day as he exclaimed what a horrible father Erickson was, he had a burst of insight about his swollen lip spasms having something to do with unfinished business with his own father. Erickson congratulated the man and encouraged him to go home and finally say to that father only what needed to be said, no more and no less. It seemed so obvious then, but it had taken nine months to dig out from all that pain and abuse and trauma. He then went home and announced quite simply but emphatically to his father that he would be making his own decisions from now on, as he was a grown man and didn't need his father telling him what to do any more. The father readily conceded and congratulated his son for this rite of passage he had successfully negotiated. And of course the swelling in the lip subsided, and he went back to moving the breath through the pipes of his vocal instrument to make the beautiful music that he loved.

After suggesting she let this arrangement be ongoing, I return to the original story and the insight that the flautist experienced as a result of holding nothing back. It was intended as a tribute to the fact that things take the time they take to honor and resolve. I want her to honor her own journey.

I am suggesting that she speak her truth directly and with kindness, letting that permission for free expression gradually open the pipes of her vocal instrument and her own breath, no longer blocked, being allowed to freely flow.

This last sequence of stories was delivered in a single session that lasted about an hour. Judy's response was profound, as was expected, considering her very literal and personal application of all previous stories. My existing ideas about therapeutic metaphor were validated, and I was reinspired with the power they can access. The answers within are, indeed, abundant and available no matter how thick and stubborn the crust of pain, scabs, and scars. It was very gratifying to be in the presence of this client's resilience and tender strength. In addition to using the metaphors described, I encouraged Judy to utilize breath work, massage, singing lessons, yoga, gardening, and reading stories to children as complementary and conducive activities to grow the seeds for personal transformation we had initiated with our work together in metaphor.

As I put the final edits on this chapter, I had a telephone conversation with Judy to follow up on her progress. I was pleased to hear how clearly and freely she spoke. Issues of the past seemed to have slipped into the past, as she appeared to be more focused in the present, explaining that she is currently suffering from a broken wrist and is taking care of herself accordingly. However, for a client who originally presented with a functional dysphonia, it seems appropriate to conclude with her own words. These are extracted from a poem she wrote early in the course of therapy, entitled "The Lost Child." Referring to herself in the third person, she speaks of her initial despair, of the therapeutic relationship, of her incorporation of concepts offered in the sessions, of growing empowerment, and of hope.

> When she came to you, she often felt she didn't have a prayer.
> Now everything is changing, just because you care.
> She deeply feels that you're her friend because now you're the one who knows
> The dark ugly secrets she didn't want to show.
> But you can watch her as she changes into something good
> And have a life full of joy like all children should.
> The timing may be off, may be a little late.
> But that's okay with her, it's just part of her fate.
> She feels a sort of comfort within herself today,
> Waiting on her friend, guiding her on her way.
> And she's so thankful for you and your concern.
> And she is very anxious, new ways to deal and learn.
> She doesn't feel as lost since you she has found.
> And awaits the day that she arrives and feels more safe and sound.

REFERENCE

Lankton, S. R., & Lankton, C. (1983). *The answer within: A clinical framework of Ericksonian hypnotherapy.* New York: Brunner/Mazel.

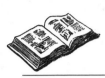

PART FOUR

Enhancing Health and Well-Being

CHAPTER 14

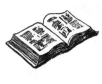

Scareless Ghost, Painless Pasta

Kids' Own Stories as Therapeutic Metaphor

George W. Burns

CONTRIBUTOR'S STORY:
A PROFESSIONAL AND PERSONAL PERSPECTIVE

George's "Contributor's Story" can be found at the beginning of Chapter 2.

PREVIEW THE CHAPTER

In this chapter, George invites you to join him on a journey of discovery that initiated and influences one of the ways he now works with metaphor. This journey began with the chance discovery of a child's own healing story, led into an exploratory study with a group of school children, and from there became a common approach in his therapy with children and, sometimes, adults. In the case of Cate, we see how kids' own stories can be engaged in the therapeutic process. She is a child facing the prospect of imminent major surgery, invasive and painful. Utilizing her school assignment in creative writing, he coaches her in writing a metaphor that parallels the problem she is about to face, that builds the resources and skills helpful for coping, and that provides her with a desirable outcome. Her story explores and employs pain management strategies with humor and playfulness, enabling her to cope with a very challenging experience.

Therapeutic Characteristics

Problems Addressed

- Pain
- Fear
- Facing an undesirable situation
- Lack of skills

Resources Developed

- Storytelling skills
- Learning skills
- Pain management strategies
- Dissociation
- Time distortion
- Hypnoanesthesia
- Positive feelings
- Future orientation

Outcomes Offered

- Competency
- Coping skills
- Feeling normal
- Pain management
- Enjoyment

Once upon a time there lived a ghost who couldn't scare a fly. He couldn't scare anyone but himself.

Sometimes you can discover something when you are not even looking for it, and sometimes that discovery can make a significant change in the way you do things. That's exactly what happened when I first read the words at the start of this chapter. I had been staying with some friends, who lent me their son's bedroom while he was away. It was one of those times when I found myself without a book to read before going to sleep, and I cast my eyes around the room for something of interest. On the bedside table was a handwritten tale, entitled "The Ghost Who Couldn't Scare," by my friends' son, Sam. It is not a story that comes from a therapeutic context, but it does, nonetheless, show us the core characteristics of a therapeutic metaphor and underscores how kids can produce stories that are essentially wise, practical, and healing. I was captivated by the first few sentences of "The Ghost Who Couldn't Scare." The story that I read is in the left-hand column, while what I saw the story communicating is recorded in the right-hand column.

Once upon a time there lived a ghost who couldn't scare a fly. He couldn't scare anyone but himself. So one day he had an idea. He was going to scare school. He had a witch as a teacher.

The problem is stated up front: There lived a ghost who couldn't scare anyone. The story engaged me with both the emotion and problem of the character. Here was something with which most kids could identify. What child has not felt inadequate, different, alone, estranged, or incapable of doing what is expected of him or her? And what child has not at least felt he or she had a witch as a teacher? I found myself wondering what the ghost would do. How would he solve his problem? What would be the outcome?

At the end of the day he went home to his father and asked, "How do you scare someone?"

His father said, "It's easy, watch me." And the father scared a girl who was walking by so much that she dropped her book. "See, it's easy" said his father.

The ghost picked up the book that the girl had dropped and read it. It was about how to scare someone.

When the ghost became aware of his problem, he began to explore ways he could resolve it. His first step reflected an important process of learning: Ask someone who knows how to do it.

Having already used a role model in his father, the ghost now seeks to discover what he can learn from a book and what other sources there are to help change his experience and build his skills in the direction he desires.

Then he puts his learning into practice.

"I'll show them," said the ghost.
Rawww!!!!
Everyone in his grade had run away except for one person—Sam.

"Rawwww!!!" This was the biggest he could do but Sam wasn't scared.

"Who are you?" said the ghost.

Sam, who has now built himself into the story, has his ghost acquire another important life lesson: Not everything we learn or try to practice necessarily works in every situation or for every person, and if it doesn't, maybe there is something important we can learn from it.

"I'm the greatest, scariest person in the school." So Sam taught the ghost all his moves.

"You are as scary as me. You and I should have lunch." So they went and the sixth graders started laughing at the ghost, but he scared them right away.

Then they went to have lunch. After they had finished Sam told the ghost to come with him to his club. He went on and saw three monsters sitting at the table: Angus, Nick, and Leigh.

"Hi" they all said.

"Guys meet our new President I've been telling you about. All Hail!"

"Now you can join the competition," Nick said.

"All right, what do I do to get into practice?" asked the ghost.

The day came and they all went to the contest. There were heaps more. After everyone had done their scare, the ghost did his.

"And now the moment you've all been waiting for. The winner is Ghost!"

The ghost finds a role model from whom he can learn how to reach his goal.

The ghost becomes as scary as his role model; he discovers a means for dealing with kids who laugh at him; and, because he has practiced and built on his skills, he is accepted among the peers he admires.

The ghost joins a club, a group of peers whose interests and goals are similar to his.

Through his efforts he begins to excel . . . and is recognized for it.

He learns the value of practicing or training in his new skills.

And, finally, his efforts pay off. He is successful.

Sam's tale is a lovely example of how a kid can create a very powerful and effective healing story. It contains the core ingredients of: (1) describing the problem, (2) building the resources or skills with which to find a satisfactory outcome, and (3) celebrating the attainment of that outcome—a process I refer to as the PRO (Problem, Resource, Outcome) approach to developing therapeutic metaphors. A more detailed explanation of this as a basis for building healing stories can be found in Burns (2001, 2005).

The problem Sam's ghost started with was that he couldn't even scare a fly. As the story develops the ghost communicates some effective strategies for solving his concerns. He asks for advice from his father, someone who knows how to scare. He looks for what he can discover in books. He finds a role model in the scariest person in school. He practices and practices and practices, building his skills as he does. He learns that his skills do not necessarily work all the time and that he still has the potential to improve. What useful abilities these are for any child to learn and possess for managing future problems. The ghost's struggle to develop these abilities results in his being accepted by his peers. In the end those efforts are rewarded. When it comes to the competition, he is the winner.

Stories reflect life, engage us, and entertain us. They inform us about the facts of life, teach us the values we need to live by, and provide models for the skills that equip us to survive and thrive. And kids love stories. If we need proof, just listen to them asking, "Tell me a story," or look at the rows and rows of books of children's stories that fill our bookstores and libraries. Stories come to life in popular children's movies, TV programs, and the tales of conflict, struggle, and victory that tend to be the theme of so many video games. As kids grow into teens the hunger for stories does not abate, although the nature of the question may change to "Can I get a new book?" or "Can we rent a video?" Given this desire to learn, to be informed, to acquire problem-solving skills and be entertained through stories, a question for therapists is how we might effectively utilize this for the young clients with whom we work.

While stories have long been communicated in words, that is not the only way to relate stories, especially to children. Our ancestors made their stories come to life visually by painting them on the walls of caves and chipping them into rocks, laying the foundations for symbols that subsequently developed into our present-day books and movies. They put on masks, decorated their bodies, and told their tales in song and dance, establishing the basis for storytelling in modern theater. Perhaps as they sat with their listeners they sketched tales in the sand, much as we now do on a blackboard or whiteboard. Shaping clay into characters, animals, and implements, they acted out their stories as kids do with toys in play today. Children's storybooks, the dramas kids watch on TV, the stories they act out in dress-up playacting, the toys that they use to model future adult-style behaviors, the play in which they engage, the humor they use, and the experiences life brings their way can all be the vehicle for metaphoric learning (Burns, 2005).

I like how Zeig (2006) describes the use of metaphor as a way of "gift-wrapping" the therapeutic goal. His metaphor about metaphors is nicely evocative of storytelling strategies with kids. Who hasn't had the experience of unwrapping a gift or watching a child unwrap a birthday or Christmas present? Who hasn't noticed the difference between receiving a gift that is unwrapped and one that is wrapped? Who hasn't taken a gift-wrapped present, felt its shape, turned it around, and tried to guess what is inside? What child who celebrates the tradition of Christmas hasn't sought out the presents under the tree, given them a shake, and wondered? No matter how humble the gift, how it is wrapped can heighten excitement and curiosity, engaging us in a process of interaction with the gift even before we know what it is.

Sam's story of the ghost who could not scare offered a rather simple goal message, but that message was wrapped in a story that engaged and captivated the reader in a search to solve the problem. It shows us how kids can develop their own empowering strategies for change through a metaphoric story.

KIDS' OWN HEALING STORIES

As I read Sam's story, questions began to form in my mind: If Sam could produce such a wonderfully wise and enjoyable story, could other kids do something similar? Would it be helpful for kids to write their own metaphoric healing stories? Would it benefit them to think and write about their problem from a slightly removed position, have a separate-from-themselves character search for the means to resolve it, and celebrate an appropriate outcome? Might they get more from the process of thinking about, creating, and penning it themselves than from a therapist or counselor telling them a story?

Curious to explore some of these questions, I became involved in a project with the generous assistance of school psychologist Susan Boyett and schoolteacher Claire Scanlon, of Helena College in Western Australia. Year seven students, approximately 12 years of age, were asked to do the homework exercise of writing a problem-solving or healing story. The written guidelines the students were given are much the same as those I use in therapy. They are presented simply, clearly and yet not too specifically:

Write me a story about
   (a) a character (such as an animal, an imaginary figure, a hero, someone your own age, or whoever you want),
   (b) who has a problem or problems,
   (c) who finds ways to fix those problems, and
   (d) who enjoys the benefits of the outcome.

The students were also given the example of Sam's story. "One child once wrote a story (a) about a character that was a ghost. This ghost (b) had the problem that he couldn't scare anyone—not even a fly. Trying to find ways (c) to fix it, he started to watch what other, scarier ghosts did and how he could copy them. Some things he tried worked, and some didn't. In the end (d) he felt so proud when he could scare off monsters that were terrifying good people."

What came from asking kids to produce their own problem-solving stories? The first was that they all did it, with varying degrees of ability and varying degrees of compliance. One boy, obviously unhappy with the task, told the brief tale of a student who loved cycling and skateboarding, and could not understand why he had to sit at a computer writing a silly story! Yet his story was helpful in that, after describing the dilemma, he reached the compromise of meeting the basic requirement to do his homework and thus allow himself maximum time skateboarding.

Second, there was an amazing similarity between the problems that the stories of this nonclinical group focused on and those I hear in my clinic. Recurring themes were parental marital problems, abuse, separation, grief, death of a parent, drug use, bullying, disability, and suicidal thoughts. Maybe these are the types of problems common to most kids and those who come to therapy are the ones who just don't cope as well with them.

Third, despite the invitation to consider a broad range of possible characters, almost all the kids in this group chose a child as the character of their story, completely avoiding fictional figures, TV and book characters, or superheroes. This I found interesting, as the literature on childhood metaphors often recommends selecting characters from a child's favorite TV show, movie, or book, but that suggestion was not supported by this sample group of kids around the age of 12 years. A story of another child might better hit the target.

Fourth, some kids showed very good problem-solving skills, and some did not. This is helpful information to observe in the stories produced in therapy. Does the child's story provide the means to reach a practical and realistically attainable outcome (i.e., is it a healthy and helpful story), or does it reach a magical outcome, offer solutions outside the character's control, or struggle to find effective resolutions (which are not so easy for the child to replicate)? Having information about how skillful clients are at problem solving enables you as the therapist to assist their development of these skills in a way that will help them cope with the current situation and also empower them to better cope with the future. The ability to solve problems successfully is, indeed, one of the core skills of a well-adjusted adult.

Finally, the project—again in a parallel of what often happens in therapy—reflected how some children produced only a partial resolution. In one tale, a child told of how a boy struggled to deal with the death of his father—a story that closely resembled his own sad loss and experiences of grief. Only after years of guilt and suffering is the child assured that the death was not his fault, and then he is still not convinced. Where such a story does not reach a clear resolution, or does not provide clear means to help the client achieve it, the therapist may seek to facilitate the search for means and solutions with questions like "What helped this boy gain the level of assurance he achieved?" "What more would the character need to feel reassured that it was not his fault?" "What else could he or others do to help ease the sadness?" With questions of this nature, therapists can help the child search for resources and outcomes within the context of the child's own metaphor, as well as permitting the child to talk about an emotionally charged experience in a more detached, third-person way.

Looking at what we learned from this project, and extrapolating that knowledge to clinical situations, it seemed that having kids create their own healing stories set up a therapeutic win-win situation. If children find a solution in the writing of their own tale, they simply need to be assisted to apply that for a successful outcome. If their story does not readily produce appropriate means or a successful resolution, the therapist can join the children in their own metaphor to ask questions that facilitate the search for resources and help shape a productive outcome. Whatever a child produces enables the therapist to further the outcome-oriented processes of the therapeutic journey for that child.

What Are the Advantages of Using Kids' Own Stories?

Using a child's own story has several therapeutic advantages.

1.   If the child is the source of the story, there is nothing for him or her to resist. Often kids are reluctant customers in therapy, brought in by parents who claim there is something wrong with the child and force the therapist into the role of Mr. Fixit. The child basically doesn't want to be there, doesn't want to talk to you, and is usually pretty skilled at undermining anything an adult offers. Often this is exactly what these children have done with their parents for a long time . . . and done very successfully. If these children produce a story, no matter how brief or incomplete, they allow you to step a little into their world.

2.   Since the child has created the story, often it is easier for him or her to identify with the message and outcome of the story than with a message and outcome that are, or seem to be, imposed by a relatively unknown adult. It is generally considered that most writers' first novel is largely autobiographical. Writing is a type of projective exercise, and this is no less so for our young clients. The protagonists they create are likely to be representative of them-selves, and so they will be able to easily identify with them. The problem they describe is likely to be representative of their own experience, and thus something with which they will identify. And here are the important therapeutic bits: First, the means, skills, and resources the character employs to overcome the problem are more likely to be identified with, and, second, the successful outcome is more likely to be accepted.

3.   If the child finds a solution or solutions to the problem in the process of creating the story, then the therapeutic exercise has been successful and the therapist has little more to do than help the child apply the solution. The therapist becomes redundant, and the child is empow-ered with a process for finding future solutions.

4. When the child's story does not find an appropriate solution—when the character remains stuck with the problem, or when the tale fails to develop adequate means for reaching a satisfactory outcome—the therapist can help guide the child toward finding a solution within the language, processes, and context of the child's own story. The child's tale provides a basis from which to work and removes the onus on you to create a wisely produced story that may or may not be effectively tuned in to this particular child.

5. If you are doing group work with kids, it is possible to request the participants to write their own healing stories in much the same way you do with an individual client. With permission, you can read their stories to the group, stopping at the point in each story where the problem has been described, and asking the group to brainstorm solutions with questions like "If you were the main character of this story, how would you go about solving the problem? What could you try? What do you think the effects of that might be? What if there are things the character cannot change? What are the best ways to manage the situation then?"

MR. PETER PASTA HELPS EASE THE PAIN

Having read Sam's story and carried out the project with the students at Helena College, I began to more actively seek stories from child clients. Caitlin, or Cate, was a bright 11-year-old girl who demonstrated how a story could help manage severe pain. Although her parents called her Caitlin, as soon as they had left the room Cate was what she said she preferred to be called. She showed the confidence of a child who had been brought up in a supportive, nurturing environment and had no difficulty communicating with this new adult figure in her life. If there was one word I would come to associate with her, it would be *brave*. She was joyful and showed no fear or anxiety about what lay ahead in the next few days.

Her parents, who demonstrated their care and support by both taking time off work to accompany her to the consultation, spoke very favorably of her and her abilities. They explained that Caitlin needed spinal surgery to graft donor bone onto her own. She had been warned that she would suffer extreme pain in the postoperative period. In addition, she would be required to lie and sleep almost perfectly still on her back. It would involve a lengthy recovery period, including at least a week in hospital, two or three months off school, and a total recovery time of three to four months. Wanting to do everything possible to assist their daughter, her parents wondered at this late stage if hypnosis would help her manage the pain and hasten her recovery.

I confess to having had doubts about what I might helpfully offer Cate when I heard the story. The operation sounded horrifically invasive and frighteningly painful. I wondered whether—despite the parents' hopes and wishes for their young child—she would have the resources to manage comfortably.

At the same time, I was mindful that Zeig and Geary described pain control as "a matter of faith" (Zeig & Geary, 2001, p. 261). They have said that there are three kinds of faith in dealing with pain. The first is the faith the therapist needs to have in his or her own ability to assist the client. Even though I have worked extensively in pain management areas, this case seemed qualitatively different from assisting someone with chronic pain or the pain of childbirth. The second, they say, is the faith the therapist needs to have in the ability of the client. Did I have this? Would an 11-year-old child be able to manage the intensity and duration of the pain that she was going to experience? That seemed a big thing to ask of a little child. Third, claim Zeig and Geary, in order for treatment to be successful, there must be faith in the therapeutic procedures as well as in the relationship between the therapist and the client. I reassured myself that there was good evidence to support the use of hypnosis in pain management (Barber, 1996) in general, as well as specifically in the area of painful, invasive medical procedures (Bejenke, 1996; Lang et al., 2000).

What resources did Cate have, I wondered, that could be employed therapeutically to enhance that faith for both of us? So I asked her, "What do you do for fun?" This can be a helpful question with clients of all ages, but particularly with kids.

"I like to write," she said. "We have to write a story about pasta for school."

"About pasta?" It seemed a curious topic. "Is this about making pasta, cooking pasta, or the history of pasta?" I inquired.

"No, it is for creative writing," she responded.

If she liked stories, then the use of metaphor became an obvious choice with her therapy. If she liked writing, then perhaps, like Sam, she could write a story that would help her explore the means and strategies she could use to deal with the anticipated problem of pain. If she had enjoyed drawing, playing with toys, writing songs, playing imaginary games, or doing dress-up plays, any of these could have been used as the medium for her to express her own story. I could just as easily have asked her to draw an outcome-oriented story, enact the resolution of a problem through toys, or borrow her parents' video camera to film a solution-focused play. Alternatively, I could simply have asked that she tell me a story, collaboratively coaching her to shape it in helpful therapeutic directions. However, putting her story in the concrete form of writing, drawing, or videoing can help consolidate and incorporate the learning while retaining a ratifying reminder.

Storing Cate's skills of writing in my mind as a possible resource to utilize later, I went on to explore what other things she enjoyed. They included playing and listening to music, as well as spending time with her dog, Hamish. The mere mention of his name brought a smile of joy to her face. She obviously had the bond of affection that most kids have with a pet.

Because hypnosis had been requested by her parents, was of interest to Cate, and, therapeutically, seemed like an appropriate tool in which I could have some faith, it provided a helpful vehicle to teach her both relaxation strategies and pain management skills. As this is a chapter about metaphor, I will not go into depth about what we did with hypnosis apart from setting the overall context of the therapy from which Cate's own healing story emerged. I chose to work with a number of questions (see the following list) that invited her to make metaphoric associations with past positive experiences, skills, and processes that could be transferred over to help deal with her anticipated pain. That single session of hypnosis, which appeared to shape the metaphor she developed, included the following areas:

1. *Dissociation.* "Are there times you become so involved in your writing, listening to music, or playing with Hamish that you do not notice Mom calling you or the sounds of your little sister in the next room?"

2. *Time distortion.* "Do you get so interested in those things that time seems to fly by and Mom says to you, 'What have you been doing? You have been in there for more than half an hour'?"

3   *Hypnoanesthesia.* "What does it feel like when an arm or leg 'falls asleep'? What are those feelings of feelinglessness like?"

4. *Antithetical, positive feelings.* "When was a time you felt really good and happy? What was something you laughed about so much you had to hold your sides or thought you might wet yourself?"

5. *Controlled attention to the pain.* "What happens when you turn the volume up or down on your MP3 player? What do you think would happen if you imagined turning up and down the volume of any pain you might have?"

More can be found about hypnotic strategies for pain in Barber (1996), Yapko (2003), and, specifically for children, in Olness and Kohen (1996).

Wanting to add every possible string I could to Cate's therapeutic bow, I also taught her a technique of self-hypnosis to help her relax and manage her pain. Additionally, I suggested a number of other exercises, which included recording as many of her favorite songs as she could onto her MP3 player and collecting her favorite photographs of Hamish. My thoughts were, first, that being busily involved in such pleasurable tasks over the next few days would help distract her thoughts from worries about the forthcoming operation and, second, that they would be things she could use in the postoperative period. With similar objectives in mind, I asked her to write up her story about pasta, and offered a little coaching.

"Will pasta be the main character?" I asked. "And what will be the problems or challenges it has to face?"

"It breaks easily and has to get cooked," she replied, "but doesn't want to be."

"Do you think the pasta might be naughty and resist getting cooked," I asked playfully with a smile, "before finding some helpful ways to cope and enjoying what it feels like to be what pasta should be?"

She nodded, reciprocating the smile, as my questions guided her toward creating a story along the lines of the PRO approach: beginning with a Problem, finding the Resources for managing it, and reaching a satisfactory Outcome. This process laid the basis not just for writing a healing story but also for managing her anticipated pain.

I next saw Cate in the hospital, a few hours after her surgery. Photos of Hamish were affixed to the wall beside her bed. Her MP3 player sat on her bed tray, the ear buds in her ears. She lay flat on her back, strapped to the bed, a drip entering her arm, and her parents sat on either side of the bed. She rolled her head slowly toward me and smiled slightly, her face reflecting her pain. As I pulled up a chair to the bedside, her father held some pages up for her to see, and she read me her story about pasta. It appears in the left-hand column that follows. I have added my comments about the therapeutic characteristics of her tale in the right-hand column.

Mr. Peter Pasta was his real name but he liked to be called Pete.

Though the main character of Cate's story is male, there is no question of her identification with him. She introduces him by an abbreviated pet name exactly as she had introduced herself to me.

Poor Pete had a problem. He was brittle and could break easily. He wanted to be soft and delicious like normal spaghetti and knew what he had to do. He had to get cooked! It was the only way but he was scared and didn't want to.

Mom put a big pot of boiling water on the stove, opened the packet and tried to shake him in. He hung on tight to the packet, refusing to let go. Mom shook harder until he couldn't hold on any longer and began to slip out. He fell out in a hurry, screamed, and leapt from the pot. He stuck to the ceiling and she had to get a chair and scrape him down.

When she tried to put him in again he jumped from the pot and landed on Mom's head. She looked like an old white-haired woman who had been out in the rain and got all wet. She was mad.

This isn't working, thought Pete. I need to get fixed. I need to be like other spaghetti that is only good when it is cooked. So Pete got brave and let Mom put him in the water. It felt so hot that he wanted to scream. Then he heard the bubbling of the water. It seemed to be singing a song. As he listened he began to sing along with the bubbles and forgot about the water being so hot.

When it started to get hot again he thought about how good the bubbles felt. It was like he was in a spa bath. The bubbles were bouncing him around. This was fun. He felt relaxed and more flexible as he enjoyed moving with the bubbles.

When it got hot again he thought about what it would be like after. He would be soft like real spaghetti. He could play with his favorite sauce. That felt good.

Before he knew it he was cooked. The hot water had gone. Mom put him in a big bowl and soon he was slopping around having fun with his favorite sauce.

Like Cate, Pete has a physical problem: He breaks easily. He wants to be normal, knows the process he has to go through to achieve it, and, like her, is both scared and reluctant.

Asking Cate what might happen if her character was naughty and resisted what he knew was necessary helped her to highlight the problems of resistance, examine her fear, and do so with humor. In her own words and images she was able to show how fear and resistance were unhelpful and lacking in a solution orientation.

The futility of his resistance leads Pete to reassess his strategies. Much as he dislikes the process, it is necessary if he wants to be "normal."

Pete adopts, and applies, some of the strategies suggested to Cate in hypnosis. Here he dissociates from the pain of the water temperature and focuses on more pleasurable sensations such as a song or music.

Cate surprised me with her understanding and acceptance that pain may not be completely, magically eliminated, but that the experience of it could be managed. Pete dissociates and focuses on antithetical feelings.

Pete takes a future orientation, thinking not so much about what is happening but how things will be when this is over.

"Before he knew it" reflects a time distortion. Sometimes things can be over more quickly than we might anticipate.

She added some cheese. Everyone liked him and said how delicious he was now that he was cooked. Pete was happy, and glad he could make others happy, too.

Postprocess, Pete felt good in himself. He could have fun and be happy, and those around could truly appreciate him.

Her parents and I laughed at the thought of Mom's head covered in half-cooked spaghetti. "Don't. It hurts," said Cate of her own inability to laugh.

"How did you feel as you were reading the story?" I asked, hoping that it had enabled her to dissociate at least a little from the pain. If it had, the question also served as a validation of her ability to do so, and a suggestion that she might be able to replicate it.

"A bit better," she answered, "apart from when I tried to laugh."

"Then do you think you can keep your enjoyment to smiling for a while and save the laughs until you are feeling better?" I inquired. "Perhaps there might be more stories you have come to mind while you are lying there, and I know you can't write them down at the moment so perhaps you could dictate them to Mom or Dad to write down for you."

She smiled and they nodded. Mr. Peter Pasta had acknowledged, incorporated, and applied some effective strategies to help Cate with a difficult and, in many ways, unwanted experience. If she could process these so effectively through her ability to tell a story, I wanted to encourage her to extend her use of such a resource.

I did not see Cate again, as I departed soon after on a national teaching tour and was away for a couple of weeks. About six weeks after I had visited her in the hospital, however, her mother phoned and told me that Cate had managed her pain "extremely well" and positively. With regard to her recuperation, she was "doing much better than expected" and had already returned to school—at least a month earlier than forecast by her surgeon. "In addition," her mother said, "Caitlin has won an award at school for her writing."

For me the stories of "The Ghost Who Couldn't Scare a Fly" and "Mr. Peter Pasta Who Helped Ease the Pain" are the most delightful illustrations of how a child can use his or her own story to learn about and build essential life skills. They demonstrate how kids' own stories may be sought and utilized in the healing processes of therapy. Working collaboratively with children to build their own metaphors, the therapist is creating a therapeutic win-win situation. If children find solutions in *their* stories it is a therapeutic success. If the child does not immediately find a solution, the therapist can join the child in his or her story to help shape an appropriate and healthy outcome. It can be a fun-filled, potent, and privileged way of working with kids.

REFERENCES

Barber, J. (Ed.). (1996). *Hypnosis and suggestion in the treatment of pain.* New York: Norton.

Bejenke, C. (1996). Painful medical procedures. In J. Barber (Ed.), *Hypnosis and suggestion in the treatment of pain* (pp. 209–266). New York: Ballantine.

Burns, G. W. (2001). *101 healing stories: Using metaphors in therapy.* New York: Wiley.

Burns, G. W. (2005). *101 healing stories for kids and teens: Using metaphors in therapy.* Hoboken, NJ: Wiley.

Lang, E., Benotsch, E., Fick, L., Lutgendorf, S., Berbaum, M., Berbaum, K., Logan, H., & Spiegel, D. (2000).

Adjunctive non-pharmacological analgesia for invasive medical procedures: A randomized trial. *Lancet, 355,* 1486–1500.

Olness, K., & Kohen, D. (1996). *Hypnosis and hypnotherapy with children* (3rd ed.). New York: Guilford Press.

Yapko, M. D. (2003). *Trancework: An introduction to the practice of clinical hypnosis* (3rd ed.). New York: Brunner/ Routledge.

Zeig, J. K. (2006). *Confluence: The selected papers of Jeffrey K. Zeig.* Phoenix, AZ: Zeig, Tucker & Theisen.

Zeig, J. K., & Geary, B. B. (2001). Ericksonian approaches to pain management. In B. B. Geary & J. K. Zeig (Eds.), *The handbook of Ericksonian psychotherapy* (pp. 252–262). Phoenix, AZ: Milton H. Erickson Foundation Press.

CHAPTER 15

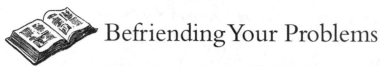

Befriending Your Problems

Metaphor with a Self-Mutilating Young Woman in Transition

Wendel A. Ray and Jana P. Sutton

CONTRIBUTORS' STORY:
A PROFESSIONAL AND PERSONAL PERSPECTIVE

Wendel Ray, PhD, is a licensed clinical social worker, marriage and family therapist, senior research fellow and former director of the Mental Research Institute (MRI), professor of family therapy at the University of Louisiana (ULM), and founder/director of the Institute for Relationship and Interactional Studies (IRIS). He lectures and conducts training internationally on brief therapy of adolescent substance abuse and Attention-Deficit/Hyperactivity Disorder, systemic therapy with family violence, and interactional theory. Wendel is the author of numerous articles and books (see Resource Section).

Jana Sutton, PhD, is a licensed marriage and family therapist, a licensed professional counselor, assistant professor of family therapy, and director of clinical services at the University of Louisiana (ULM). Her expertise is in the application of systemically focused models of treatment to domestic violence, adolescent substance abuse, and group therapy. While describing herself as in the very beginning stages of her career, she has published and presented internationally on interactional approaches to brief therapy with children, youths, and families.

PREVIEW THE CHAPTER

With Jana in the role of therapist and Wendel as supervisor and principal author, these two contributors combine their skills to bring us the case of a young woman who has been raped, has engaged in wildly promiscuous behaviors, is severely self-mutilating, and lacks sexual satisfaction with a husband she loves. Her story is one of an intimate relationship with her problem of "cutting"—more intimate than that with her husband. Rather than pathologizing the mutilation, as other people in the client's life have done, the authors join her story of cutting as her best friend, explore it with strategic questioning, use it as a metaphor for her relationship with her husband, and facilitate a shift to a healthier, happier story. Underlying this approach is the premise that, rather than being a problem, a presenting symptom may "make sense," be adaptive for the client, and offer the solution to a more helpful adaptation. The case clearly illustrates how the client can own the story of the future as much as the story of the past.

Therapeutic Characteristics

Problems Addressed

- Self-mutilation
- Depression
- Hurt
- Sexual dysfunction
- Past trauma
- Rape
- Disempowerment
- An unhealthy relationship

Resources Developed

- Making sense of a symptom
- Seeing a problem as a friend
- Utilizing externalization
- Reexamining the symptom relationship
- Modifying problem processes
- Creating desired outcomes

Outcomes Offered

- Self-caring
- Pleasurable sex
- Association of love and sex
- Focus on pleasant present and future experiences
- Empowerment
- Meaningful relationships

When working with a family, I find myself thinking of Don Jackson. What comment would he make? Don managed to have the idea that there is nothing wrong with the patient, which is quite a feat. He accepted a lot of behavior as being communication instead of physiological, which made a whale of a difference in the therapy he was doing. —JAY HALEY, 1988

Jane came into therapy initially saying she was depressed, ostensibly due to the recent divorce of her parents. Referred by her parents, this 18-year-old young woman did not know where she belonged: where she should live, which college she should attend, which career path she should take, which parent she should be loyal to and when, and which intimate relationship she should be involved in. Jane was lost.

Initial conversation was kept light, as Jane revealed only the parts of her life and information about her relationships that she felt safe sharing. All the while, I suspected Jane was not sharing something vital to successful therapy. She would say, "Everyone keeps telling me what I should do. They believe I am not capable of making decisions that are right for me, and I am."

Listening to your client will inevitably give you direction in therapy, and Jane was no exception. Not pushing, we believed, would later allow her to share her deepest secret of all, which she did after several sessions. Jane was self-mutilating, or "cutting" as she referred to it. Shifting away from the pathological and negative connotation implied by "self-mutilation" to the client's term of "cutting" in our discussions made sense given the context in which the behaviors occurred and our nonnormative/nonpathological conceptual framework.

Jane was delighted to raise the leg of her jeans and the sleeve of her heavy sweater to show her wounds, stating, "I am not ready to tell you why this is a part of my life, but I am ready to show you what it is." While the revelation of cutting was not shocking, the extent of it was. Gruesome scars on her legs and arms, both new and old, were apparent: thick, open, red, and numerous.

With as much calm as I could muster, I responded, "Jane, I feel privileged that you could share this with me." A composed therapeutic response was conveyed for several reasons:

1. *All behaviors make sense.* Jane had stated, "I get so tired of having to explain some of the things that I do. I know that I do many things differently than others, but they have not walked in my shoes. I'm used to being called crazy and insane, but I hate it. I'm not crazy or insane. They are all crazy for believing that I am." While Jane may not have been specifically referring to cutting or to our therapeutic relationship, the implication for our relationship was clear. I had to be sure not to react in a way that would give Jane the impression that I, too, thought some of her behaviors were abnormal. Central to this therapy and to this use of metaphor is the belief that all behaviors make sense given the context in which they occur.

2. *Shift thinking about symptoms.* Essential shifts in thinking, to be found in the work of Bateson and team (Bateson, Jackson, Haley, & Weakland, 1956, 1963; Jackson, 1957), in the early years of the Mental Research Institute (MRI), are prerequisites for any therapist attempting to incorporate metaphor and story into his or her therapy in a manner consistent with the therapeutic use of metaphor in the case of Jane. These shifts in thinking include the following:

    ■ Therapists' preconceptions and biases are as much a factor in therapy as what the client brings into the situation (Cecchin, Lane, & Ray, 1994; Jackson, 1955; Weakland, 1967).

- Symptoms make sense in the present context(s) and relationship(s) of the client, as opposed to only being understandable as a product of past experiences (Jackson & Haley, 1957; Ray & Crawford, 1991).

- Therapists need to understand and work within what the MRI Brief Therapy Team refers to as "patient position," or the language and worldview of the client (Fisch, Weakland, & Segal, 1982).

3. *Expect the unexpected*. Human beings are naturally adaptive and adroit in bringing attention to untenable relationship circumstances in ways that avoid open, explicit accusation of others. Never think you have seen everything; never think that you have heard everything. Rather, expect the unexpected. Jane's revelation was her way of assessing whether the therapist could assist in ridding her of cutting as a response to pain. Jane announced, "I am very capable of leaving relationships and acting like people never existed if they want more than I can give or get in my way. I know what I want and can do without people that do not share my dreams or philosophy of life."

Indeed, a few years later when Jane returned to therapy, she recalled my reaction to her revealing her butchered arms and legs: "I am now ready to tell you why 'cutting' is a part of my life because I know that you will not judge me and will accept what I tell you as the truth. You did it once before, and I will never forget how you reacted to me showing you my legs and arms. I thought you would be appalled, not just by my arms and legs, and you weren't."

THE SECRET BEHIND THE SECRET

Jane made good initial progress, enrolling in college and moving away from home, but soon discontinued therapy. When she returned to therapy a few years later, she did so because she had developed a brand-new set of challenges. She was now married, and her cutting was causing problems in a manner that it had not previously. Her husband was now privy to the secret, but not to the secret behind the secret: Jane had been raped.

Jane's passion for literature, reading, and writing became evident as she told a chilling story, narrating it as though it were someone else's, with little to no emotion. I observed that this capability for externalization could become a primary resource and metaphor in our work together. In a very moving narrative, she revealed, "I was date raped when I was seventeen. It was the first time I had ever had sex. It is not a big deal. It didn't hurt then and it doesn't hurt now. Really, I believe it happened to someone else. When I think back, it was not me lying there. I was there, but I was watching me from the upper corner of the room. It was like I was my guardian angel, but I could not work my magic. My magic is now worked in the form of a best friend, but I will tell you about him later."

I was curious about several things Jane disclosed in this emotionally subdued narrative, such as rape being "no big deal." Jane's describing herself as being a guardian angel unable to work her magic was also noteworthy. My impression was that Jane had indeed been hurt, beyond either my or Jane's comprehension, but I decided not to pursue that line of questioning given Jane's earlier warnings of being leery of people assuming they knew what was best for her. She said her only difficulty in dealing with the rape was that it had been her first sexual experience. As a young girl, she had envisioned that her first sexual experience would be the romantic event of a lifetime, but it turned out to be one she had not even consented to. She dealt with the emotional turmoil of the rape by cutting herself and by becoming promiscuous.

"I don't think the rape would have affected me if it had not been my first time," she said, "but since it was, I decided, 'What the heck. I've already had sex, so there is no point in saving myself any longer. That's already been taken away from me.' So I slept with who I wanted, for whatever reason I wanted, and when I wanted."

An underlying theme in her conversation was that since the rape Jane had not thought very highly of herself, and therefore she felt she did not have to protect herself from dangerous situations as she had done previously. She had been violated, so she was worth nothing, and since she was worthless she described herself as "needing" to be harmed, destroyed, and used. "I decided I might as well sleep around. I wasn't worth anything anyway. And besides, who would care?"

"What did you gain from sleeping around?" I asked.

She responded, "Well, I didn't care about any of those guys, just like that guy hadn't cared about me, and I realized I could hurt guys by sleeping with them once and refusing to do it again. It was like a game."

"That makes sense to me," I commented. "It sounds as though you were getting back at men by deciding to put yourself in control."

"Well, not only was I getting back at men, but I was also ensuring that I got what I deserved too . . . to be treated like trash. Having sex all the time, with lots of people, gave me the same satisfaction as I get when I cut. It's as though I needed to cause myself harm, but not initially. I never feel pain when I cut, and I never felt pain when I slept around. I always enjoyed myself. The sex was great. Just like when I cut myself . . . it's euphoric. It was always after I had another one-night stand that I started to feel bad, in much the same way as I feel bad after I have cut myself . . . when it really starts hurting. I so want to stop cutting. It's really starting to get to Michael [her husband] . . . and so is our sex life."

THE NONEXPERT, ONE-DOWN STANCE

To clarify the direction of therapy, I said, "It seems as though you would not want to stop cutting or do anything about your sex life if it wasn't for Michael. Is that correct?"

"Exactly," said Jane. "Now that Michael and I are married, things are different. I no longer enjoy sex anymore like before when I was sleeping around, and the cutting really upsets him. He doesn't know what to do."

As therapists, we prefer to adopt a nonexpert or one-down stance throughout therapy, for two reasons. First, it allows us to meet clients within their own frame of reference. With Jane, this involved respecting her insistence that she knew which direction her life should take. Second, we see therapy as a collaborative cocreation of solutions, rather than a hierarchical interaction in which the therapist knows more and has better ideas than clients have.

"I love Michael," she continued, "more than I have ever loved anyone, and both issues bother him tremendously. The problem with our sex life is that it is not meaningful to me, and I don't understand this. How can I have great sex with people that I don't care about, but I can't have sex that means anything with someone I love so much?" She said it was as though she was looking down upon the sexual activity of which she was not a part—just as she had described her rape—without feeling anything, physically or emotionally. Her ability to detach and externalize had become a primary technique she used to cope and move forward in life.

"Why do you think that you can't even 'be there' or enjoy yourself when you have sex with Michael?" I asked. "You have described sex before marriage as being extremely enjoyable."

Jane hesitated, then responded as though she was having an epiphany. "It seems obvious now that you have asked. I never equated sex with love. In fact, sex and love do not go together. If I love Michael, I cannot have sex with him. Sex is to be had with people that you don't care about, so I go somewhere . . . up into the corner of the room . . . and watch, but I don't feel. Sex has never meant anything to me. Now Michael does mean something to me, and it seems wrong to do with him the things that I did with people I thought nothing of and wanted to hurt. I don't want to hurt Michael, I want to be closer with Michael than I've been with anyone before, but I can't seem to relax with him in the bedroom. I know it hurts him."

The pieces of the metaphorical puzzle came together: Jane could not enjoy sex with someone she loved.

EFFECTING METAPHORIC CHANGE

Having used the change-evoking effect of empathic inquiry to join and gather information, I felt that in the next session it was time to start intentionally effecting change. Understanding and working within the worldview and language of the client is a core concept in effective systemic brief therapy (Sutton, Ray, & Cole, 2003). Aspects of Jane's worldview included: (1) her belief that cutting was not pathological, (2) her confidence that she could find her own direction in life, (3) her belief that she loved her husband, and (4) her inability thus far to have meaningful and enjoyable sex with him. Speaking Jane's language involved adopting her use of elaborate narratives that presented herself as an outsider to the story as though it were not hers. It was also important to be mindful of Jane's reference to out-of-body experiences, both while she was being raped and while she was making love to her husband. These descriptions fit logically with the manner in which she described other experiences, with little emotion and as though they had happened to someone else. It was considered that such aspects of Jane's worldview, language, and experience would be used to cocreate a hopeful solution and story line for the future.

One last bit of information would ultimately become the largest piece of the metaphorical puzzle: the riddle Jane had dangled in an earlier session when she said, "My magic is now worked in the form of a best friend, but I will tell you about him later."

Madanes has noted that "Metaphorical communication is central to therapy. If we did not express ourselves metaphorically, people would state their problems clearly and therapists would have no difficulty in understanding them" (1990, p. 18). In light of this, I decided to fish for information that could be important but that Jane had not yet elaborated upon. This could be a key to open the door to Jane's life as she envisioned it, free of cutting, with a happy marriage and bright future.

Reflecting back on Jane's words, I began to wonder if cutting was what she described as her best friend. I tested this hunch by mirroring back to Jane how she had described cutting in earlier conversations in which she had said, "Cutting allows me to release pain. It doesn't cause me pain as some would assume. I call it a way of life, strangely comforting. Maybe if cutting hurt I would stop."

"Please correct me if I am wrong," I began, "but I'd like to ask you more about your best friend. He brings you comfort, understands you, has never hurt you or caused you pain, and he is always there for you—no matter what time of day or night it is—no matter why you need him. Cutting is your best friend, is he not?"

Earlier, Jane had referred to her "best friend" in the masculine gender. In keeping with her language, I intentionally personified cutting to externalize the problem, as she had been doing. I invited her to correct me if I was wrong, first, to be respectful of Jane's expert position on herself, and, second, to indicate that further progress depended on her as much as it did on the therapist.

Using self-disclosure to make Jane more at ease, I mentioned that my best friend was my husband. Jane gazed at the floor with tears in her eyes and was silent. I, too, remained silent, although the turning point in our therapy was palpable. Jane raised her head and whispered almost inaudibly, "I want Michael to be able to fulfill me, not cutting. I want to be able to turn to him instead of a knife or razor blade. I just can't."

FACILITATING A CHANGE OF BEST FRIEND

If Jane accepted the metaphor of cutting as her best friend, she could continue the conversation in a way that would surely bring about change. Metaphor allows for discussion without having *the* discussion and for comparison without mentioning *the* comparison. At a literal level our conversation focused on cutting, while by implication it addressed Jane's present and future relationship with Michael—albeit indirectly, as a *topic of Jane's thoughts.*

Jane was self-driven and did not like anyone leading her in a direction that required her to be a follower. Once I understood the benefits of Jane's having cutting as her best friend, I was able to discuss the benefits of *not* having cutting as her best friend and of Michael stepping into cutting's shoes (Jackson, 1967).

Listening attentively to clients—their language, metaphors, presuppositions, tone, and pacing—provides many essential tools for effective therapy. Once cutting was understood not as pathology but rather as Jane's best friend, Jane's ability to discuss it offered a pivotal moment in therapy. Toward the end of the session in which Jane first showed the scars and cuts, she provided a clue as to how to speak freely of her relationship with cutting. She did not want expressions of sympathy that did more to reassure others than to help her, nor did she need the therapist to act as if the truth was too unbearable to hear. Cutting and scars were part of Jane's intimate world, a very important part.

It is our belief that metaphors work most effectively when cocreated by the client and therapist, rather than being imposed from the therapist's ideas and ideals. The metaphorical designation of cutting as Jane's best friend was a primary therapeutic tool that allowed the conversation to deepen, and allowed us to discuss her problems in a way that did not address Jane and the "problem" as being one and the same. Indeed, according to Gale and Long (1996), "From a postmodern perspective, human experience can only be expressed (and understood) metaphorically" (p. 15).

"What would you miss about cutting if he was ever to abandon you?" I asked.

"I would be lost," she replied. "I would have no one to turn to with my most intimate thoughts, and most importantly, I would have no one that truly understands my need to cause myself pain in order to release it. It's like I've found a way that allows all of that anger inside of me to be released. I watch it being released and it feels good . . . like nothing else, in fact."

"What else does cutting do for you that no one else can?" I pursued.

After thinking for a moment, Jane replied, "He allows me to be in control of my own emotions, actions, and outcomes. He understands that sometimes I need to be down on myself, and that that is easier than being happy all the time. I can't be happy all the time, and he allows me to be sad. It's okay to be sad around him. It's not acceptable around others, who keep telling me to cheer up, whereas he is perfectly okay with me being down in the dumps. He likes it that way, even."

Dialoguing with Questions

As our dialogue continued I asked Jane a series of questions: "What about you does cutting understand that no one else does? What is going on when you choose to invite cutting into your life rather than anyone else? When are you most likely to invite cutting to visit you? Do you always invite cutting to spend time with you, or does he at times invite you to spend time with him?"

She responded, "He understands my need to be alone . . . no one else understands that about me. When I want to be alone, or don't want to be with my family, they assume something is wrong and try to get me to be sociable. I wish they wouldn't do that. Cutting does not care if I want to be alone. He prefers it that way—in fact, he insists upon it, and I like that. I like being alone. That way I don't have to be in conversation with anyone, make small talk, or pretend that everything is all right. I hate doing that. They don't want to hear what's wrong anyway, so why ask?"

"How could you and cutting get any closer than you are now?" I inquired.

"If Michael and I were to divorce, I would certainly rely on cutting even more than I do now. There are times when Michael intercepts my relationship with cutting. Those times have been very emotional for me and Michael. He has caught me in the bathroom with cutting before, and he has to force his way in, and he just crumbles and holds me and we cry. That has happened more than once."

This was helpful information. An exception emerged to the hold that cutting had on Jane: Michael did, indeed, prevail at times. In retrospect, this was the point at which the line of inquiry should have changed in order to allow Jane to verbalize the advantages of having Michael become her best friend, but the opportunity temporarily slipped by, as it sometimes does in therapy.

Instead, the focus remained on Jane's closeness to cutting. The intention was to have Jane's anger connect with how cutting was affecting her marriage in ways similar to a relationship with another man. I asked Jane, "How could you and cutting get closer than you are now? What would change if that added closeness occurred? How do you feel after cutting has visited you?"

She responded irritably, "I want to get all the anger out, but no one else wants to hear it. When I've had it with everyone around me and I just want to be mad, for the time being he makes it all all right."

Jane's earlier comment "I want Michael to be able to fulfill in me everything that cutting does and to be able to turn to him instead of a knife or razor" provided the context for inviting her to think about how her life would be different if Michael were to fulfill these needs.

Jane continued, "That's one thing that disturbs me. It's as though he [cutting] wins over Michael every time. Michael desperately wants to be there for me, but I push him away. It's almost like Michael is jealous of cutting as though he were another man. It's really not good for my marriage."

I pressed her to consider the preferred outcome of Michael being the one who fulfilled her needs rather than cutting, underscoring the relational ramifications of depending on cutting.

In a hostile voice, Jane responded: "That absolutely cannot occur. It has just dawned on me that if I were to get closer to him, my husband and family would just give up on me. They can't cope now—never mind if it gets worse. You've made this guy out as having complete control over me. It's not like that; no one has that amount of control over me. I'm stronger than cutting, and if you want me to declare war with him, I'll win. If you don't believe me, just watch."

Inquiry turned from the advantages of being close to cutting to the advantages of Jane's being closer to Michael. My questions invited her to express some downsides to having cutting as her best friend, to make space for life without cutting, and to replace cutting as her best friend with Michael. She was encouraged to show anger toward me for daring to suggest she was not as powerful or in control as cutting.

"Who would be your best friend if cutting were to ever abandon you, even temporarily?" I asked.

"I don't know what you are implying," Jane replied, "but I already told you he is not stronger than me. If there is any abandoning to be done, it will be me abandoning him, not the other way around."

Developing a Game Plan

It is our belief that this line of dialogue was successful with Jane largely because of the solid therapeutic alliance built with her. This challenge aimed at utilizing the client's position in order to effect change. On more than one occasion, she had said she did not take kindly to anyone's implying that she could not do something. Deliberately inciting clients in such an openly provocative way may not always be the wisest road to travel, yet Jane's response indicated that the goals of therapy had, for the most part, been accomplished. What remained was to assist her to develop a game plan for reducing time spent with cutting and instead turning to Michael for support.

"What would you gain if you were to abandon cutting, even temporarily?" I asked her.

"I would gain a closer relationship with Michael. That would make him very happy, and if I had a happier marriage I'd try harder to please him in the bedroom," Jane said.

"Would you gain closer relationships with anyone else?"

"Oh yes," said Jane. "My family loves Michael. They hate the way I treat him. He talks to my mother and brother about my problems and our relationship more than I ever would. All they see is I have a loving husband that wants to meet my every need, and they despise the fact that I push him aside. Of course, they love me and are afraid. They think cutting is extremely dangerous, and I understand that."

To suggest how Jane could begin replacing cutting with those around her who truly cared about her welfare, I asked, "Who else has some of the characteristics that you trust in cutting?"

"Whenever I give them the chance, they listen . . . especially Michael." She continued, sobbing, "I just hate that I don't give him that chance very often."

To elicit elaboration, I asked Jane, "When do you choose to turn to anyone other than cutting to ease your pain?"

"When I'm feeling loving and when I am not depressed," she responded.

"So cutting and depression collaborate with each other? Is that a way cutting lets you down, Jane, by encouraging depression to visit you?" I wondered.

"That's one way. But there are so many . . . when he comes around I'm more depressed, I'm more angry, my relationships with others are shit, and I end up feeling totally bad about myself. I don't even feel pretty or sexy. How can you feel pretty or sexy when you have to wear huge clothes to cover the scars? I can't wear sexy clothes, a bikini, or shorts . . . and I don't feel sexy. That's probably why I can't have a satisfying sexual relationship with Michael. I just don't feel sexy. He deserves more than that." Jane sobbed uncontrollably.

"Is that how cutting has you feeling about yourself, Jane . . . not sexy, not pretty, not worthy of Michael?"

"Yes," she replied, with her head down. Despite her feelings, though, she was a beautiful young woman, both inside and out. Michael and her family members obviously thought so, too.

Lax (1992) has commented that "In therapy, new narratives/perspectives can arise through the interplay of the client's metaphors and phrasings with those of the therapist. Thus, the therapist can attend to what is not said by the clients and offer a different view back to them as a reflection" (p. 72). The therapeutic conversation with Jane became a combination of shared metaphors, phrasings, and thoughts. She was encouraged to make verbal the nonverbal, which allowed different meanings to emerge.

"Michael thinks I'm beautiful, even with my scars . . . and he hates that I wear all these dowdy clothes," Jane said. "He wants me to show how sexy I am and to be proud of it. And I will. Just wait and see what I look like next session."

Applying the Metaphoric Outcome

At the next session, Jane looked great. Vibrant in colorful, body-hugging clothes, she had brought Michael with her. She announced that she had decided to wage war against cutting, saying he was only a friend on the surface and that she had successfully replaced him with her husband. Once Michael claimed his rightful place, and Jane allowed him to claim it, the rest of Jane's problems dissipated. Jane and Michael described their love life as bringing "a new meaning of what pleasurable sex is." Jane continued, "I will not be watching myself having sex with Michael any more. It is too much fun to miss out on." Her depression subsided; she became more involved in her college classes, stopped confining herself to her apartment, and renewed meaningful relationships with both of her parents and her brother. She revitalized her involvement with writing, another source of pleasure and pride.

Roth and Epston (1996) have noted that "Seeing oneself as in a relationship with a problem (through its objectification or personification), rather than as having a problem or being a problem, immediately opens possibilities for renegotiating that relationship" (p. 149). It was just that possibility we hoped Jane would discover for herself. Not only did she do so, but, additionally, she inspired us with her ability to renegotiate it in such a positive and determined manner.

When interviewed at a one-year follow-up session, Jane confirmed this. "Everything goes back to that day I was raped. I lost all self-respect and hope. While he took everything from me that day, he gave me everything back by making me stronger." She described herself as being "extremely happy" with Michael, and announced the joyful news that they were expecting their first child.

At the two-year follow-up, Jane was a proud mother and wife, describing her life as one without pain or regret, full of meaningful relationships that did not include cutting. She had developed a new passion, voluntarily reaching out to others who were compelled to enter into relationships with cutting. She said cutting still existed, was a friend to many, and temporarily visiting and befriending others. "I know he can come back at any time. He's only a friend on the surface, [but] still he is a friend and will be there if I need him again, but at this point I can do without him. I will do all I can to help others do without him, too."

A CLOSING COMMENT

In our work with clients experiencing serious difficulties, such as the self-mutilation that was a temporary part of Jane's life, we have found that the use of metaphor is an effective way of working within clients' frames of reference to find safer ways to handle their relationships and the pain that they feel. Constructing metaphorical relationships to "problems" allows therapists to engage in conversations devoid of problem- or disease-saturated language, and to remove any doubt that the problem is not within the client. Clients are enabled to discover a path to preferred realities in which they are not crazy or pathological, and to find solutions without altering who they are as people. Previously impossible possibilities can now be entered into, discussed, believed, and lived. Clients can leave therapy without their "problem" and with themselves intact. Solutions can be found without our tampering with their being, personalities, characteristics, or whatever else they hold dear (Hoyt, 1996; Ray & Keeney, 1993; White, 1989; White & Epston, 1990).

REFERENCES

Bateson, G., Jackson, D., Haley, J., & Weakland, J. (1956). Toward a theory of schizophrenia. *Behavioral Science, 1*(4), 251–264.

Bateson, G., Jackson, D., Haley, J., & Weakland, J. (1963). A note on the double bind. *Family Process, 2*(1), 154–161.

Cecchin, G., Lane, G., & Ray, W. (1994). *The cybernetics of prejudices in the practice of psychotherapy.* London: Karnac Books.

Fisch, R., Weakland, J., & Segal, L. (1982). *The tactics of change: Doing therapy briefly.* San Francisco: Jossey-Bass.

Gale, J. E., & Long, J. K. (1996). Theoretical foundations of family therapy. In F. P. Piercy, D. H. Sprenkle, & J. L. Wetchler (Eds.), *Family therapy sourcebook* (2nd ed., pp. 1–24). New York: Guilford Press.

Hoyt, M. F. (Ed.). (1996). *Constructive therapies 2*. New York: Guilford Press.

Jackson, D. (1955). Therapist's personality in the treatment of ambulatory schizophrenics. *AMA Archives of Neurology and Psychiatry, 74,* 292–299.

Jackson, D. (1957). The question of family homeostasis. *Psychiatric Quarterly Supplement, 31*(part 1), 79–90.

Jackson, D. (1967). Pain is a prerogative. *Medical Opinion and Review, 3*(11), 110–114.

Jackson, D., & Haley, J. (1957). Untitled (unpublished original audio recording and transcript). Palo Alto, CA: Bateson Research Project.

Lax, W. D. (1992). Postmodern thinking in clinical practice. In S. McNamee & K. J. Gergen (Eds.), *Therapy as social construction* (pp. 69–85). London: Sage.

Madanes, C. (1990). Strategies and metaphors of brief therapy. In J. Zeig & S. Gilligan (Eds.), *Brief therapy: Myths, methods, and metaphors* (pp. 18–35). New York: Brunner/Mazel.

Ray, W., & Crawford, A. (1991). The function of symptoms in institutionalized adolescents. *Louisiana Counseling Journal, 2,* 61–65.

Ray, W., & Keeney, B. (1993). *Resource focused therapy.* London: Karnac Books.

Roth, S., & Epston, D. (1996). Consulting the problem about the problematic relationship: An exercise for experiencing a relationship with an externalized problem. In M. F. Hoyt (Ed.), *Constructive therapies 2* (pp. 148–162). New York: Guilford Press.

Sutton, J., Ray, W., & Cole, C. (2003). The ties that bind: Breaking a relational impasse. *Journal of Brief Therapy, 2*(2), 109–118.

Weakland, J. (1967). Communication and behavior. *American Behavioral Scientist, 10*(8), 1–3.

White, M. (1989). The externalizing of the problem and the reauthoring of lives and relationships. In M. White, *Selected papers* (pp. 5–28). Adelaide, Australia: Dulwich Centre.

White, M., & Epston, D. (1990). *Narrative means to therapeutic ends.* New York: Norton.

CHAPTER 16

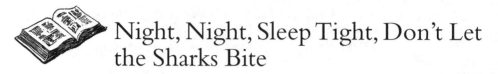

Night, Night, Sleep Tight, Don't Let the Sharks Bite

"What's Missing?" in Metaphors

Robert McNeilly

CONTRIBUTOR'S STORY:
A PROFESSIONAL AND PERSONAL PERSPECTIVE

Robert McNeilly, MBBS, had a medical training and practice in Melbourne, Australia, before becoming interested in counseling and hypnosis to provide patients with more than investigations, referrals, and pills. Drawn to Milton Erickson's therapeutic style, he spent several weeks learning from him over the last years of Erickson's life.

Rob has been associated with a number of professional hypnosis, psychotherapy, and counselor organizations, and is director of the Centre of Effective Therapy and the Milton H. Erickson Institute of Victoria. The author of two books, he is currently releasing a series of DVDs of counseling and hypnosis demonstrations (see Resource Section).

Rob considers himself blessed with seven children from two marriages and three grandchildren. Hiking in the Australian bush and playing the violin sit in the background of his awareness but will have to wait, as his life is increasingly full of the pleasures of teaching, conversing, and learning in Australia and overseas.

PREVIEW THE CHAPTER

In this case Rob describes working in a single, brief hypnosis session with a nine-year-old girl learning to let go of her night terrors. In doing so, he offers a clear example of how a solution-focused approach to the use of therapeutic stories can be delightfully effective. Working to build a collaborative metaphor, he emphasizes that, because the source of the story and the steps toward outcome came from the client, she was capable of easily owning the benefits provided in the metaphor. At the core of Rob's work is the question "What is missing?" An understanding of what the client needs to resolve the presenting problem can bypass lengthy history taking and problem analysis, more effectively targeting the metaphoric interventions toward the client's desired goal. The conversation presented here took place in a light and playful mood, adding to the likelihood of the learning becoming permanent for the client, as well as adding to the professional and personal satisfaction of the therapist.

Therapeutic Characteristics

Problems Addressed

- Anxiety
- Separation anxiety
- Parent-child relationships
- Limited peer relationships
- Thumb sucking

Resources Developed

- Understanding how to make things happen
- Learning to make choices
- Taking control
- Learning to relax
- Developing playful learning
- Enhancing positive relationships
- Enhancing pleasurable experiences

Outcomes Offered

- Reduced anxiety
- Greater independence
- New friendships
- Freedom from thumb sucking

A participant in a hypnosis diploma brought her nine-year-old niece to see me. Angela was a quiet little girl with a cute smile, and was comfortable enough as she climbed into the chair and we began to talk together for the first time. Her eyes softened, and there was an easy smile as we began to get to know each other a little. She had been waking, screaming, every night for several months, terrified by nightmares of sharks eating her. Awake and scared, she would go into her parents' bedroom and climb into bed with her mother and father. They were concerned about their daughter's obvious distress in spite of their cajoling, reassurance, and even discipline, and were becoming desperate to get some peace and some sleep themselves. This all began after Angela had watched a video of the film *Jaws* several months previously.

I asked Angela, "What can you do just before you go to sleep that would put you in a safe mood?"

"I have been reading Harry Potter during the day," she answered. "Maybe I could read this at night."

When we spoke together about her enjoyment of reading the Harry Potter books, her eyes lit up, her face relaxed, her whole body became still, and she smiled. I took this as an indication that we were on the right track for her. We were talking about her and what was enjoyable for her. We weren't talking about some boring adult stuff having to do with problems and how she should be. Her mood was very different from the mood when her aunt was telling me about the nightmares and the film that had frightened her.

We were speaking together, sharing conversation, and starting to enjoy our interaction. Here I want to emphasize the importance of her being the source of the content of the conversation. It was her book, her enjoyment, and her choice, entirely. I was imposing nothing. In addition, because she had chosen this topic related to my question about safety, there was already a mood of safety created as we spoke together. The missing resource—for her, safety—began to emerge in the room, in our conversation, and in particular, in *her* experience.

A PERSONAL INITIATION INTO STORYTELLING

My introduction to using stories in therapy began with my first visit to Milton Erickson in 1977. I was still in general medical practice, had been using traditional hypnosis for five years or so, and was increasingly enthusiastic about the way hypnosis could help people. I was initially paralyzed with fear when I approached Erickson, having sat at the feet of "the master," feeling in awe of his perceptiveness, his flexibility, the wisdom he had distilled from 50 years of intense personal and professional learning. How could I ever do what he was doing? How could anyone match his simple and effective grasp of a seemingly impossibly complex situation? And then there was his ability to tell stories, from an endless collection and with a multitude of subtle variations. I retreated into my previous habit of reading scripts to clients after "putting them into hypnosis."

In that first visit with Erickson, on the very first day he asked me what I wanted to learn. I said that I didn't understand how hypnosis could be used for pain management. He had me sit on an uncomfortable stool, assisted me in going into my own experience of trance, and told me a series of stories. I can still recall some of them. The mood and the point of them have stayed with me for nearly 30 years.

After more than three hours in an increasingly painful position, I had the opportunity to experience my own ways of dealing with pain. Coming out of hypnosis, I asked Erickson for some explanation of what I had just been through. He distilled the experience of the three-hour session into a single sentence: What we experience depends on how we direct our attention. If I'd only heard that short version, my experience would have been very different. The stories he told me added texture, substance, context, and meaning to the ideas I was learning. They allowed the ideas that he was offering me to sink in, to make their own complex connections that were both individual and personal. As a result, they remain personally memorable to this day.

Erickson always encouraged people to be who they were as clients, as therapists, and as people. He was offended if anyone tried to ape him, his words, his phrases, his accent, and would even wryly insist that it was no use anyone trying to copy him, because they couldn't even if they wanted to. The twinkle in his eye as he spoke these words dissolved any suspicions of arrogance and left the listener feeling challenged yet encouraged.

Even with this assurance, I was still feeling only slightly hopeful that I might be able to find some capacity to tell stories that were useful. Stories were not part of my childhood. I read very little. Looking back, I recognize now that I thought there were two kinds of therapists: those who could tell stories, and those who could not. I had myself pigeonholed in the group that could not. When I read books about therapeutic metaphor, I was further overwhelmed by my relative incompetence compared with the skills of the authors. I moved between hoping and feeling hopeless about the process.

CREATING EXPECTANCY IN THE CLIENT

I mention my introduction into therapeutic stories because it was a formative factor in the style in which I now work with cases such as that of Angela. When Angela self-initiated the idea of reading Harry Potter at the time of going to bed, I asked, "Can we play a game of pretend?" She agreed with enthusiasm, closing her eyes so she could pretend even better. I then suggested, "Imagine that you are Harry Potter's sister. Since he is a wizard, you could also be a wizard, not a muggle." She was very interested to go along with this game, and became increasingly absorbed in her experience.

I offered Angela another idea. "As a wizard, you can cast spells." Then I asked her, "What kind of spell do you think you can create that would be helpful to protect you from the sharks?" I emphasized that I didn't know what would be the best way, the best spell, or how she might do this. "You could enjoy discovering how you might enjoy playing with this experience," I added.

Her joyful engagement showed on her face, as she became increasingly absorbed in her experience. She was amazingly still for a nine-year-old, seemingly oblivious to both me and her surroundings as she wove her magic—and it was her magic that she was weaving!

By asking clients to create their own experience, you ensure that the experience they create will be theirs. Asking, as compared to telling, is likely to connect clients with their own search and generate their own unique associations that will fit them individually.

WHERE CAN WE LOOK FOR A METAPHOR?

Several years ago I was teaching a hypnosis diploma and found myself totally devoid of stories to tell when I was demonstrating how to include them in a hypnotic session. Being blank is trouble enough at any time, but being the teacher, and being expected to have some abilities in the area that I was teaching, compounded the embarrassment even further. In the absence of any magical, inspirational, imaginative ideas, I found myself stuck. And is this not a position in which our clients often find themselves? So I chose to tell a story from the position of my current experience, a story about someone I knew who found himself speechless when he had to speak. He felt embarrassed, smiled humbly to himself, took a breath, and found that a few words came to him, then a few more, and then a flood. As I spoke these words, an idea for a story came to mind, then another, and then a flood. The day was saved, and my reputation as a teacher remained intact. In fact, the participants seemed to enjoy hearing of my crisis, identified with the experience, and learned something about how they might deal with a similar situation while working with a client.

I began to realize that stories were useful therapeutically if they met criteria relating to the client's needs and experiences. Knowing this, I could then begin to explore with clients the question "What's missing?" For me, this question above all others clarifies what might be a useful theme for a story. If clients are anxious, and what is missing for them is a trust in themselves, it seems obvious to look for a story that communicates something about learning to move from anxiety to self-trust. If what is missing for someone who is depressed is a purpose for continuing to live, then a story about finding purpose will obviously be relevant.

There are many sources of potentially helpful therapeutic metaphors. Therapists may look for stories in classical mythology, literature, television shows, or films. One source I particularly enjoy exploring is within the client. Asking clients what they like to do, what they enjoy, or what is fun for them predictably results in a cluster of stories around these activities. Because these activities are enjoyable, they have a personal relevance for each individual client, and they are activities with which the client has dealt without any conflict. By engaging in pleasurable activities, we build the skills, resources, and coping strategies that are integral to that experience.

If someone likes fishing, for example, what he might like is getting away from the pressures of everyday life, spending time by himself, being in nature, or enjoying a time of tranquility. Knowing this can add to the stories we could create around his favored topic of fishing. If someone likes walking through the woods, and what she enjoys most is the feeling of freedom, then freedom could emerge as an emotion to add interest or relevance to stories about hiking in nature. These stories would make sense to the clients, since they were already an important part of their lives and an individual expression of the individual human being that each of us is.

Asking a client "What's wrong?" will lead us on a search for causes and pathological explanations of why the person has the problem, whereas asking "What's missing?" leads the client in a different direction. It is a question that has a solution orientation. This solution-oriented approach emphasizes strengths and abilities to be recalled, reconnected with, or learned. Finding an individual client's resources and reconnecting the client to these resources is a pivotal component of any solution approach. The solution approach assumes that we don't have a problem because of a pathological defect caused by some past trauma, but rather considers problems the result of a disconnection from some preexisting resource. The process of any solution approach is that of reconnecting (McNeilly, 1994, 2000, in press; O'Hanlon & Weiner-Davis, 1989).

In a personal conversation, Michael Yapko told me that he was concerned that, all too often, stories were left on the doorstep of a client's experience, like an abandoned baby, with the hope that someone would take them in. Tailoring the therapy to each individual client is one of Erickson's multitudinous contributions to our learning, and it follows that tailoring therapeutic stories to the individual client will result in the story being taken in, connected with, owned, and used in a way that enhances learning.

ACCESSING AN INDIVIDUAL CLIENT'S UNIQUE RESOURCES

As Angela played with the image of being Harry Potter's sister and creating spells that could protect her from sharks, a wide smile spread over her face. She proudly informed me, "I have surrounded myself with a white light!" She looked totally confident, totally certain, and totally definite that this was a genuine experience that was happening for her.

When I expressed my doubt, asking "How might that help?" she was emphatic in stating that the white light would protect her. Her certainty was impressive. To prove it to me, she brought the sharks into the game, and grinned even more widely with even more obvious satisfaction and authentic self-confidence. Then she told me, somewhat condescendingly, "The sharks are trying to get at me through the white light, but they can't because it is a protective spell. They are getting frustrated and bored because they can't bite through the white light. Now they are going away." Her mood of being in charge of her own experience, rather than feeling controlled by the fear of sharks, was palpable.

It was such a pleasure for me to see her smile. What better validation can there be of a client making a connection or really "getting it"? Such physical ideomotor responses confirm that the learning is in the client's emotions and body, not just an intellectual understanding. It was Angela who created the white light, not me. I would never have thought of doing this, but it was obvious to her, and plainly satisfying for her.

There are times in therapy when, rather than being too encouraging, I like to play the doubting Thomas. This throws the responsibility on the clients to convince me of the effectiveness of their solution, and in convincing me they add to their own conviction that the solution is real for them. When I asked Angela "How might that help?" she spontaneously had the idea of testing the light by bringing the sharks into the picture. Her willingness to do this was already evidence that an important change had taken place. The images of sharks had so recently been terrifying. Now she was displaying an obvious omnipotence by consciously and voluntarily choosing to bring sharks into her own imagery. For me—and, more important, for her—there could be no more substantial evidence of her reclaimed control.

When she reported that the sharks were going away, it was a "ho-hum" kind of comment, as if she found it almost a boring thing to say. It was like a full stop marking the end of a sentence—a full stop to mark the end of her problem.

"WHAT'S MISSING?" IN THERAPY

A Sufi story tells of the Mulla, Nasrudin, who is down on his hands and knees looking for his house key under the light from a streetlamp. His long-suffering neighbor comes to his aid, but after some time neither of them has found the key. The neighbor asks if Nasrudin is sure he dropped the key here. Nasrudin replies that he didn't drop the key here, under the light, but over there, in the dark. When the surprised neighbor asks, "Then why are we searching here?" Nasrudin explains, "Because the light is better here."

During my medical training and my career as a family doctor, I learned the importance of asking about what's wrong when a patient came with a problem. This led to the gathering of information, making a diagnosis, and developing a treatment plan that could be applied and monitored. This approach continues to be the backbone of medical practice and has become a methodology in many therapeutic approaches.

From Milton Erickson, I began to learn another approach. Among his many contributions was the invitation to explore not what was wrong but what *does* work in a client's life. On the basis of this the therapist can help clients do more of what is effective, rather than focusing on the defects that have not worked. Like Nasrudin, many clients have been looking for a result without success simply because they are looking in the wrong place. A question that can open exploration in a different direction is "What's missing?" When we ask this question, a client has an opportunity to look for where the key to the solution really is.

Questions of "What's missing?" can take many forms: "What is something that, if you had access to it, would enable you to feel okay?" "If you could have anything you wanted, what would you have so that you would be okay?" "If you were at a supermarket, and the shelves had things you might find useful, what would you choose so that the problem wouldn't be there?" "If you could make a wish, and wish for anything that would be helpful, what would that be?"

Just asking such questions can be a delightful beginning to an exploration of experiences that a client has not explored for some time. When we have a problem, our vision can become so blinkered that we see nothing but the problem. The question about what is missing brings a mood of curiosity, wonder, and possibility as opposed to the mood of resignation, resentment, and hopelessness that often accompanies problem exploration. This change of mood is therapeutically useful even before the answer to the question becomes apparent.

The missing experience may be a feeling of confidence, a way of managing, a sense of future, calmness, quietness, sleeping better, or any number of thoughts, emotions, and behaviors. Having defined what resource we are looking for, we have a better likelihood of finding it. My Irish ancestors remind me that if we don't know where we are going, we might end up in a different place! When we do know where we're going, we can often find the missing resource in abundance within the client's pleasurable activities. Creating stories within this context is where the everyday magic of therapy can happen.

The conversation that Angela and I shared was very much that—a conversation. When I reflect on how the conversation unfolded, I note that I did not ask specifically what was missing for her, but in asking what would be more helpful for her before she went to sleep, I enabled her to identify for herself that the missing resource was in the magic of the book. This did not need to be made explicit, but rather was fostered in her as a result of my questioning and our conversation. The fact that she had been able to create the nightmare alerted me to her skill at imagining in a creative way, so I knew that if she could imagine sharks and have a real problem, then she would be able to imagine something else and create a real solution, which she did with elegance. The dialogue was a conversation where I asked questions to add detail and texture to the experience of her created solution. Our conversation connected her with her magical abilities—powerful, yet everyday magic.

BRINGING THE LEARNING TO LIFE

After Angela had described how the sharks were going away, she spontaneously opened her eyes. I took this as her message to me that she was finished with the process, and that she was absolutely definite she would now be okay. I also took this as evidence that she was now back in charge of her experience. She did not need to wait for me to instruct her or guide her.

Wanting to help her build effective discriminatory skills and ensure her safety in regard to sharks, I spoke with her about the unlikely event that she might encounter one while swimming in the sea. "If a real shark were to appear," I began, "you would get out of the water, and not waste time surrounding yourself with a white light?"

"I know that!" she told me disdainfully.

She had opened her eyes without any cue from me, contributing even further to her own autonomy. She had done what she needed to do, in her own way, in her own time, with me as a gently guiding onlooker. Then, when she was satisfied, she let me know of her satisfaction by opening her eyes. She demonstrated again that therapy is an experience that happens for the client within his or her own experience, and all we can do is do our best to influence the experience in a way that is helpful to each individual client.

Her obvious disdain in helping me with my concern about real sharks further added to her own dignity and strength, as well as placing her previous fear in a realm different from reality. Our conversation only lasted about 20 minutes.

REFLECTIONS AFTER THE SESSION

It's always a pleasure to know that we have been able to assist someone. I particularly like assisting children. Helping them to deal with the particular problem that they bring creates the possibility that this learning can generalize and become a future source of learning to deal with other problems, or even prevent them. This applies to adults as well, but seems more obvious to me in working with children.

Children are so delightful in part because they have not yet learned how they "should" behave, think, or respond. They are more ready to play and learn while having fun. We adults have learned, as part of our socialization, what is expected of us. As therapists we can discover a lot from working with children about how to assist adults to play more, have more fun, be more creative in using their imagination, and build flexibility—all so helpful for any learning process, including learning how to let go of a problem and connect with resources that will allow a solution to be created or discovered.

Because the metaphor in this case came from the client, she could relate to it, be in it, and connect with it, far more easily than if I had offered her a metaphor from my experience. Any story from me would have required her to translate my words into her meanings, my hopes and wishes into hers—an additional effort for her when she was already struggling with her problem.

Any time we have a problem, we feel overwhelmed, a lesser person, and small in relation to the huge problem. By allowing clients to create their own metaphors, from within their own areas of strength, we can help them reconnect with these resources. This, in turn, may help them feel more aware of who they are, feel larger or stronger in relation to the problem, and be better able to begin the process of change. From this strengthened position it may be easier for them to overcome a problem that previously seemed so massive.

CONCLUSION AND INVITATION

Over six months later, Angela's aunt reported that, after that one 20-minute conversation, Angela had not had a single problem with waking during the night. She had climbed into her parents' bed on only one occasion, for an unrelated reason. Gone were the nightmares and insomnia. Gone were the sharks.

Working with clients by using metaphors from within their own areas of strength and enjoyable activities adds to the effectiveness of the therapy by restoring each client's own individual autonomy, individual possibilities, and unique dignity. It also relieves therapists of the need to pretend that they are the source of wisdom and change.

Next time you are working with a client, of whatever age, I invite you to consider the following steps. First, ask the client what he or she likes. Second, collaboratively explore what is missing from that person's problem experience. Third, ask the client to tell you a story, or create one together, where the missing resource is found in the client's area of likes. Finally, be willing to be surprised, delighted, and intrigued by how a client, faced with some problem, can create his or her own individual solution—if we simply give them the opportunity.

REFERENCES

McNeilly, R. B. (1994). *Healing with words.* Melbourne, Australia: Hill of Content.

McNeilly, R. B. (2000). *Healing the whole person: A solution-focused approach to using empowering language, emotions, and actions in therapy.* New York: Wiley.

McNeilly, R. B. (in press). *Learning solutions in counseling and hypnosis: A series of DVD demonstrations.* Carmarthen, UK: Crown House.

O'Hanlon, W. H., & Weiner-Davis, M. (1989). *In search of solutions: A new direction in psychotherapy.* New York: Norton.

CHAPTER 17

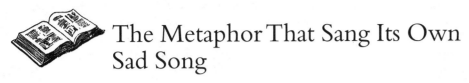

The Metaphor That Sang Its Own Sad Song

Therapeutic Storytelling in Pediatric Hospice Care

Roxanna Erickson Klein

CONTRIBUTOR'S STORY:
A PROFESSIONAL AND PERSONAL PERSPECTIVE

Roxanna Erickson Klein, PhD, has master's degrees in both nursing and urban affairs and a doctorate in public administration. Being the seventh child of the eight raised by Milton and Elizabeth Erickson, Roxanna found that storytelling, metaphors, and creative use of resources were an integral part of her upbringing, as her father, Milton H. Erickson, MD, is, of course, well known for his innovative techniques in psychotherapy, including the use of metaphors.

Roxanna has lived in Dallas, Texas, for the past 27 years. For seven years, she worked for a nonprofit hospice organization whose mission was to orchestrate home care for terminal patients. Currently she is dedicated to advancing the archives of the Milton H. Erickson Foundation, a non-profit organization preserving the professional work of her father and advancing education for health professionals. She is a published writer (see Resource Section) and was coeditor of the Neuroscience Editions of 11 books her father wrote with Ernest Rossi.

PREVIEW THE CHAPTER

This heartfelt story by Roxanna shows us the applicability of several types of metaphor in the context of home care nursing with a courageous young girl facing the prospect of death. Roxanna begins her work by asking the client's family to tell their stories, thus eliciting client-generated metaphors that enable them to explain their own understandings and perceptions of their current difficult circumstances.

A second style of metaphor is the use of children's storybooks to present therapist-generated metaphors that parallel the child's problem and demonstrate potential means for coping.

Third, using an experiential metaphor, Roxanna presents us with the challenge of what happens when the therapeutic intent of an intervention goes awry, with potentially untherapeutic consequences. What do you do when you give a dying child a pet bird to cheer it up only to find that the bird is dying, too? Among the many things this case clearly highlights is the value of listening carefully to clients, no matter how young, for the potential solutions they hold within themselves.

Therapeutic Characteristics

Problems Addressed

- Significant illness
- The prospect of death
- Lack of open discussion
- Lack of helpful coping skills

Resources Developed

- Building strength within weakness
- Increasing empowerment
- Learning to face reality
- Learning to plan for the inevitable
- Learning from the wisdom of a child
- Being prepared

Outcomes Offered

- Acceptance of the inevitable
- Openness of communication
- Strength
- Helpful coping skills

THE HOMECOMING

Violeta looked tiny and frightened as she peered out of the back of the ambulance that blocked the street in front of her home. Her Spanish-speaking parents had waited a very long time for this moment, which they described as "the joy of bringing their daughter home." Hearing their words struck me with a sad irony, as I wondered if the parents had any idea what "hospice services" implied, or whether they were aware that their eight-year-old daughter was only expected to survive "days to weeks."

After a long absence from clinical nursing, I had joined an agency that provided home visits to terminal patients. Hospice care addresses the palliative needs of those who are facing serious illness from which recovery is not anticipated, and thus it involves a broad range of interdisciplinary support. It attends to fundamental matters of food, shelter, and transportation. In addition, hospice arranges for medical equipment, medications, and supplies and offers a variety of emotional support services for all family members as well as a 24-hour phone service safety net, which provides on-the-spot guidance from a nurse. The goals of hospice care include healing rather than curing, facilitating family involvement, and, most important, capturing as much as possible of life's pleasures. The hospice stay is a short and delicate interval in life when stress is very high, and only one opportunity arises to make choices that remain in survivors' memories forever.

Once the hospital bed was assembled and the oxygen and other supplies set up, Violeta was welcomed with a new fluffy pink blanket. The aroma of cooking beans wafted through the modest home as the hospice director and I settled down to explain the procedures and complete the paperwork, but here problems arose. No one in the family spoke English. They had no friends or local relatives, they had not yet joined a church, they did not know their neighbors, and none of the father's coworkers spoke English. At that time I was the only person in the agency who spoke Spanish; thus my role was transformed from that of a supportive observer to a key player in the care of Violeta—she became my first case on the new job. The combination of the family's pleasure at having Violeta home and my own self-satisfaction with the role led to a good-natured, friendly, even happy exchange of information.

Violeta's parents arranged the chairs in a semicircle at the bedside. They explained that they had made a commitment to include Violeta in all conversations about her—her care, her needs, her illness, or her prognosis. With the challenges of translation and the child listening, it seemed unlikely that the opportunity for an open discussion about terminal care or funeral needs could be approached.

The happy scene of the parents sitting at the bedside and Violeta all tucked in with her fluffy pink blanket was cozy, but left our hearts aching. As we walked down the street on the way back to our cars, the director made a remark that has echoed in my ears: "We have a lot of work to do here, and not very much time to do it in."

Violeta overcame the odds. Even though she remained seriously ill and at risk for precipitous demise for her two years in hospice, she did well in the bosom of her family. Her extended survival was not a matter of misdiagnosis, but rather an expression of the healing power of comfort and love.

TELLING THEIR OWN STORIES

Over the first few visits I encouraged the family to tell me their stories. This is my way of learning about the dynamics, the hardships, the joys, the sorrows, and the strengths that sustain them. Not only does this ensure that I have all of the information that the family wishes to share, but many times families have told me that I am the only medical person who has listened to their whole story.

Violeta's mother, Pureza, and father, Eternidad, had been blessed with four children, including two teenage boys and Violeta's 10-year-old sister, Lucy. Their tale focused on three and a half years of a desperate search for treatment for the youngest child. Tearfully, Pureza touched the corner of her apron to her nose as she described the small town in Mexico where they had once lived contentedly, just across the field from her elderly parents. Violeta had been a healthy and energetic child, happy and always close by. She liked to play in a gully behind the house, and she waited eagerly each day for her siblings to return from school and for her father to come home from his work as a butcher. When Violeta unexpectedly became ill, the serene scene changed into an ordeal of consulting one physician after another.

As her parents related this disturbing story, Violeta wiped her own eyes and blew her nose several times using a wad of tissue from the roll of toilet paper kept on her bed. The awkward gesture required the removal of her oxygen face mask and glasses. It required both her attention and ours to get it all put back together.

In their aggressive, desperate, and mostly futile search for help, the family gave up their home and livelihood, left behind their family and community, took their children away from school and friends, and embarked on a journey that culminated with illegal migration into the United States. They explained that they knew that if help was available, it was here.

THE ILLNESS

Violeta's primary diagnosis was a devastating course of hepatitis with severe lung involvement. She required such high levels of oxygen that she could not be without it for more than five minutes. Additionally, she had experienced an episode of bleeding from veins in her esophagus, a serious complication that is hard to treat and has a high probability of recurrence resulting in death. She had spent many months at the Children's Medical Center, where she was found not to be a candidate for transplant surgery.

In response to my inquiry, the parents accurately related the prognosis doctors had given: Nothing more could be done for Violeta, and she was not expected to survive for more than a week. I asked whether the parents understood or disagreed with the distressing diagnosis Violeta had been given. Carefully, and with a measured harmony, they explained that they realized now that nothing could be done *in* the hospital, but they remained hopeful that God might perform a miracle.

Violeta appeared younger than her age of eight years, and was considered to be fragile but stable from a medical perspective, with a necessary but unpalatable handful of twice-a-day medications. She was gaunt, unable to stand without assistance, without appetite, and markedly jaundiced. The health care team knew from experience that over the first few days Violeta would either gradually adapt or rapidly decline. Either way, being at home was a desire that both the client and the family expressed. Everyone involved was hopeful that Violeta would live longer and more comfortably at home than she could have in the hospital.

Years of health care delivery and intensive measures to find a cure inevitably bring with them trauma, especially to a seriously ill young child. That trauma leaves a wake of scarring that is difficult to penetrate and even more difficult to overcome. It is not unusual for children who have spent much of their lives in health care settings to associate health care workers with painful procedures, bad news, and separations from loved ones. Violeta was no exception. Though alert and oriented, she was reluctant to speak to me. She turned away and behaved as if she could not hear or understand me. It took weeks for Violeta to finally look at me, speak to me, and trust that I would not hurt her. Her mother would nudge and prod her, and provide Spanish translation, and Violeta would answer in a whisper so soft that her oxygen mask had to be removed so that Pureza could hear. It was not until I began to bring books, metaphors chosen for her, that I made a difference and helped her to begin to look forward to my visits with eager anticipation.

SETTING GOALS

During the initial assessment I inquired about the goals that each individual in the family held. I believe that it is important to communicate the expectations and desires of the client as well as the individuals involved in caretaking. Eternidad spoke broadly. He wanted to give all of his children an opportunity to live together as a family. His hope was to reclaim some semblance of a normal family life, where he could go to work and provide for his family. Pureza remained fully focused on her daughter and expressed an eagerness to attend to daily care needs. She exuded confidence in her abilities, and explained she would like to help Violeta to grow and gain weight. Lucy looked puzzled, as if she could not imagine that her wishes or desires had anything to do with anything. Violeta turned away, and refused to speak or to express herself. I identified my own goals of supporting their adjustment to needs and changes as they arose. I emphasized my hope that I would earn their respect and trust, and that they would be willing to share their concerns with me.

Happily, Violeta thrived during the first weeks, which stretched into months and finally into two years. The family eased into routines, but it took a long time for Pureza to realize that her efforts to build up Violeta's weight were in vain. For nearly a year Pureza would describe her weight gain strategy for Violeta, and often she would cry when the scales showed a lack of progress. She finally accepted that her tears were not helping and put her tactics aside when I urged her to let Violeta set her own goals. Together the three of us agreed that the scales would not be used as a measure, but rather Violeta's own sense of well-being and comfort. Violeta set very realistic and practical intake goals, and this pleased her mother, as well as making for more comfortable and pleasant interactions throughout the days. From there, Pureza began to focus on making every day the best that it could be. She became a model in appreciating little moments of joy.

RELATING THROUGH STORIES

To build my own relationship with Violeta, I started reading storybooks to her. At that time, her sister Lucy was not yet enrolled in school, and Pureza could not leave the house to go to the library. The two girls often played together, and our social worker already brought art supplies. I wanted to introduce another level of interest into their lives, and I hoped that the mother and sister might discover that literature resources can be comforting and useful. I suspected that their travels were not over, but books can generally be found in any community. In making them aware of that, I hoped to strengthen the resource options for not only the client but her mother and sister too.

I developed a routine of reading a story each visit after completing the physical exam and addressing needed modifications in medications and care. I chose children's books from my own collection, selecting ones with beautiful illustrations and simple stories. With Lucy and Pureza crowding around the bedside, I would put the book in Violeta's lap and read it first in English, then tell the story in Spanish, and finally tuck the book under the covers, giving charge of it to Violeta for the week. Each week I would pick up last week's book and discuss the stories with Violeta. It worked wonderfully. By the end of the week Violeta was able to give me her own versions of stories based on the illustrations. Sometimes the stories matched the text, and other times they were delightfully inventive. Some of the traditional stories were familiar to Pureza, while others were not.

It was my intention to give Violeta control over a small part of her own life. I chose a variety of books: Some had metaphors of their own, some stories had favorable outcomes, and some ended with the loss of beloved characters. It is my own philosophy that the stories that have lived in our culture for many years speak deeply to healing within, in ways that we do not understand. Unquestionably, Violeta enjoyed listening to the trials and tribulations of characters in unfamiliar circumstances; Hansel and Gretel, Goldilocks, the Three Pigs, Rapunzel, and many others captured her fascination and connected her with a history of others who had faced and endured trials. But rather than selecting stories just for their content, I also chose those that had intriguing illustrations. Violeta listened carefully to the stories as I read them, and then developed her own tales as if the written text were only one possibility of what could have been written. She smiled and laughed as she told the stories, clearly making them up as she went along. She could "read" the same book many times and come up with different plots each time, some happy and some sad. The spontaneous creativity with which she did this delighted her mother and was a clear demonstration of the spirit of childhood unfettered by harsh circumstances.

Over the many months that the reading activities went on, other changes came as well. Lucy started school, and Violeta brought up the question of whether she too could attend school. As she was not physically capable of doing so, with the parents' permission I arranged for home schooling. A couple of times a week, a volunteer Spanish-speaking teacher began to visit. The teacher brought her own stories and texts, and, more important, Violeta began to learn the alphabet and to write her own name. For hours at a time she would sit on her bed practicing the letters in the scrawled handwriting of a beginner, brimming with excitement and pleasure.

STRENGTHS WITHIN WEAKNESS

The circumstances that defined Violeta were a tangled mesh: weakness within strength and strength within weakness. What was a barrier for the health care team gave power to the family, and efforts to untangle or enhance the resources could also jeopardize the fabric that nurtured family togetherness.

For instance, the family clung almost proudly to their limitation of speaking only Spanish. It was a barrier that interfered with their ability to access needed resources, including the hospice after-hours phone lines. For a long time, language interfered with Lucy's willingness to attend school. And yet the same cultural resource base enabled them to find a rental home, furnishings, a vehicle, and jobs. Later on it gave them a church and a group of fellow compatriots who were better able to offer emotional support than we were as professionals. However, a sense of social isolation was pervasive and affected all of the family. They had spent years moving from community to community, never staying long enough in any one location to establish friendships. Their extended family was left in Mexico, and they frequently did not even have the means to keep in contact. Eternidad worked long hours, driving himself and his sons to work in the family's only vehicle. Pureza was emotionally if not physically confined to the bedside of her sick daughter. The 16- and 14-year-old brothers worked to provide needed income. Though it was clear that the two sisters treasured each other, Lucy needed to develop a life outside of the home, and Violeta could not. Violeta had spent such a large part of her life in the hospital that she had no young friends other than her siblings, and had only fleeting interactions with other sick children.

At the same time, the family's experiences on their journey together brought with them an unusual unity and harmony. Although they had individual needs, and at times seemed to be eager to break away, the priorities at home were clearly defined and they all seemed to graciously participate in the roles asked of them. Most striking to me was the family agreement to speak of matters that involved Violeta only at her bedside. The implicit respect for her, at such a tender age, was unique, powerful, and remarkable.

PREPARING FOR DEATH

What finally emerged as the most difficult problem was the preparation of both Violeta and her family for her death. As a hospice nurse, I was familiar with the complications of planning a funeral that involves an international border. I also knew that Mexicans have traditions, like sitting with the deceased overnight, that require special arrangements in this country.

Although Violeta had a reprieve, I knew that the probability of her recovery was nil. If her parents chose to ignore this, they would still be forced to plan a funeral. I was aware that such arrangements are much less problematic if dealt with in advance of need. Yet each time I tried to approach the topic, Pureza shushed me, stating that they did not want to think about that possibility. With the child as a participant in the conversation, I felt helpless to advance the discussion further. Week after week, I felt as if I had not fulfilled my responsibility to provide needed education.

A COMPANION WITH A METAPHOR

The social worker was the first to notice that Violeta liked looking at the birds outside the window. When I commented on Violeta's interest to Pureza, she told me about a parrot that Violeta's grandmother had kept. Violeta was thrilled with the conversation and remembered the parrot, too.

This led the social worker to propose a bird as a companion for Violeta. The therapeutic intent was to provide Violeta with companionship, a friendly relationship that was special to her. Additionally, we thought that Violeta would be strengthened in accepting responsibility for caring for a dependent who was smaller and weaker than herself. With agency and parental permission, the social worker and I brought richly illustrated books, magazines, and pamphlets so that Violeta could select a bird. With the pictures littering her fluffy pink blanket, Violeta excitedly asked many questions about the variety of birds on display, finally selecting a yellow parakeet and announcing that she would name it "Tweety." Mother and daughter worked out an agreement about the caretaking of Tweety. Eternidad would bring home newspapers from work, Violeta would keep an eye on the food and water, and Lucy would speak to Tweety in English. Laughter erupted through the household at the prospect of Tweety becoming bilingual.

For the first month Tweety's presence was all we could have hoped for. He learned to sit on Violeta's finger and did so for hours at a time. She related to him fully and said that he loved her too. She read to him from the books that I continued to leave with her. The companionship Tweety provided gave her a window into the joy and value of a relationship outside her immediate family. It gave her the special gift of personal responsibility for another living being who needed care and nurturing. The friendship was her very own yet something wonderful she could share with others. Over the next few weeks, we celebrated the bonding and the many positive elements we saw emerging.

AN UNEXPECTED SONG

Slowly we began to realize, however, that something wasn't quite right about Tweety. He didn't seem to grow, and his energy level seemed insufficient. Despite the loving attention showered on the bird, he became less responsive. In a hospice team conference we discussed the horror and irony of the gift becoming another tragedy for the client and family to endure. Though the bird had been checked by a veterinarian prior to our giving him to Violeta, something was clearly wrong.

Unwilling to take the risk of further demise without discussion, I broached the topic of Tweety's health immediately and directly. I asked Violeta if she had noticed that he looked weak. She had. I asked whether she had thought he might need a doctor's care. She had thought about this, and concluded that the bird should stay with her at home rather than go to a hospital without her. I asked whether she had considered, since we didn't know what was wrong with him, that he might get worse. She replied that she knew he might die.

Pureza sat mute during the conversation. I had carefully respected their sensitivities and not talked about death before, but because of Violeta's responsiveness I continued. "It would be really sad to wake up one morning and to see him lying at the bottom of the cage," I commented to Violeta. When I then asked what would be the best thing she believed could be done for Tweety, Violeta answered, "Let him live here, with me, and I will take care of him. I will give him the best care that I can. And when Jesus calls him, he will go."

I was in awe of her outspoken clarity, and at that moment I knew that I had an opportunity for discussion that might not come again. "What next?" I asked, pausing only momentarily while I went on to explain, "When people die, you have to do something with them. You can bury them, or cremate them and have an urn of ashes." I was relieved that I had finally spoken the words the family needed to hear—even in an indirect, metaphoric manner.

Violeta listened carefully, and asked a number of questions, before she finally admitted that she had already planned to bury him. She pointed to a bush outside the window as the site she had selected. The revelation startled Pureza, who asked incredulously if Violeta had really made those plans or whether she had thought of it just now. Quietly, Violeta reached under the bed and produced a small box. "See," Violeta said, holding up the box that contained a lovely white lace hanky, "I will put him in here." At this, Pureza burst into tears. She sat at the foot of the bed, her face covered with her hands, sobbing.

My question about burial was asked about Tweety, but I was metaphorically addressing the same questions about Violeta. I was certain that Pureza knew, and perhaps Violeta did too. The conversation between Violeta and me was soft, gentle, and frank; we modeled for Pureza that this conversation was healthy, needed, and even comforting. I told Violeta how much I admired her for letting Tweety see what loving care she had waiting for him, in case he needed it. I carried the discussion another step, saying, "You know, you and your family will not live in this house forever. Your family may move, may go back to Mexico. If you bury Tweety here in the backyard, it will be difficult to leave him behind." I offered the possibility of cremating him and taking the ashes to Mexico, to the grandparents' home. It was understood that the family would not return to Mexico while Violeta was alive, so by inquiring about Tweety, I encouraged Violeta to express herself about the problem of leaving a deceased loved one when the family relocates.

After thoughtful consideration, Violeta said, "He lived here, and if he dies here, this is where he should be. His spirit can fly on down to Grandmother's home." Pureza remained awash with tears, but listened attentively to the lucid clarity of Violeta's guidance. I held Violeta's small hand and praised her for thinking ahead and being ready for even the worst of times. I admired her practical, forthright manner, her willingness to talk about hard subjects. I applauded her decision to give him such loving attention, even if love and care could not extend his life.

I appointed Violeta the official "hospice nurse" in charge of Tweety and gave her an eyedropper to offer water to him. I let Violeta record my home phone number in her little address book, telling her it was a special "24/7 on-call" number for sick birds. The family had asked for my home phone number before, but I had respected the agency policy and not given it out. Sometimes it is all right to break the rules.

When I returned the next day to see how Tweety was doing, Pureza told me, with great excitement, that Eternidad had discovered the bird had a small imperfection in its beak, a crossbill, that made it difficult to pick up seeds. He had performed "surgery" with an emery board, and the bird was now picking up seeds again. We celebrated the hope that Tweety might actually recover, but I did not lose the opportunity to express that it is good to be prepared for the worst while hoping for the best.

AN UNINTENTIONAL METAPHOR

The metaphor in this case was not one that was planned or intended, but effective therapeutic work entails responding to the windows of opportunity as they arrive. Hospice tasks include preparation for death, and that job had not been done. Now I knew that Violeta was ready to discuss death, even if her parents were not. Once the words were spoken and the practical issues put forth, it became clear that direct discussion can be comforting and helpful to the bereaved as well as to the dying. By the time we had the discussion, the mother was ready to learn from her daughter.

Integral in this particular case is the child's propensity to tell the story as it came to her; her family admired this strength. Moreover, the family respected what she had to say, and treated her as an equal in serious conversations.

Tweety was expected to bring pleasure, participation, responsibility, and interaction to Violeta's life. He was a tiny helpless creature who depended on her, needed her, and responded to her. Initially he seemed to be an answer to many of her needs. When we realized that Tweety was tiny, undernourished, shy, and like Violeta in more ways than intended, it was still a scenario that seemed acceptable. But when his demeanor became frail, sickly, and withdrawn, he mirrored the weakness of his little owner. Anxiety and worry overtook the pleasure of the intervention. Violeta, wanting him to gain weight, felt her mother's angst. She worried that each time she played with him might be the last.

Through her conversations with Tweety, Violeta showed her mother that involving the dying in needed decisions is desirable, appropriate, and comforting. Violeta had demonstrated that planning for what needs to be done does not jeopardize well-being but rather is an expression of love that can heal both the sick and the grieving. She also understood that sometimes health slips away for reasons that no one can understand.

Under Violeta's tender care, Tweety thrived and became a robust adult bird, with whom she spent over a year of happy companionship. During that time the family moved to a new home. Looking out the window, Violeta saw irises in bloom outside her window and initiated conversation about finding a new plot for Tweety. At this time, I felt that Violeta offered me the opportunity to speak with her about her own burial. Though her remark implied that she expected to outlive Tweety, it also showed her acceptance of the inevitability of death. It is frequently easier to broach these topics when the need is not pressing, to gather information that allays indecision and confusion of how to best honor a loved one. Pureza participated in this conversation, even mentioning that the family might need to move again in the future. Violeta announced it was "all right to go on and leave me in the flowers."

In another delicate conversation with me, Violeta expressed that she would like a lacy white dress for herself. A few weeks later the dress appeared, hung on the wall where Violeta could admire it. Violeta and Pureza told of their efforts to select the right dress for Violeta, which involved arranging for several to be brought to the home for her inspection. The dress, I noted, was several sizes too large, an indication of hope that Violeta would live to achieve that stature. The dress on the wall invited discussion about many happy occasions on which it might be worn. She wore it when the chaplain arranged for her to receive her communion. After that she dressed for her birthday, again when the family moved to a larger home, and once more to celebrate her sister's graduation from middle school. While Pureza was never comfortable speaking of the dress as Violeta's personally selected shroud, she never again resisted occasions to discuss choices to be made in the event of Violeta's death.

Later, seeing signs of Violeta's decline, I sat down with her and her parents one final time. We discussed the difficult topics, practical issues of when and whether to return to the hospital, what final measures of care were desired, and wishes for funeral and burial. With Tweety on her finger, Violeta answered all of the questions herself. She spoke with words and ideas that seemed far beyond her young age, and eternities removed from the shy child who previously would not even look at me.

The family decision to not speak of Violeta outside her presence initially seemed to be a barrier, but it turned out to be the greatest strength. As she neared the end of her life, she was able to provide precise and specific guidance to her family in regard to her needs and preferences. When she finally died, it was at home with her family at the bedside and Tweety close by.

Violeta's strength sustained the family, and her grace and peace affirmed in an elegant manner that illness is not a personal failure; it is something that defies comprehension. Joy did flourish in the most barren of circumstances. The metaphor was a song that needed to be sung and found its own tune—a sad song that was also sweet.

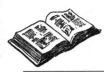

PART FIVE

Developing Life Skills

Chapter 18

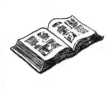

Reclaiming Poise after Persecution

Client-Based Cultural Stories in Trauma Therapy

Angela Ebert and Hasham Al Musawi

CONTRIBUTOR'S STORY:
A PROFESSIONAL AND PERSONAL PERSPECTIVE

Angela Ebert is a psychologist and social worker in private practice and a lecturer at Murdoch University, Perth, Australia. With 20 years' experience as a trauma specialist, she has published papers and presented at international conferences on the topics of refugee trauma, cross-cultural counseling, and recovery. Aware of the limitations of Western psychological approaches with different ethnic groups, she looked at how other cultures provide counsel and guidance, discovering a very simple, gentle, and yet powerful tool: storytelling.

On a personal note, she is happily married and shares with her husband a passion for good food, good company, and walking their two dogs.

Hasham Al Musawi, the client whose case Angela describes, is a refugee from the Middle East who now lives with his wife and three young children in Australia. He holds a bachelor's degree, graduate diploma, and master's degree in information and library studies, and is starting work on his PhD in librarianship. He is an avid reader and a rich source of knowledge about Arabic literature.

PREVIEW THE CHAPTER

Distrust, suspicion, depression, anger, and a loss of the sense of self are just some of the issues encountered by Angela with a traumatized client from a vastly different cultural background. How do you bridge such a potential gulf to establish an effective healing relationship? Angela describes the ways she and Hasham worked together to elicit and employ his cultural stories in the therapeutic process. These tales are interspersed and integrated with approaches to trauma therapy that include behavior modification, mindfulness therapy, interpersonal therapy, and cognitive behavioral therapy. The stories quickly tap into the client's resources and are easily incorporated by the client because they are brief, client generated, culturally relevant, and therapeutically directed. By reflectively collaborating in writing this chapter, therapist and client consolidate their therapeutic journey, and share the tale in the hope of its being helpful to others.

Therapeutic Characteristics

Problems Addressed

- Posttraumatic Stress Disorder
- Major Depressive Disorder
- Anger
- Nightmares
- Suspicion and lack of trust
- Cultural differences

Resources Developed

- Learning to discuss issues openly
- Becoming aware of own behavior patterns
- Changing patterns of behavior
- Staying calm in adversity
- Finding purpose and meaning

Outcomes Offered

- Openness of thoughts
- Forgiveness
- Calmness
- Anger management skills
- Self-trust
- Confidence
- Self-worth

A rich man who was well respected in his village was unhappy with his life and was complaining all the time. The people around him advised him to go and see a wise man who lived in the next village. He listened to their advice and went to see the wise man. When he reached there, he approached the wise man and told him that he was sad and unhappy with his life. The wise man looked at him and said, "Why should you be unhappy? You are rich and knowledgeable. Come with me; I will show you something."

He took the man to a place where people with disabilities lived. The wise man said, "Look at these people; they are happy the way they are. You have so much more than them, you should be happier."

The sad man said, "May God forgive me. I really have everything and I should be happy." From that day on, whenever he felt sad, the man brought the picture of those people to his mind.

Once upon a time, a Muslim man of Arabic background and a Caucasian woman of European background met on a therapeutic journey. That man, Hasham, shared many stories from his cultural background, like the one just relayed. The stories that reflected his experiences and opened options for change were short and pithy, as befitted their cultural origins. They were not as lengthy as some therapist-generated metaphors may be, but nor were they as brief as Japanese koans, Taoist sayings, or some Zen tales. Each contained a clear, pointed message or moral that we could work with in therapy. This chapter outlines how such metaphors can help bridge a cultural divide, establish connections between different worldviews, and promote healing. Despite our differences, stories have the potential to enable us to connect in the basic and essential process of being human.

I will include just a few of the many stories Hasham brought into therapy and describe how some of these were employed to further the therapeutic process of healing the aftereffects of the multiple traumas he suffered from being persecuted in his country of origin. Hasham has generously written this chapter with me, so, rather than seeing the story solely from my perspective, you will find his words and insights woven through it. Through sharing in the writing, we wanted to show you, the reader, the way metaphors sculpted the therapeutic journey from both of our perspectives. We also felt that writing the chapter jointly reflected a key element of the therapeutic process, namely, working in close collaboration toward change and recovery. This collaboration was a reflection of trust rebuilt over time, of sharing our humanity and wisdom of how to be well, and of developing resources.

A LITTLE OF HASHAM'S BACKGROUND

"What do you hope will change through therapy?" I asked Hasham when we first met. Given that hope is a significant factor in building resilience and overcoming trauma, I wanted to direct his attention immediately toward the future, realistically and hopefully (Hubble & Miller, 2004; Snyder, 2000).

"I want to be well again, but how I do not know," he answered, looking away and glancing sideways out of the window. "I am sad," he continued, "and have a lot of anger inside me. Sometimes I feel that I could kill someone without realizing it. I am sad knowing that I lost many years of my life without achieving anything. I had many dreams that I couldn't fulfill yet and time is passing by. On top of this, the language barrier is another challenge for me, as is the Australian culture. I feel lonely most of the time, scared, and depressed."

While Hasham spoke, he continued looking sideways, but I did not call attention to it, aware that for cultural reasons he was not supposed to make eye contact with me as a woman. Little did I know that his behavior in fact meant a lot more. Much later he revealed that he was so worried and so distrusting during our first sessions that he was constantly checking out the room to see where the tape recorder or video camera was hidden. "I was feeling depressed and came from a place where trust is a big issue," he told me. "I thought I was being recorded, and watched, so I was not saying everything. It took me a long time to relax and talk about my past and be open about it. Even if I were asked how I was feeling about trusting you, I would have said, 'Yes, I trust you,' but I didn't."

Hasham is an intelligent, soft-spoken, and polite man who has suffered a great deal in his life—much that he does not want to see in print. He sought refuge in Australia because his life was in serious danger in his country of origin. As a consequence, he was haunted by memories of the traumas to which he had been exposed and was struggling with intense feelings of anger, sadness, and depression. At the same time, he was highly motivated to get better.

"I migrated to Australia and I was lucky enough to go to the trauma service for refugees," he says now. "I visited there on regular occasions. I felt there was some hope for me to recover and enjoy life again. I was made to feel special, and I didn't feel that I was just a client, any client, which I believe was very important for me to continue coming to the sessions."

Over time, Hasham slowly started to tell the story of his life experiences, including his upbringing in a caring family that taught him important values and gave him guidance and counsel about how to be a good man in this world. He also talked about his studies and then the beginning of his decline: being recruited into the army and put through training at a military university. In his country, to just leave the army was not an option. He struggled to maintain his values and beliefs amid a system that was crushing. Some officers tried everything to make him submissive and turn him into a nicely oiled cog in their machinery, but he refused to submit and, consequently, suffered considerable hardship and mistreatment. Nevertheless, he coped with these challenges and stayed well both physically and mentally.

"In the Army University I was able to control my anger and gain respect from the people that knew me and liked me, as well as from my enemies. I used to be strong and in control. I survived and still remember myself as the strong man who didn't let the superiors at the university make him feel low, and I gained their respect. But at the beginning I had suffered. I had to stand up for myself, and that was the key for success, standing up for myself no matter what. Having said that, there the culture and the language were familiar to me, and I had experience in how to deal with this kind of people and this kind of situation."

Later on, Hasham became involved in an uprising against the reigning dictatorship. When the uprising was crushed, he had to flee, finding refuge in a camp where he had been promised a safe haven and a new beginning. Instead, he found himself trapped in a place with no rights, no choice, and no freedom to determine his everyday living. Everything was ruled and regulated. It was like a prison, in which he was confined for three years—an experience that wore down his strength and belief in himself.

"The camp was the worst experience in my life. I then thought about what I had learnt in the past, and I had come to a stage in the camp when I believed that whatever I had learnt in the past was wrong, or was useless. I thought of committing suicide many times but, thank God, I did not."

When Hasham finally left the camp and settled in Australia, his mind remained troubled. He thought he had found freedom, and yet the mental unsettledness and memories of his experiences stayed with him like a shadow. Among other symptoms, he suffered frequent disturbing nightmares.

"I used to have nightmares about the camp, and every morning when I woke up I thought that I was in the camp, or in my country of origin, mainly at the Army University. I often dreamt about being sent back to the camp again from Australia. In the dream I had problems with the immigration papers, and had to go back to the camp for another six months. The dreams were like real and upset me a lot. It took me a long time to stop seeing those dreams."

In addition, Hasham found himself in a confusing culture with very different values. Certain behaviors appeared offensive to him. He was very confused about the way people spoke and acted. Some interacted with him in a patronizing way that felt belittling, demeaning, and devaluing. Others appeared coarse and rude, ignorant of the social etiquette that was part of his heritage. Equally, though, he spoke of being amazed at the kindness of some of the people he encountered. But he was plagued by a lingering suspicion that he could not trust that it was real.

Through all the ordeals Hasham had suffered, he had become a man who was reactive, whose anger was sparked easily and burned fiercely. He reacted irritably and angrily to people and situations that triggered memories of the mistreatment he had suffered, and he was very concerned about his short fuse. He had become a slave to his troubled emotions and the memories that intruded into his life, day and night. While he was desperate to change this, he was also fearful that he couldn't. He felt confused and lost in the space in which he found himself, to the point of contemplating suicide. The symptoms Hasham reported indicated that he suffered from Post-traumatic Stress Disorder with a comorbidity of Major Depressive Disorder (American Psychiatric Association, 2000).

THE INTERVENTIONS

What Therapeutic Goals Did Hasham Want to Achieve?

"I went to the sessions and there was one thing on my mind, to recover," says Hasham in reflection. When initially prompted to elaborate his goals, Hasham described to me the kind of person he once was and said he wanted to become that kind of man again: a man who was able to feel calmer, maintain control in the face of adversity, cope with people even when their behaviors were challenging, choose his behaviors, and have an overall sense of control over his life. His overarching goal was to rebuild his life and come to terms with his past. His immediate goals were to control his anger, cope with his disturbing emotions, and gain hope for the future.

What Therapeutic Models Informed the Interventions Used with Hasham?

In deciding what models would be most suited to help Hasham achieve his goals, I considered the core issues presented: a high level of distrust, out-of-control emotions (especially anger), a series of traumatic experiences that made no sense to him, and a loss of personhood and life opportunities. The breadth of these issues suggested that a one-size-fits-all approach was not likely to be effective, and I decided that I needed to combine different models for greatest therapeutic benefit. Metaphors seemed a salient vehicle for promoting change, while the different models of therapy described in the following sections informed my ways of working with metaphors.

Learning from Cultural Stories

> *Once there was a young man who used to beat up his aged father. One day this young man started beating his father in the market and continued until they reached the front door of his father's home. Only then did he stop the beating. Time passed, and this young man in turn had a son. When this man too became aged, his son started beating him up. In fact, his son beat him all the way from the market to the front door of his home, but when the son wanted to continue beating him, the father said, "That is enough, my son. I got my father to the front door and stopped, so now leave me in peace here."*

This was the first metaphor Hasham told me when I invited him to consider stories from his cultural background that were relevant to his problem and the outcomes he wished to attain.

"What does this story tell?" I asked Hasham.

"I am afraid one day when I get old and get to the stage when I can't defend myself, I would be attacked by someone who, like me, can't control his anger. Whatever you plant now you will get later. So if I attack someone now I will be attacked later," he replied.

It seemed that the story put his problem in a nutshell. As we continued to talk about the metaphor I recognized a sense of hopelessness in Hasham. He was afraid to be stuck in a powerful and highly repetitive pattern of reacting angrily to the world. Given that his anger posed a threat to himself and potentially others, we set containment of the anger as the first priority. The therapeutic models that guided this part of therapy were behavior modification (Craske, Barlow, & O'Leary, 1992) and mindfulness therapy (Kabat-Zinn, 1990, 2005). Behavior modification identifies behavior patterns, triggers, and maintaining factors for behaviors, and develops alternative behaviors. The story of the old man and his son illustrated this process for Hasham to some extent. In his words, "We explored ways to control my anger through discussions, examples, and stories from the past that I have read or experienced." Like every good metaphor, Hasham's story offered an indication about the path to a better outcome and an image of what that better outcome could look like.

"What else do you think this story is telling?" I queried.

His response was prompt: "I have to do something about my anger, think before I act, and when I act, don't overreact."

Hasham's interpretation of the story was that it signaled the point of change when the father speaks up and says, "It is enough." At that point the son stops beating him up. The father achieves his desired outcome by making himself heard. Similarly, by voicing the issue and making it more visible, Hasham had started along the path of change. He took the messages of the metaphor into his real life, wanting to become more aware of his behavior and more determined to change.

In order to aid this change process, I was interested in helping Hasham reconnect to his existing resources and, additionally, to utilize anxiety and stress management techniques that were already part of his makeup. For example, Hasham had mentioned that he had enjoyed exercise in the past and that he prayed regularly. These activities offered themselves as means for relaxation and stress management. He summarizes this phase of therapy by saying, "I felt that my therapist was serious about treating me and was interested in what I had to say. We had very interesting conversations, and I was interested in what she had to say about me and the stories and subjects we were talking about. She advised me about slow walking meditation, relaxation exercises, regular exercise and how to breathe slowly. What we did was of great help for me."

Accessing and Utilizing Hasham's Resources

As Hasham had previously and successfully coped with many adverse events, I expected, first, that a stronger side of himself was hidden under the rubble of his damaged sense of self and, second, that he had inner abilities and resources he could again tap into. Keen to get to know his strengths, wisdom, and resources, I encouraged him to tell me about his life before his troubles started. What were his dreams and aspirations? How had he coped with persecution and living in danger? I was particularly interested in accessing what had previously enabled him to withstand challenging encounters with other people, such as those at the military university and during the three years in the camp. My hope was that activating and utilizing these resources would enable Hasham to return to these behaviors and resume a calmer, more comfortable position when encountering others, particularly in situations of conflict. We went about this task by: (1) reflecting on his previous coping repertoire, (2) assessing how certain coping mechanisms could be utilized in his current life, and (3) considering how to put them into practice.

Validating his coping ability and resources rekindled a sense of strength. "We never spoke about my weaknesses," he recalled as we worked on this chapter. "What we did was always positive, not overdoing it, but it showed me the strength in me that I had lost during the times of suffering. Through this I was able to build up my skills and abilities to be strong and develop them more, as they had been weak and nearly gone."

Accessing and utilizing Hasham's resources was important for a number of reasons. First, it was an expression of my respect and trust in his strength and potential to recover. Second, it was likely to communicate hope to him. Third, it allowed for faster progress, because identifying and tapping into existing resources was quicker than building new ones. Fourth, it sought to rekindle Hasham's trust in himself. Finally, it aided the purpose of rebuilding an intact sense of self.

In the process of doing this, I asked him, "Can you think of a story that gives you a sense of support and strength?" Rather than telling me a story from his cultural heritage, this time he told about an experience that had deeply impressed him.

> *I was walking in the street during the war, and to make my way home shorter I had to cross a football field. But something inside me stopped me and I decided to go the longer way. Without clear reason I went through another street which leads home. As I was in the street parallel to the football field, a missile hit and exploded on the field. I was stunned and shocked, but I realized that someone is looking after me, and that I don't have total control over things that might happen to me. Therefore, I don't need to worry. My life was planned for me by someone greater than I can imagine. I didn't choose my parents nor the time I live in; someone else did. Just thinking about this story gets me to be relaxed, and I always remind myself about it.*

With this metaphor, Hasham related a salient part of his inner makeup. He talked about a higher power looking after him and keeping him safe. He deeply felt that he was not alone and that there was a bigger plan for his life. In practical terms, his faith, as expressed in the metaphor, was an important source of strength. It helped him to rebuild trust, allowed him to feel safer and less worried, and gave him a sense of purpose and meaning.

When exploring the meaning of his story further, I learned more about Hasham's faith and the role of prayer in his life. Interestingly, what he described reflected the core principles of mindfulness therapy (Kabat-Zinn, 1990, 2005): to become more of an observer of one's thoughts, feelings, and sensations and less reactive to inner or outer processes. This was exactly what Hasham wanted to develop again. Given that his daily routine of prayer already included some forms of mindfulness practice, I asked him whether we could extend this with other mindfulness exercises to find more peace and calm. He began practicing slow walking meditation, physical exercise, and other relaxation strategies, during which he became more observant of his thoughts, actions, and feelings.

When I asked him during one of the subsequent sessions how he was coping with his anger, he replied, "A few things happened at the gym that got me thinking about myself. For example, I went to use a machine, took the weight out of it and put the new weight in, then I started training. As I was using it another person came, looked at me in a friendly way, and left. After I finished with that machine, the same person came and put the weight back in that was on it at the beginning and started training. I went to him and asked, 'Were you using that machine before?' He said, 'Yes.' I said to him that I was sorry and that I didn't know he was using it. I left and that incident got me thinking, if that had been me, what would I have done? I would probably have got angry and shouted at that guy and maybe even worse, bashed him up. But what that gentleman did was quite simple, and got my respect, and showed that he is polite. Why can't I do that, I wondered. I wanted to be like that, too, and so I started to practice what to do in the same kind of situation or in similar kinds of situations."

REBUILDING TRUST

In the aftermath of human-made trauma, a loss of trust is one of the most pervasive and debilitating consequences (Sadavoy, 1997). The erosion of a sense of choice and free will, connected with an experience of mental defeat (Ehlers et al., 1998; Ehlers, Maercker, and Boos, 2000) or even mental death (Ebert & Dyck, 2004), frequently features in severe trauma resulting from experiences such as long-term human rights violations. Rebuilding a positive sense of self, choice, and control is thus an important task in therapy. In this context, the sharing of metaphors can greatly enhance the sense of control, particularly when the stories are client generated. Choosing and discussing the stories Hasham wanted to share underscored the cooperative nature of therapy and created experiences of choice and control.

Being very mindful of the fact that trust would only form gradually, I was prepared to walk at Hasham's pace. Therefore, the approach I chose to guide the therapeutic process during this stage was interpersonal therapy (Andrews, 2001), rather than exposure therapy, which is commonly used for trauma (Foa, Steketee, & Olasov-Rothbaum, 1989). In some cases of severe and complex interpersonal trauma, exposure therapy has been found to be contraindicated as the first form of intervention (Ehlers et al., 1998, 2000). If I pushed for the quick disclosure of traumatic experiences to process through exposure therapy, I thought Hasham would not continue with therapy. Therefore, I paid close attention to the delicate process of building a therapeutic alliance by validating his experiences and being aware and respectful of his strengths and resources. As trust grew, he slowly unpacked the parcels of his life story, allowing me, in very small increments, to learn about his more distressing life experiences, about his suffering, and about the way the aftereffects of his experiences had come to rule his life.

As Hasham began to tell me about his life, sharing his feelings of despair and loneliness, I recognized the rift between his former and current perceptions of himself. Such a rift, or discontinuity of self, is a common feature in people who have been exposed to complex interpersonal trauma (Ebert & Dyck, 2004). Recovery from this requires several steps, such as: (1) reconnection to the former self (Ehlers et al., 2000), (2) reconnection to the once-held assumptive world (Janoff-Bulman, 1989, 1992), and (3) the cognitive processing of the traumatic experiences and subsequent changes in selfhood (Herman, 1992; Horowitz, 1999). Because cognitive restructuring is an important tool in rebuilding damaged identity and facilitating the integration of traumatic experiences (Linehan, 1993; Linehan, Heard, & Armstrong, 1993), I chose the cognitive behavioral therapy (CBT) model (Beck, 1976; Beck & Freeman, 1990) as one of my key tools.

As we continued sharing stories, I asked which cultural stories spoke of the type of thoughts or cognitions that might help him process his past trauma. Hasham told me of a very famous author in his country who centuries ago had written a volume of stories known by many people in this country. "These stories are parables," he said. "They give information about how to live a good life. They are part of our culture and religion, teaching life values and life instructions."

By now Hasham had made it clear that he wanted more than anger management. He wanted to again become the kind of man he once was, a man "who was respected by his friends and enemies alike." He told a story that pointed this out beautifully.

A Tale of Respect

Once there was a community leader who was known for his wisdom, patience, generosity, and humbleness. A man in the marketplace approached him. That man was paid to test the community leader's patience, so he approached and vilified the leader in front of everyone. However, the community leader kept walking and didn't say anything to the man. Nonetheless, the man was not to be deterred. He followed the leader and vilified him again and again, but the community leader kept walking and didn't say anything back. Eventually the man confronted the community leader and said, "I am talking to you!" The community leader responded, "And I am ignoring you!" The leader went on to add, "Whoever asked you to vilify me, go ask him to pay you. You have done what you were asked to do!"

The story tells of a man who, despite being persistently harassed, remains calm, true to his values, true to his chosen path, and able to see through the other person. In maintaining such a high level of control over his behaviors, he even earns the respect of his opponent. Hasham's tale clearly expressed the very goal he sought to achieve. "Who doesn't want to be like that community leader?" he asked.

"He managed to control his anger and showed how wise he was. He even gained the respect of the man who was vilifying him."

Hasham took this story to heart and subsequently made an effort to take a few steps back from his anger, gain a larger perspective, suspend judgment, and better control his reactions. In doing this, he returned to a previously well-established behavior pattern that allowed him to deal with difficult situations more calmly and more effectively. Not long after, he told about an event that indicated his ability to replicate what the community leader had demonstrated.

"Recently, when I was at the gym, there was a situation when someone did something I didn't like and found really offensive. I was angry, but I was able to go and ask him why he actually did that. He replied that he was not aware of what he had done and didn't mean to be offensive. He apologized and was very kind with his words. I felt really embarrassed, as I realized there was no need to get angry with him."

A LITTLE OF HASHAM'S OUTCOME

With time, Hasham became calmer and more relaxed. His ruminative, worrisome thoughts settled. Even though he still got frustrated or angry at times, he was better able to control his reactions. His focus became more future oriented, and, while he still remembered the past at times, Hasham started to build a future. He completed a postgraduate degree, got married, and now has three delightful children. As we discussed his reflections on therapy and penned this chapter together, I asked if he would sum up what made the difference for him.

"What has helped me along the way? There have been several things. I have learnt more about the Australian culture and language. That has put me more at ease. In therapy, I was shown a few techniques to relax. I joined a gymnasium, and was able to get myself tired doing all the exercises . . . and got all my frustrations and anger out. Also, my nightmares became much less. The only dream I still see, every now and again, is the one in which I dream about going back to the camp for another six months.

"We talked about stories to learn from, and how to apply them into the real world that we live in. Some of the stories were real. The purpose of the stories was of interest to both the therapist and me. One important thing about sharing the stories was to enable her to understand the way I was thinking and my culture. They were a bridge across our cultures. But also the stories were a source of knowledge: They showed what kind of person I was and how she could deal with me.

"In regards to the therapy, what was the overall outcome of my journey there? I used to lose my temper easily, and reacted irrationally when I was angry, without thinking. I could have killed someone without realizing it. I did overreact every time I got angry. I was worried about losing my freedom, sad, scared, could not think straight, my thoughts were mixed up, my brain was thinking all the time even when I was asleep, and I was talking to myself in the street. In the counseling sessions, I got to talk about my thoughts and what was happening inside my brain. I was able to put my foot on the right track and kept moving with time. I started to build trust in myself and other people. I felt more confident, and I was able to do further studies. It took time but I was getting better every time—well, nearly every time—we used to meet. I was able to gather my thoughts and started to think clearly. The only thing I couldn't achieve, or we couldn't achieve, was to forgive the people who made me suffer. Forgiveness was the only problem left, if we can call it a problem. I still find it hard to forgive those people."

Hasham left me with a story that reflected his new understanding and attitude.

THIS TOO WILL PASS

A powerful king, a ruler of a large kingdom, was in such a strong position that he could employ the wisest of men. One day, he felt confused and upset and called the wise men. He told them he felt strongly compelled to find a certain ring, a ring which would enable him to feel happy and calm. "I must have that ring," he said. "The ring that will make me joyful when I am unhappy. Equally, it must make me sad if I look at it when feeling happy."

The wise men thought about this deeply, consulted each other, and finally reached a decision regarding the characteristics of the ring that would fit their king's request. They devised a ring inscribed with the words "This too will pass."

REFERENCES

American Psychiatric Association. (2000). *Diagnostic and statistical manual of mental disorders* (4th ed., text rev.). Washington, DC: Author.

Andrews, H. (2001). Back to basics: Psychotherapy is an interpersonal process. *Australian Psychologist, 36,* 76–92.

Beck, A. T. (1976). *Cognitive therapy and the emotional disorders.* New York: New American Library.

Beck, A. T., & Freeman, A. (1990). *Cognitive therapy of personality disorders.* New York: Guilford Press.

Craske, M. G., Barlow, D. H., & O'Leary, T. (1992). *Mastery of your anxiety and worry.* Albany, NY: Graywind.

Ebert, A., & Dyck, M. J. (2004). The experience of mental death: The core feature of complex posttraumatic stress disorder. *Clinical Psychology Review, 24,* 617–635.

Ehlers, A., Clark, D. M., Dunmore, E., Jaycox, L., Meadows, E., & Foa, E. B. (1998). Predicting response to exposure treatment in PTSD: The role of mental defeat and alienation. *Journal of Traumatic Stress, 11*(3), 457–471.

Ehlers, A., Maercker, A., & Boos, A. (2000). Post-traumatic stress disorder following political imprisonment: The role of mental defeat, alienation, and perceived permanent change. *Journal of Abnormal Psychology, 109,* 45–55.

Foa, E. B., Steketee, G., & Olasov-Rothbaum, B. O. (1989). Behavioral-cognitive conceptualisations of post-traumatic stress disorder. *Behavior Therapy, 20,* 155–176.

Herman, J. L. (1992). *Trauma and recovery: From domestic abuse to political terror.* New York: HarperCollins.

Horowitz, M. J. (1999). A model of mourning: Change in schemas of self and others. In M. J. Horowitz (Ed.), *Essential papers on post-traumatic stress disorder* (pp. 253–273). New York: New York University Press.

Hubble, M. A., & Miller, S. D. (2004). The client: Psychotherapy's missing link for promoting a positive psychology. In P. A. Linley & S. Joseph (Eds.), *Positive psychology in practice* (pp. 335–353). Hoboken, NJ: Wiley.

Janoff-Bulman, R. (1989). Assumptive worlds and the stress of traumatic events: Application of the schema construct. *Social Cognition, 7,* 113–136.

Janoff-Bulman, R. (1992). *Shattered assumptions: Towards a new psychology of trauma.* New York: Free Press.

Kabat-Zinn, J. (1990). *Full catastrophe living: Using the wisdom of your body and mind to face stress, pain and illness.* New York: Delta.

Kabat-Zinn, J. (2005). *Coming to our senses: Healing ourselves and the world through mindfulness.* New York: Hyperion.

Linehan, M. (1993). *Cognitive-behavioral treatment of borderline personality disorder.* New York: Guilford.

Linehan, M., Heard, H., & Armstrong, H. (1993). Naturalistic follow-up of a behavioural treatment for chronically parasuicidal borderline patients. *Archives of General Psychiatry, 50*(10), 971–974.

Sadavoy, J. (1997). Survivors: A review of the late life-effects of prior psychological trauma. *American Journal of Geriatric Psychiatry, 5*(4), 287–301.

Snyder, C. R. (Ed.). (2000). *Handbook of hope: Theory, measures and applications.* San Diego, CA: Academic Press.

CHAPTER 19

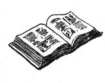

Of Goths, Fairies, Dragons, and CBT

Joining the Client's World with an
Evidence-Based Metaphor

George W. Burns

CONTRIBUTOR'S STORY:
A PROFESSIONAL AND PERSONAL PERSPECTIVE

George's "Contributor's Story" can be found at the beginning of Chapter 2.

PREVIEW THE CHAPTER

Cognitive behavioral therapy (CBT) and positive psychology have revealed, and continue to reveal, much about the attitudinal and behavioral attributes that contribute to depression and happiness. Yet how do you communicate such research-derived information to an adolescent client who has aligned herself with a subcultural group that has turned depression into both an art form and a lifestyle? This is the question George explores with a 16-year-old client. Weaving the metaphor (told in italics) through the unfolding case story, he illustrates how the healing story evolved from an exploration of the client's goals, exceptions to her depression, and client resources that are utilized in the metaphor. The evidence-based intervention provides cognitive strategies for modifying thoughts, feelings, and patterns of behavior—all in the language, imagery, and world of the client. A collaboratively developed therapist-generated metaphor offers choices for establishing and enhancing new cognitive patterns.

Therapeutic Characteristics

Problems Addressed

- Loss of loved ones
- Major depression
- Suicidal ideation
- Unchangeable circumstances
- Inadequate coping skills
- Rumination
- Global thinking
- Pessimism
- Lack of choices
- Powerlessness

Resources Developed

- Managing loss
- Assessing alternative attributional styles
- Thinking specifically
- Thinking positively
- Being optimistic
- Becoming action oriented
- Learning to make choices
- Developing empowerment

Outcomes Offered

- Grief/loss management skills
- Effective cognitive skills
- Specific thinking
- Optimism
- An action orientation
- Choices
- Effective communication skills
- Enhanced happiness

THE ASSESSMENT

Her 16-year-old head hung forward on our first meeting. Dyed jet-black hair tried to conceal a pale, milky complexion. She was dressed in black, with black mascara, black lipstick, a wide black leather wristband and matching choker studded with silver spikes, like an ancient knight's armor, announcing long before she told me, "I'm a goth."

While wanting to assess the direction that Reyna and I might proceed in, I was also aware that she would be assessing me, that she would be doing so on the basis of my first communications with her, and that her assessment would be a strong determinant of the therapeutic outcome. She had previously seen a number of counselors and therapists, and I guessed this meant she had already talked about her problems at some length. If things were to be different this time, we needed to tread a different path. In addition, a successful outcome to the therapeutic process would be better assured if we were working together rather than pulling in different directions. I sensed that one step in the wrong direction at this point could easily result in our being opponents instead of teammates.

So the first question I asked Reyna was not about her problems but "What do *you* want to achieve from the time we spend together?" I hoped this would put the ball in her court, empowering her to make some choices, rather than giving the appearance that I was accepting what her mother had already told me.

"I have always been depressed," she answered, indicating in her "always" the global style of thinking common in people who feel depressed (Yapko, 1997, 2006). Certainly she had a long history of battling depression—over 50 percent of her young life. However, her mother had indicated she had been a happy child prior to that, and there had also been times when she felt better over the last eight years. Had she been thinking more specifically, she might have concluded that depression had occupied a larger than desired part of her life *and* that there were also times when she felt happier.

"It's gone on for so long and nothing has made any difference," she continued, with an orientation that was both fixed and past focused, as if she expected that because it had previously been that way it would always go on being that way. Her words held a sense of helplessness and a lack of personal power, as though her thoughts and feelings were outside of her realm of control and thus unchangeable.

It is not uncommon for clients to answer a goal-oriented question in the negative, stating, as Reyna did, not what they want but what they do *not* want to be feeling. Research into the goal-setting patterns of depressed people shows they often hold avoidant goals ("I do *not* want to be depressed, constantly fighting in my relationship, or gambling when stressed") and strive to reach conditional goals ("I will not be happy until I finish my degree, my partner loves me, or I win a million dollars"; Emmons, 1991, 2003; Street, 2000, 2001, 2002).

"If you are not wanting to feel so depressed, how would you rather be feeling?" I pushed gently, wanting my question to open up the possibility of hope that her experience could be different. While the hopelessness and helplessness that Reyna had expressed are characteristic of depression, hopefulness is strongly associated with happiness (Seligman, 1975, 1990, 2002). If I, as her therapist, am practically and realistically hopeful, I model and communicate hope to my client. Hope is not only a core element in successful psychotherapeutic processes but may even be more closely correlated with outcome than the actual therapeutic interventions used (Frank, 1968, 1975; Hubble & Miller, 2004; Lopez et al., 2004; Snyder, 1994, 2000, 2002).

"I want to feel happier," came the response.

"When have you felt happier?" I explored, hoping for some exceptions to the generalization she had previously stated of "always" being depressed. Inviting the client to be aware of those occasions on which the problem-saturated story has been different validates that the therapeutic goals are attainable (as they have already been during those exceptions), opens up the possibility for further change, builds hope, and provides possible directions to follow in therapy (Berg & Dolan, 2001; Berg & Steiner, 2003; Linden, Chapter 4 in this volume).

She looked up a little, her stark white skin and heavy dark makeup as high in contrast as a black-and-white photograph, and expressed surprise. "I am a goth," she replied, with the assumption that I should understand the full implications of what that meant in relation to my question. Goth is a modern subculture that first became popular during the early 1980s, when it arose as a subgenre of the postpunk rock music scene. The subculture is associated with a mood of horror, darkness, death, and the supernatural—characteristics of the gothic literary tradition from which the name derives. Adherents usually wear black clothing and makeup—often inspired by horror films and television series such as *The Addams Family* and *The Munsters*—and listen to gothic rock or death metal music. When I sought to learn more about the subculture from younger friends and family members, one young woman who had been a goth herself described them as "late adolescents with a maudlin fascination in depression." Fortunately, I was not aware at the time that happiness and fun were the antithesis of the whole goth subculture and so was able to push Reyna by asking, "So, what do you do for fun?"

"I go on the Internet. I'm into nu-metal things. Oh, and I'm a fairy."

"You're a fairy?" I asked, both curiously and almost incredulously, upon which Reyna went on to describe the secret life of a public goth. From childhood she had been interested in fairies, collecting a library of illustrated fairy stories, posters of fairies, and statues of winged dragons. Figurines of colorful fairies and cute dragons apparently cluttered every flat surface in her bedroom. Then there was the secret that she hid from her goth friends: She had a job in which once or twice a weekend she dressed up as a fairy—frilly skirt, ballet shoes, sparkling tiara, gossamer wings, and magic wand—to entertain at children's birthday parties with games and stories. Her face lit up in a smile as she told me, "Some kids and parents are jerks, but most are good fun. I enjoy it."

"What is it you enjoy about being a fairy?" I inquired, seeing an exception I had hoped we might find to the always-depressed story she had initially communicated about herself.

"When I put on my fairy costume, it is like I become a fairy. Fairies want to make wishes come true, to see the children smile. I have to actually *be* a fairy, and enjoy what I am doing, to bring joy to the kids whose parties I go to."

Already cues were forming as to potential characters and processes for using metaphors in therapy. First, Reyna liked, collected, and worked with fairy stories, telling them to children in her persona as a fairy. Second, there was something secret, special, and enjoyable for her about characters such as fairies and cute dragons. Third, fairy stories are often rich in themes of magic and change, as well as processes for reaching a desired outcome.

In addition, I was obtaining very useful information about Reyna's resources and abilities—a process whose importance has been underscored with practical examples by many contributors to this volume. Gregory Smit considers the searching for, finding, and utilization of a client's resources one of the most important functions in the assessment process (Chapter 8). It is easy to think of such resources, strengths, or abilities as the positive attributes or characteristics a client displays, the exceptions to the problem when he or she appears strong, capable, or confident. These might be a client's athletic skill, like mountain climbing (Hildebrandt, Fletcher, & Hayes, Chapter 5); the ability to express oneself in poetry (Hicks-Lankton, Chapter 13); or the knowledge of one's own cultural stories (Ebert & Al Musawi, Chapter 18). However, resources may also be found in the seemingly negative. For Ray and Sutton (Chapter 15) the "problem" of self-mutilation is seen as a strength that can be mobilized toward the resolution. Mills (Chapter 11) considers a child's "obsession" with keys as a resource with positive potentials and possibilities, while Garcia-Sanchez (Chapter 20) utilizes the hostile resistance of a disruptive group participant as an energy to be redirected with therapeutic advantage. In fact, all chapters contain examples of how the practitioner found a resource in the client's ability to express, understand, and process metaphors, whether in a story told by the client (Erickson Klein, Chapter 17), a descriptive metaphor that communicated his or her problem (Kopp, Chapter 4), a willingness to create a new story (Nel, Chapter 9), or the ability to simply listen and learn (Yapko, Chapter 9; Hicks-Lankton, Chapter 13).

So what were the resources I saw in Reyna, and how did I see that they might be employed toward attaining her therapeutic goal? In donning her fairy costume, Reyna also donned the fairy persona. She not only played the role of a fairy but *became* the fairy. She *was* the positive, cheerful, entertaining qualities of the character she enacted. And so I began to ponder: Did she engage in a similar process when donning the clothes and makeup of a goth? Did dressing for the role, being the characteristics of the role, mean that she took on the mood of that role, whether goth or fairy? Perhaps her ability to do this could be utilized to role-play, and live, more helpful, less depressive cognitions and behaviors.

Thank you for telling me about your secret. I am fascinated to know that you are interested in fairies and fairy stories, too. I similarly have an abiding interest in fairy stories and, as I am sure you are aware, they have long been used not only to entertain children and adults but also to educate us about some of the important issues of life. What young girl hasn't been fascinated by the story of Cinderella, of the fairy godmother who teaches her how it is possible to move from an unhappy situation where others are treating her badly to a situation where she can feel good about herself and enjoy greater happiness?

And as you have shared something with me I would like to share a fairy story with you, which may help us as we work together to achieve the goals you have identified for therapy.

"Who would you like to be the heroine of our story?" I asked.

"Tinkerbell," she replied without hesitation. "I have always liked the Peter Pan story, so I chose Tinkerbell as my name. She is the fairy I play."

"And we will need a second character, someone Tinkerbell can help. Who would you like to choose?"

"Puff."

"As in Puff the Magic Dragon?" I asked.

"Yes," she said. "I had him as a soft toy when I was a kid, and of all the dragons I have collected, Puff still remains my favorite."

Well, perhaps we can have a story in which Tinkerbell and Puff are friends who lived in a turreted fairy castle along with their family and friends. One day Tinkerbell and Puff flew off to a valley where they played by a stream, linked daisy chains together, and did those things you might imagine a young fairy and dragon playfully do on a day out. It may sound strange, but one of the games they liked most of all was dressing up as people, pretending they were people, putting people expressions on their faces, behaving like people behave, trying to think like people. So absorbed were they in their game, so good were they at being people, that time flew by and it was already dusk when they reached home to find a shocking surprise.

The fairy castle was empty. Their family and friends had disappeared without a trace, the ones they loved were gone, all their possessions were gone too, and it felt like they had never existed. Tinkerbell and Puff were shocked, and scared, and sad, and maybe some other emotions as well. Why had they gone? Had someone driven them away? Was there anything Tinkerbell and Puff could have done to prevent it? They sat on the corner of a stone wall and looked out over the empty castle feeling forlorn, stunned, and despairing.

THE BACKGROUND

The metaphor began with a problem that matched Reyna's. Initially she had been brought to the appointment by her mother, perhaps a little reluctantly, and both mother and daughter considered that Reyna had been depressed for half her life. She had previously been on antidepressant medication and received counseling on several different occasions without improvement.

The story emerged that this was her mother's second marriage. A half brother and sister from the first marriage had lived with them but were in constant conflict with their stepfather, Reyna's dad. She was 8 years old when her father ordered her 15- and 17-year-old stepsiblings out of the house, never to return. For Reyna, that was the turning point. Given this background, I hoped having Tinkerbell and Puff come home to an empty castle—with all the associated confusion and emotions—would be an experience with which Reyna could identify.

Following the departure of her stepsiblings, she began to display some of the many different styles of coping associated with depression (Elliot, Sheldon, & Church, 1997; Emmons & Kaiser, 1996; Lyubomirsky & Nolen-Hoeksema, 1995; Street, 2000; Vaillant, 2004; Yapko, 1997, 2001, 2006). First, she became angry with her father. As a result, they had virtually not spoken in eight years. Second, she avoided the unpleasant conflicts and loss in her young life: She retreated from pressures, refused to go to school, complained of being unwell, shut herself in her bedroom, avoided friends, and did little else apart from sit in front of the television. Of course, at eight years old, there was little she could do to change the circumstances or prevent her beloved siblings from being exiled from her life. Nonetheless, her strategy for coping was not helpful in that it was neither problem solving nor solution focused, and simply left her feeling powerless.

When she reached her early teens, she displayed the ultimate of avoidant behaviors, attempting suicide several times by cutting her wrists and swallowing pills found in her mother's bathroom. She had improved for a few years, but her mother was deeply concerned that Reyna was now slipping back into depression, becoming avoidant, and possibly having suicidal thoughts once more.

Reyna displayed a second characteristic coping style typical of depressed individuals, namely that of rumination—a cognitive pattern in which a person engages in a constant mental rehashing of negative thoughts about bad past experiences, especially those incidents associated with guilt

(Nolen-Hoeksema, Grayson, & Larson, 1991; Street, 2000). Reyna had gone over and over in her head countless times the exile of her siblings, the loss of her connectedness with them, the change in the family structure, and her continuing experience of grief. She blamed her father for doing it, her mother for allowing it to happen, and herself for whatever indefinable things she might have done to contribute to it. As with any repetitive task or thought, usually the more we do it the better we become at it, and the better we become the easier it is to do, whether studying material for an exam, practicing an athletic skill, or repeating a negative thought. Ruminative patterns of negative thinking are associated with more frequent depressive symptoms, longer depressive episodes, and more vulnerability to relapse (Lyubomirsky & Nolen-Hoeksema, 1995; Street, 2000). It may be easy for a person to think that going over and over an unresolved issue will eventually provide a better understanding and hopefully a solution, but the reverse seems to be true. As Segal, Williams, and Teasdale (2002) have observed, "In fact, in this state of mind, repeatedly 'thinking about' negative aspects of the self, or of problematic situations, serves to perpetuate rather than resolve depression" (p. 36).

Reyna revealed that she had recently broken up with a boyfriend and considered that to be the source of her current depressive feelings. She was also supporting a goth friend whom she described as more depressed than herself. As I listened to these aspects of her story, I found myself thinking that perhaps it would be helpful to include a relationship in the metaphor, to have the two characters illustrate the different types of thinking styles that are more helpful and less helpful.

Then Tinkerbell thought of the first thing that any good fairy was likely to think about: She took out her magic wand and tried her best spell for making things reappear. But nothing happened. Sometimes, she discovered, no matter how much you try, some things cannot be changed.

Puff the Magic Dragon found that he was a dragon without magic, for without hope there is nothing to wish for and without wishes it is unlikely that a wish will come true. "This is hopeless," said Puff. "They are gone and there is nothing we can do about it."

"It certainly does look bad," said Tinkerbell, feeling a distinct and understandable sadness. "I agree that the things we have been doing aren't working. Maybe there is something different we can do—maybe there is another way that might be helpful," she added thoughtfully.

THE INTERVENTION

Tinkerbell reflected that the things Reyna had been doing were not working, and that magic, unrealistic wishful thinking, and avoidant behaviors were not likely to solve her problems. She needed to look in new directions, to try to experiment with different approaches. To offer helpful suggestions for Reyna about those skills and directions, there were still several questions I needed to address in my mind.

1. *What is (are) the client's specific therapeutic goal (goals)?* For Reyna there appeared to be a couple of core goals. First, she wanted to be happier; she had clearly illustrated that she already had both existing and potential ways to feel better. Second, I considered that if she adopted different cognitive styles she might experience those greater levels of happiness that she desired.

2. *What therapeutic model might best help her achieve those goals?* Reyna's current cognitive style

was counterproductive to the achievement of her goal of happiness. If Reyna changed her thinking, she might also change her experience. So my choice was to work from a CBT model, at least initially.

3. *What interventions within that model will be most beneficial?* My thinking was that it would be helpful to show Reyna the evidence-based differences between the thinking styles of people who generally feel depressed and people who generally feel happier. If she had the choice to adopt and become the joyful, positive character of a fairy, perhaps she could also adopt and incorporate the cognitive characteristics of people who generally cope well with life.

4. *How can this be communicated most effectively?* Citing the research to Reyna, telling her what she *should* do, or setting homework exercises for a 16-year-old who is depressed and not highly action oriented was not likely to be effective. When most clients arrive at our office, they have already been told many times by well-intentioned friends, family, physicians, or therapists—often on sound bases—what they need to do. If the advice or information was sound then it probably had not been communicated effectively for this particular person. Fortunately, with Reyna I had a clear indication of how this might be done. Given her interest in and use of stories, metaphor seemed an appropriate means for communicating the cognitive skills that might be beneficial for her.

5. *What type of metaphor will best help her reach her goal(s)?* Reyna was engaged collaboratively in defining the characters and general theme of the metaphor, but there were particular cognitive skills that I considered helpful for Reyna of which she may not have been aware or able to access herself. Using experiential metaphors was also a possibility that I considered might be better employed later in the therapy once the rapport that can develop with storytelling had been established. This led me to choose a therapist-generated metaphor as a vehicle to communicate specific cognitive skills.

"I don't know how we can do anything different," said Puff, the corners of his dragon mouth drooping sorrowfully and his eyes looking doleful. "This is the worst thing that could happen to anyone. How will we ever get over it?" And as he spoke he looked even sadder.

"It certainly is terrible," said Tinkerbell. "But aren't we lucky that we were out playing and haven't disappeared like the rest of them?" There is no doubt that she, too, felt a deep sadness about the loss, but being aware of their fortune enabled her to feel perhaps just a little less sad.

Puff continues to think globally and pessimistically, leading him into greater sadness, while Tinkerbell models a more specific and optimistic style of thinking. Here the story acknowledges her grief, invites an awareness of the positive, and shows the benefit in lessening the sadness.

THE METAPHOR STRUCTURE

Every story is said to have a beginning, a middle, and an end. Similarly, therapeutic stories usually have their beginning in a problem, challenge, or task that parallels that of the client and that the character needs to resolve, such as Tinkerbell and Puff coming home to find their loved ones gone. The middle is where we are in the current story. It is where we address the question that Rob McNeilly poses in Chapter 16: What is missing? It is where the character adopts the missing resources, acquires the knowledge, builds the skills, or finds the means to effectively resolve or manage the problem. Here Tinkerbell models effective cognitive skills juxtaposed against Puff's less helpful style of thinking. The end (which we have yet to reach in Reyna's metaphor) will be the client's desired therapeutic outcome. I refer to the three elements of a therapeutic metaphor—problem, resources, and outcome—as the PRO approach, as mentioned previously in this volume (Chapter 14) and discussed more fully in *101 Healing Stories* (Burns, 2001) and *101 Healing Stories for Kids and Teens* (Burns, 2005).

> *"We have lost everything," moaned Puff. "All our family, our friends, everything is completely gone."*
> *"It could be worse," said Tinkerbell, trying to reassure Puff and finding that the reassuring attitude was reassuring for herself as well. "We have still got each other. We still have the castle for shelter, and there is plenty of food and water to help us survive. Maybe we can rest overnight and begin a search tomorrow."*

Puff is the one who sees the glass as half empty, while Tinkerbell has the half-full perception. Puff is pessimistic, Tinkerbell optimistic, and that optimism permits her to make plans for the future.

As with this tale, telling a metaphor usually begins with the problem, moves through the appropriate resources, and concludes with the desired outcome. However, when planning the metaphor you want to tell, it may be easier to start at the end. When planning to go to work, for example, we first decide where we want to go (the outcome or destination), then how best to get there (the means: bus, train, car, bicycle, or feet), and finally what problems we need to overcome to get there (such as arising from a warm bed on a cold morning). Of course, in carrying out the plan we follow the reverse order: arise (face the problem), take the appropriate transport (engage the resources to resolve it), and arrive (reach the outcome). So in planning Reyna's story, I was first aware of her desired outcome to be happier. I then asked myself what means, skills, or resources would be most helpful for her to get there, concluding by deciding on appropriate cognitive styles.

> *"I don't care about the others," said Puff angrily. "I am just hurting too much to be bothered about anyone else. Why does this always happen to me? Why is it that I am the one who always seems to suffer?"*
> *"Let's get some rest," said Tinkerbell, "and see how it looks in the morning. I have heard my mother say that nothing stays the same forever, that even in the worst of times things can change and get better."*

Puff is focused on his own hurt, and his talking of "always" shows that he holds the perception that the current experiences are permanent or constant. Contrastingly, Tinkerbell sees that things may look different in the light of a new day, that things do change and don't remain constant.

Juxtaposing the two styles of thinking between Puff and Tinkerbell, and the consequences of thinking in that style, the metaphor presents examples of coping styles that are likely to be helpful and coping styles that are less likely to be helpful. An important learning for Reyna was that it was not so much *what* had happened to her in the past, or would happen in the future, but *how* she perceived and handled those happenings or events that made the difference between satisfactory and unsatisfactory adjustment. Knowing this and making choices about how we respond to circumstances is a key determinant of how well, or poorly, we adjust to life's many challenges.

"It never will get better," said Puff, almost defiantly. He felt the heaviness and bleakness of his own words. He knew that being so pessimistic wasn't being helpful, but still he couldn't see anything to look forward to and began to feel even more bleak.

"Things sure have changed," agreed Tinkerbell. "They won't be the same again. If our friends and family don't come back or we can't find them, life will certainly be different for both of us. If they do come back, life will be different, too, because we now know the pain of loss and suffering. But let us not lose hope for the future. Without hope we have nothing. We can hope for their return, and if it doesn't happen, we can hope that there may still be things in life that we can do and enjoy."

The thought of taking some positive action, and the possibility of joy some time in the future, permitted Tinkerbell's sadness to fade just a little more.

Puff holds an inflexible attitude toward what has happened, and the story reveals the consequences of that on his mood. Tinkerbell is more flexible, exploring the options, making choices, and seeing the consequences of those choices.

Throughout Reyna's metaphor, my emphasis was to highlight the different styles of possible coping skills through Puff and Tinkerbell, hopefully modeling in Tinkerbell styles that would be helpful for and accepted by Reyna. In using Tinkerbell, Reyna's own fairy character, I hoped to facilitate Reyna's identification with the more desirable, functional, and adaptive skills.

In the next part of the metaphor, Puff continues to ruminate on the past, reflecting the style used by Reyna to that point in confronting the loss of her siblings, while Tinkerbell models an alternative, more action-oriented approach.

"Why are you talking about hope when things couldn't be worse?" asked Puff. "I have lost everyone and everything. There is nothing we can do; nothing is working out right anymore." Puff didn't seem to be aware that the more he said these things, or the more he thought them over and over again in his head, the worse he felt and the less he felt like doing anything except just sitting on the stone wall, looking out over the empty castle, and feeling even more miserable.

"Come on," said Tinkerbell, springing to her fairy toes and giving Puff the very unmagic dragon a nudge. "We need to do something. We need to find a place in the castle to make ourselves comfortable, to cook a warm meal, and to plan what we are going to do."

As she got up and began to move, Tinkerbell was surprised that she started to feel a little better still. Moving felt better than sitting around doing nothing. The action helped to lift her feelings, to help her think a bit more clearly.

As Tinkerbell began flying back toward the castle, she realized it was going to take time for her and Puff to adjust to this huge loss that they had both experienced. You don't lose someone or something close to you without feeling it, and feeling it strongly at times.

Perhaps, thought Tinkerbell, it isn't just a matter of time, but also what you do and how you think in that time that determines how happy or unhappy you feel. Even though the same thing has happened to each of us, she reflected, we have each responded in different ways. Perhaps it is possible to make some choices about how I think and feel, just like I do in the games we play pretending to be people. As we play the role of being people, we start to think and behave as though we are people.

"Because this is our story," I said to Reyna, "we can make up the ending just like we made up the characters. So I am wondering, of all the things Tinkerbell thought and did, what you think might be the most helpful for her to get on with her life, and how she might go about it."

THE FOLLOW-UP

I saw Reyna for four appointments, with Puff and Tinkerbell making an appearance at each appointment, each time communicating a little more about skills that might be helpful to Reyna. Two months later she made another appointment of her own initiative, and this time it was she who brought her mother and father to therapy, saying that she wanted to "tidy up the edges." The makeup around her eyes was still dark, yet on her lips she wore a soft pink lipstick. She was dressed in a style that, in a crowd, would not have distinguished her from most other teenagers: faded blue jeans, a white polo shirt, and an unzipped grey sweat top. Gone were the armorlike metal studs. Gone was the dress of the goth. She had ceased going to weekend parties with her former goth friends and was seeking to build new friendships at school. On her feet were a pair of soft ballet-like shoes, part pink, part white, with delicate floral patterns, befitting any good fairy.

Her mother described Reyna as "happier and lighter," saying she was in "a better mood most of the time." Specifically, her mother emphasized how Reyna's relationship with her father had improved, describing her as "open and friendly" toward him, with the result that he had "warmed more toward her," and the positive aspects of this had become mutually reinforcing. She said she had even observed them joking and laughing together—something that had not happened over the last eight years. Her father smiled and nodded in agreement.

"I really am an optimist," Reyna said, almost dismissively, as if her mother's comments related to something from the distant past and were not even in the realm of relevance. She wanted to get down to the business of the current session: working on the parent-daughter relationship. And she was clear about what she needed to do: "I want to see more well-being between all of us."

REFERENCES

Berg, I. K., & Dolan, Y. (2001). *Tales of solutions: A collection of hope-inspiring stories.* New York: Norton.

Berg, I. K., & Steiner, T. (2003). *Children's solution work.* New York: Norton.

Burns, G. W. (2001). *101 healing stories: Using metaphors in therapy.* New York: Wiley.

Burns, G. W. (2005). *101 healing stories for kids and teens: Using metaphors in therapy.* Hoboken, NJ: Wiley.

Elliot, A., Sheldon, K., & Church, M. (1997). Avoidance, personal goals and subjective well-being. *Personality and Social Psychology Bulletin, 23,* 915–927.

Emmons, R. A. (1991). Personal strivings, daily life events, and psychological and physical well-being. *Journal of Personality, 59,* 453–472.

Emmons, R. A. (2003). Personal goals, life meaning, and virtue: Wellsprings of a positive life. In C. L. M. Keyes & J. Haidt (Eds.), *Flourishing: Positive psychology and the life well-lived* (pp. 105–128). Washington, DC: American Psychological Association.

Emmons, R. A., & Kaiser, H. (1996). Goal orientation and emotional well-being. *Social Indicators Research, 45,* 391–422.

Frank, J. D. (1968). The role of hope in psychotherapy. *International Journal of Psychiatry, 5,* 383–395.

Frank, J. D. (1975). The faith that heals. *Johns Hopkins Medical Journal, 137,* 127–131.

Hubble, M. A., & Miller, S. D. (2004). The client: Psychotherapy's missing link for promoting a positive psychology. In P. A. Linley & S. Joseph (Eds.), *Positive psychology in practice* (pp. 335–353). Hoboken, NJ: Wiley.

Lopez, S. J., Snyder, C. R., Magyar-Moe, J. L., Edwards, L. M., Pedrotti, J. T., Janowski, K., et al. (2004). Strategies for accentuating hope. In P. A. Linley & S. Joseph (Eds.), *Positive psychology in practice* (pp. 388–403). Hoboken, NJ: Wiley.

Lyubomirsky, S., & Nolen-Hoeksema, S. (1995). Effects of self-focused rumination on negative thinking and interpersonal problem solving. *Journal of Personality and Social Psychology, 69,* 176–190.

Nolen-Hoeksema, S., Grayson, C., & Larson, J. (1991). Explaining the gender difference in depressive symptoms. *Journal of Personality and Social Psychology, 77,* 1061–1072.

Segal, Z. V., Williams, J. M. G., & Teasdale, J. D. (2002). *Mindfulness-based cognitive therapy for depression: A new approach to preventing relapse.* New York: Guilford Press.

Seligman, M. (1975). *Learned helplessness: On depression, development, and death.* San Francisco: Freeman.

Seligman, M. (1990). *Learned optimism.* New York: Alfred A. Knopf.

Seligman, M. (2002). *Authentic happiness.* New York: Free Press.

Snyder, C. R. (1994). *The psychology of hope: You can get from there to here.* New York: Free Press.

Snyder, C. R. (Ed.). (2000). *Handbook of hope: Theory, measures and applications.* San Diego, CA: Academic Press.

Snyder, C. R. (2002). Hope theory: Rainbows in the mind. *Psychological Inquiry, 13,* 249–275.

Street, H. (2000). Exploring relationships between conditional goal setting, rumination and depression. *Australian Journal of Psychology, 52,* 113.

Street, H. (2001). Exploring the role of conditional goal setting in the etiology and maintenance of depression. *Clinical Psychologist, 6,* 6–23.

Street, H. (2002). Exploring relationships between goal setting, goal pursuit and depression: A review. *Australian Psychologist, 37*(2), 95–103.

Vaillant, G. E. (2004). Positive aging. In P. A. Linley & S. Joseph (Eds.), *Positive psychology in practice* (pp. 561–578). Hoboken, NJ: Wiley.

Yapko, M. D. (1997). *Breaking the patterns of depression.* New York: Random House/Doubleday.

Yapko, M. D. (2001). *Treating depression with hypnosis: Integrating cognitive-behavioral and strategic approaches.* New York: Brunner/Routledge.

Yapko, M. D. (Ed.). (2006). *Hypnosis and treating depression: Applications in clinical practice.* New York: Routledge.

CHAPTER 20

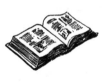

That's Not a Problem

Metaphor with a Disruptive Client in Ericksonian Group Therapy

Teresa Garcia-Sanchez

CONTRIBUTOR'S STORY: A PROFESSIONAL AND PERSONAL PERSPECTIVE

Teresa Garcia-Sanchez, MA, ECP, is the founder and director of the Instituto Erickson in Madrid, Spain; founder of the Asociación Española de Hipnosis Ericksoniana; chairperson of the European Association of Hypnosis and Psychotherapy; and a board member of the European Association of Psychotherapy. She has presented her work internationally at various congresses and universities in Cuba, Mexico, the United States, Spain, Poland, Lithuania, Malta, South Africa, and the United Kingdom, and was on the invited faculty of the 25th anniversary International Congress on Ericksonian Hypnosis and Psychotherapy.

Her father's dinner-table stories absorbed her childhood interest and curiosity with their humor. Continuing the tradition, she used stories with her own two children "to play, to educate, to help, or just to have fun with them" before she started to work with stories in therapy, for similar goals.

When not either doing or teaching therapy, she most enjoys time with family and friends. Traveling, painting, reading, and flower arranging are also high on the list.

PREVIEW THE CHAPTER

We all meet challenging clients at times: the clients who don't follow the textbook examples of how therapy should work. When this happens, as it inevitably will, what do you do? Teresa gives the example of a male client in a group therapy session who was disruptive of the group process and disrespectful of others' issues, yet had some very challenging existential questions of his own. She describes the structure she uses in group work, gives examples of brief experiential metaphors that she calls two-minute metaphors, and then provides a transcript and explanation of the therapist-generated metaphor she used. Her exercises and tales quickly engage a potentially resistant client by metaphorically letting him see her understanding of his issues. From there the therapist-generated metaphor gently and joyfully guides him through processes that open up the prospect of a reframed perception.

Therapeutic Characteristics

Problems Addressed

- The search for answers
- Questions of life
- Hostility
- Anger
- Denigration of others
- Confusion
- Lack of enjoyment

Resources Developed

- Learning flexibility
- Accepting limitations
- Accepting incomplete answers
- Enjoying the process
- Learning to be more relaxed
- Knowing when to stop the search

Outcomes Offered

- Playfulness
- Appreciation of the good times
- Enjoyment of the experience rather than the result
- Appreciation of relationships
- Fun

"**T**hat's not a problem," said Vicente,[1] loudly. This was any group therapist's worst nightmare: a member who was not only not participating in the group processes but who sat at the back of the room actively and verbally denigrating others when they began to discuss their problems. "That's not a problem," he would cry out when various members presented the issues that were so deeply concerning and critical to them. Sometimes it was just a remark to himself; at other times it was a complaint that he wanted heard: "THAT'S NOT A PROBLEM!"

The first time he spoke, I thought, *How strange!* Then with each subsequent interjection my responses, thoughts, and emotions changed. *What lack of respect for the person who is now speaking. Should I allow him to go on like this? What impertinence! All problems have their own importance.* I began to conclude, *Well, it certainly seems that he has a problem. I am going to have to talk to him.* Then I wondered, *Should I intervene? Does he want to provoke me into intervening? What does he think is a problem?* What was clear is that this session certainly had the potential to turn into a problem!

What was I to do? To help answer that question, I will first give some background on the way I work with groups and the context in which the metaphoric interventions were used in this case.

WHY WORK IN GROUPS?

My beginnings as a psychotherapist found me specializing in group therapy from client-centered (Rogers, 1970) and Gestalt models (Perls, 1969; Ginger & Ginger, 1987/1993). Learning about the work of Milton H. Erickson, I decided to follow his example of taking advantage of the power of naturalistic hypnosis and indirect suggestions (Erickson, Rossi, & Rossi, 1976; Geary & Zeig, 2001). It is not the usual practice to apply Ericksonian hypnosis in the context of groups, since Erickson had emphasized the importance of the therapist adapting to the individual client. Trying to individualize therapy and keep several persons together in the process at the same time is not an easy task. However, it occurred to me that, when treating one person and making general comments, it might be possible to make suggestions that were addressed to members in the group, as I have seen Dr. Erickson do in the videos of his training sessions.

With this aim, my group therapy sessions usually follow a simple format. After allowing time for discussion, in which different personal situations commonly come to light, I usually ask for a volunteer for a more individualized intervention. There are several reasons for this individual intervention. On one hand, that person receives complete attention during the meeting, and on the other, the intervention centers everyone else's attention on that person, allowing me to give general or "elastic" examples, metaphors, and suggestions, which may help other members of the group. I finish with a group hypnosis induction, with ingredients that may be useful for everyone as well as for the specific individual's issues.

Not only is group work a practical and inexpensive method of therapy, but it can also accelerate changes and encompass more aspects than the first problem that the client brings up as the main one. Since the participant volunteers present their concerns in public, in front of others, this is a unique experience that often achieves surprisingly effective results. In this volume, Lewis and Perry discuss the values of witnesses and reflecting teams in the enhancement of therapeutic outcomes, while Nel goes so far as to wonder whether any challenge to old, unhelpful discourses can be sustained at all without an audience (Chapters 7, 10 and 9, respectively). Rossi has remarked that he believes a synergy happens when a problem is dealt with in public, and has even talked about a parallel with the healing practices of faith healers (Rossi, 2004).

THE STRUCTURE OF GROUP SESSIONS

Group Composition

The formula I have put into practice is to form a mixed group that contains both people who wish to receive treatment and students who are participating in my training course at the Milton H. Erickson Institute of Madrid. Obviously, all participants are duly informed of the composition of the group.

The Intervention

Each group receives a brief presentation about the format of the forthcoming session in which I seek to explain and clarify the concept of hypnosis as an integral part of the therapy. I like to inquire about what people believe about hypnosis, what they expect from a treatment with both hypnosis and Ericksonian psychotherapy, and how much fantasy or misconception there is in their expectations.

Preparation for Metaphorical Interventions

Disappointment may occur if participants anticipate directive hypnosis, expect a deep and stuporlike trance, or associate the fact that we talk in metaphoric terms with a simple relaxation devoid of explicit therapeutic references. Consequently, I want them to be certain that, even though their problems or desired solutions may not be mentioned directly during the formal hypnosis intervention, they may still obtain positive results. Taking time to demonstrate how a metaphor is effective and how it even has an influence on the client's body usually prepares the participant for the session, increases the efficacy of hypnosis, and heightens a state of curiosity and surprise.

A Two-Minute Metaphor

Exercises are offered that demonstrate how, after listening to a brief metaphor, physical changes can be achieved. These exercises give the participants the opportunity to discover that transformation can take place in bodily experiences after a couple of minutes during which a tale has been told or some images described.

To demonstrate how a metaphoric exercise can influence flexibility, the participants are asked to establish a baseline for their flexibility by standing, then rotating the torso to the right, with an arm outstretched so that they have a reference as to how far they can reach. They are then asked to imagine holding a rope in a vertical position with one hand about 15 inches below the other. I also do the exercise simultaneously with the attendants so that I can join them in their experience and keep my verbalization more coherent with the exercise. I thus guide the visualization, asking them to twist the imaginary rope, turning one hand to the right and the other to the left. Then I ask that they close their eyes so that they "will be able to see the rope better." This paradoxical suggestion (of eyes closed yet seeing better) allows me to observe their responsiveness. Continuing the description of twisting and turning, needing to put in a big, bigger, effort for one or two minutes, often results in a decreasing space between their fists. At that point, I ask them to open their eyes and observe how their hands have moved closer to each other. In doing so, they often think this was the single purpose of the demonstration, so I then say, "Now turn again with your arm outstretched as you did at the beginning, and see if you are able to rotate further."

They are usually surprised by the realization of how much more flexible their bodies have become. They are told that this has demonstrated how the unconscious mind knows how to make the translation between the symbol (the rope in this case) and the application (the flexibility when turning). Despite the absence of direct suggestions about greater skeletal and/or muscular flexibility, the outcome has occurred as the result of listening to a simple metaphor.

Different Exercises for Each Case

I propose different exercises for every person, case, or group session. I choose exercises that will provide a foretaste of the therapeutic metaphors that will come along later during the session. All exercises are short and chosen on the basis of what symbolic and metaphorical value the exercise contains. For example, I may choose the exercise of the imaginary rope for people who are rigid and not willing to incorporate any changes, or for someone in pain who does not believe in the relationship of mind and body. Other exercises would be appropriate for other issues.

The Opportunity to Make Indirect Suggestions

After the demonstration exercise, the group is generally more receptive. They exchange surprised looks and naive smiles, and ratify the changes obtained by sharing the results of the experience with each other. This is a good time to make indirect suggestions in the form of general remarks such as "It is easy to change and to grow," "The most unexpected changes are often carried out effortlessly," "The body can be much more responsive than we think," and the like.

A CHALLENGING CLIENT

Vicente actively continued with his exclamation of "That's not a problem" whenever other participants discussed their concerns—which, not surprisingly, they were becoming reluctant to do. When the time came to choose an exercise to demonstrate metaphors' efficacy, I wanted it to be something that was useful for this person who kept interrupting from the back of the room.

Would I select the rope exercise described earlier, or would I choose one about growth? I thought, *Vicente could do with a metaphor about growing up, one that perhaps communicates that he should stop behaving like a spoiled child.* I hesitated because it seemed to me that I was beginning to project my metaphors onto him and that I also had to be more flexible when respecting the problems of the others—including his. So I chose the rope exercise with its suggestions of flexibility. The exercise appeared beneficial for everyone, and even though it was addressed specifically to Vicente, at no time did I look at him directly or exclusively.

After the coffee break, it seemed as if the echoes of "That's not a problem!" were still thundering in the room as we resumed our seats. It was certainly very much present in my mind, and I felt like it had predicted that *we* would have a problem. This feeling was heightened when I called for a volunteer to work personally with me in front of the group. Vicente was the one who got up! Had he, perhaps, made his attitude more flexible after the rope exercise, or had the change in his bodily experiences intrigued him by activating his need to know so that he wanted to delve some more into this form of therapy?

In truth, I felt a certain relief. It did not seem right to me that such an unsettled member of the group would go away without having explored his concerns in greater depth, especially as he had expressed them so vigorously, loudly, and repeatedly. Besides, I felt somewhat curious and challenged as well.

Without further ado, he left his seat at the back of the room in a sudden and energetic manner. Not waiting for my acceptance, he got up, went to the armchair habitually reserved for volunteers, and sat down. He was tall and thin, with slightly stooped shoulders, just like an adolescent who has grown too quickly and not yet adjusted his eye level. His face was a mixture of disgust, suppressed smile, and inquisitive eyes, and the whole of him expressed tiredness mixed with some rebelliousness.

He sat in the armchair, or rather slid along its surface, again adolescent-like, until he rested on his lumbar region rather than his pelvis. He was able to lean his head on the back of the chair, adopting a spectator stance. This passive attitude was a contrast with the challenging look he threw at me, turning his face toward me when my silence upset him. While I continued absorbing the sensations transmitted by his body, he had both hands on the arms of the chair, and his attitude was both open and wary. He seemed to be saying, *Give me something . . . but it certainly will not be what I want.* And, in that unspoken sentence, I found the "end of the ball of string" from which I could start. He reminded me of an impatient child, almost in a tantrum, a child who cannot be comforted with what he is asking for.

"This is typical!" complained Vicente after I had been silent for a while. My silence was not a therapeutic strategy so much as a need to absorb all the information that was being transmitted. "Typical of certain therapies . . . and, at the same time, it represents very well what is happening to me, what happens to us all! All we have is silence! There are no answers! What the devil are we doing here? I mean in life, in what we call life . . . and, on top of it, we perpetuate ourselves . . . because even I have a daughter!"

His hands, which he flapped without moving his arms, brought to me a whole sentence implicit in his gestures: *"Blah, blah, blah, you are not even giving me any words. You see, this is not going to do me any good . . . once again!"* For a moment, I was afraid that he might be right and that I would have nothing to offer him. And, as if he had guessed my thoughts, he made to get up, saying, "I just never learn. I never learn not to get in these messes . . . not even after so many therapies and therapists."

NOT SEEING WHAT IS

On my notepad was a blank sheet of paper. I picked it up and handed it to him. My first thought was to interrupt his pattern of action: the incipient standing and leaving. However, there were four other reasons as well. First, at that moment it became clear to me that this therapy had to be different. To make it different I had to start by not taking any notes, and I let him know this by handing him the notepad. Second, I had just thought of an experiment to propose to him, and he would need a sheet of paper. Third, giving him the sheet of paper responded to his request, *Give me something.* Finally, if he "won" the challenge he had created, he would lose an opportunity to resolve an issue for which he was clearly, and audibly, seeking help.

What told me, in that fraction of a second, that this was the best stimulus to achieve a different therapeutic result? How is one able to think about so many things in a specific moment? I am not sure I know how to answer that. Perhaps it has something to do with our well-trained thinking about therapy, or maybe it was just a response to a situation of need.

He grabbed the paper and looked at it, and not just with his eyes. His whole face posed a question. His question was silent, and, above all, it was different. There was something closer, more familiar, more immediate, and less transcendental that was asking, *What do I do with this paper?*

I inhaled, felt my body straightening, leaning more on the front edge of the chair. He now had a request, not a demand. He was now more receptive. He was now expecting an indication, an everyday suggestion rather than a transcendental one. The emotion present in that moment was totally different. He was no longer rejecting what I offered but ready to accept the next suggestion. He was asking me to give him direction. It was the time to give him something that was simple but that held a sufficiently important impact to make him open to receive more.

I leaned over the sheet of paper that Vicente was holding and, with a pencil, drew a one-inch-wide black circle and filled it in. This Vicente allowed me do without breaking the silence. I then drew a black cross, the two figures being about four inches apart, center to center. (This drawing is reproduced in Figure 20.1, and this and similar exercises can be found in Maturana and Varela, 1988, pp. 16–23.)

With a mixture of paradoxical intent and therapeutic seeding, I asserted, "You believe that what you can see and touch exists . . . but sometimes you cannot see everything that exists. Your body is a limited instrument."

He raised his head and looked at me, almost expressionless, wanting to check the certainty I was expressing with those words. "Cover your left eye and hold the page about fifteen inches away from you," I continued. "You still see the dot and the cross. Fix your eye on the cross. Notice what happens to the dot. Then slowly move the paper closer to your face. Then further away."

He did so, several times. He was so surprised that he was unable to express his incredulity. His reaction was so frozen that I had trouble identifying the fact that Vicente was repeating the exercise several times because it *was* working for him. When moving the paper back and forth, he had discovered that there was a certain distance where he could *not* see the dot.

And yet the dot was still there.

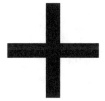

Figure 20.1

I thought, *I should not be surprised that he is careful and discreet in his reaction when realizing that something that is there disappears from his sight. He is an intelligent person, and he is processing the meaning of the experiment. This is not the time to leave him alone. He has already spent years trying to "understand" what is "not understandable."* I gently took the paper away, looking kindly at him.

Vicente crouched slightly, bent his head a little, and gave me a trusting and resigned look, bringing forth in me that protective affection that a child makes you feel when you are taking away his storybook at bedtime and he asks, with that slightly spoiled or dependent attitude, that you stay and tell him the end. My training as a therapist allowed me to identify this as a time to offer self-confidence, courage, joy of living . . . but I also saw his request for certainty and honesty in whatever I would say.

Suddenly *I* was the one who felt childish. It was *not* a matter of increasing his self-esteem, of getting him to focus on the here and now, or of instilling courage. Vicente already had all of these. And with abundance! One needs a lot of courage, strength, and ability to see reality and to face the most basic question: What are we doing here? Even though most of us may have contemplated this at some time, even though we have all vibrated with the emotion of not understanding, we have only had the courage to hold that vertigo for a very brief instant. We have protected ourselves from that total loneliness by setting the whole question aside, or by taking refuge in an already established belief, lacking the courage to continue the quest by ourselves.

A PUZZLING METAPHOR

I saw Vicente as an isolated being, misunderstood because he did not understand what he wanted to understand. In that moment he seemed like a child who wants to reach out and take hold of the moon or who wants answers that are impossible to reach. In a calm, sure, and trusting voice I told him the "end of the story"—the story that had started with a dot he *saw* disappear, even though he *knew* it remained on the paper. Seeing him as a lonely child looking for a response reminded me of an experience I had two weeks before when I shared almost an hour helping a young boy, Ignacio, who, like Vicente, was looking to complete a puzzle. The extraordinary lesson I learned from this child was profound: We can *enjoy the process* even if it is impossible to reach the goal.

What happened with Ignacio and the puzzle was a true story. How I used and emphasized the language, details, and processes is my way of remembering to utilize every opportunity to ratify the responses from the client, and to direct those responses toward the client's goals. With this in mind, I need to be very attentive to the different levels of communication, because a lot of words and images may have several interpretations, connotations, and symbolic meanings. I need to be a very critical observer of every idea that comes to me so that I can assess it and decide if it is going to be useful for the client. Consequently, I improvise the way I tell the story even if the story is based in a real experience, like the one I used with Vicente, choosing what aspects to mention and what not to mention.

In the following metaphor, I chose to add that I sat on the floor. I did so with the clear intention of showing that while seeking to resolve the puzzle I was, myself, at the same level as Ignacio and metaphorically at the same level as Vicente, too. This meant I was not positioning myself in a superior stance or preaching to him about any "truth," for the fact is that I did not have the answers any more than he did. What we were dealing with had more to do with the processes for handling his questions than the answers to those questions. My intention was that joining the character of the metaphor at his level would increase rapport with Vicente, moderate his expectation that I would give him an answer, and seed the outcome that it was possible to enjoy the process even if there is not a prescribed solution. At the same time the image of playing on the floor modeled a joyful and a cheerful experience, while inviting Vicente to engage in and accept what was going on in the process.

The story as I told it is in the left-hand column, and some explanatory notes about my thinking and rationale for using various aspects of the story are provided in the right-hand column.

Not everything you do not see is not there (1). The other day, at some friends' home, I sneaked into their son's room. He had a nearly completed puzzle on the floor (2), with a shoebox almost full of puzzle pieces. Looking closer, I discovered that the pieces belonged to several different puzzles, all of them scenes from a Walt Disney film, *The Little Mermaid*.

They were all mixed up (3). I sat on the floor (4). Ignacio gave me a look: first curious, then enticing. He was encouraging me to play. Yes, because the puzzle was a game, a form of enjoyment. Enjoyment with every little piece located, enjoyment with the thrill of finding, or believing to have found, the missing one (5). Analyzing each shape, comparing it with the empty space, wondering whether it would fit (6). Full of hope, anticipating that you are going to complete it (7) . . . checking, turning it around. It seems to fit, and sometimes it does . . . but you look closer and see that, even if the shape has filled the space, the picture is different. The image has not been completed or is distorted. You have not found what you sought (8). But the thrill of looking comes back, and refills you with energy (9). That whole that you can only see partially in this moment (10) . . . will you be able to get the complete picture? Will you like completing the search? It is so thrilling, it is constantly renewing the process of creating new paths (11) . . . of seeking new ways to go forward, enjoying the path that you create while in the process . . . in the process of finding. And there we were, Ignacio and I, patiently, pleasurably sharing the adventure, an adventure that was even more interesting because we were not alone. Each one of

(1) I began with a paradoxical sentence because Vicente (hereafter referred to as V.) was asking for certitude, because it linked with the previous exercise, and because it activated surprise and curiosity.

(2) I wanted V to associate himself with the child, a nonrationalizing attitude, and completing a metaphoric puzzle.

(3) "Mixed up" parallels V.'s situation.

(4) Sitting on the floor brings associations of caring, playing, sharing, and loving—feelings that I wanted V. to accept from me in an indirect way, as his prior experiences with therapists had not been the best.

(5) Focusing on the joy of process.

(6) Paralleling what V. had been doing.

(7) I was giving V. the chance to recover feelings of hope and experience them again now, orienting them prudently to the process of searching rather than that of finding.

(8) "You" is purposeful, allowing V. to identify with the experience of the main character.

(9) I used an enthusiastic tone, even with the failure to find the right piece, to seed the suggestion that the best game was to play, not to find.

(10) "This moment" invites V. to be in the present of the story, and of life.

(11) The tone of voice communicates enthusiasm about having new options to exercise creativity.

us would search in the pile. Soon, without words, we took different searching paths (12). I would separate the corner pieces of other puzzles. It was a question of eliminating elements and reducing the number of pieces, of uncertainties. He seemed to be selecting the contents, piling up the different colors. After a while, I had become specialized in the edges, backing myself up in the belief that it would be easier to find the missing piece in the puzzle's edge because one of the ends was straight, easier to identify. He continued selecting the details (13), looking for pieces that showed his idol, the Little Mermaid. He discarded other pictures and symbols, such as a starfish, a chest, some pearls. He was not interested in all those treasures; they did not fit in the empty space (14). When one of us thought that we had found *the* piece (15) that we were looking for, we would breathe out, slightly relaxing the bated breath that had accompanied the thrill of the search (16). We would make a soft sound, calling the other's attention. Sensing the importance of the moment, "Has he found it?" we exhaled. Relaxing and stopping the search, we would concentrate on the experience of checking the find. We would both pretend to grant a unique and great value to that moment.

While the other looked on, patiently and expectantly, the piece would be placed in the space. When it did fit, and before the last check, before focusing on the logic of the drawing satisfactorily completing the image, we would enjoy a slight pause, full of complicity, as if, for a moment, we were pretending to want to believe (17) . . . to, perhaps, savor the hope of having obtained an answer . . . giving ourselves the opportunity to savor it, to feed our expectations. And, if we had not achieved it, it would allow us to remain steeped in something like the flavor of success, to strengthen our determination to search (18).

After that shared instant of hope and advance congratulations, after some smiles, we would look at the details (19). No, that was not the piece . . . and we would be cloaked in a subtle and secret caress of relief. We did not have to stop playing! (20) We still had to continue with this process, this complicity, this search!

In that way, I believe we tested all the pieces . . . and

(12) This validates the different ways of looking for a metaphysic answer: the more rational and scientific method versus the more emotional and analogical one.

(13) The emotional way of searching can incorporate "symbols" or "idols," which may be a real treasure chest.

(14) Reminding V. of the need to fill an "empty space."

(15) Emphasis on "the" matches V.'s expectation that there could be only one correct answer.

(16) Matching my breathing to the suggestions of the story modeled those changes for V., added realism, and enabled me to observe his altered respiration as a sign that he was "living" the "adventure" of experiencing the process.

(17) These comments are designed to increase the suspense and communicate a contradictory emotion: We want to find the piece yet we don't want to stop looking for it. At the same time, a slower rhythm and tone of slight sadness anticipate that the puzzle and story are going to finish. (18) With a change in tone, I start talking about "strength and determination" to go on. Even if we do not find the answer, we will be looking for it together. (19) This paragraph introduces the hope of finding a new path. (20) "We did not have to stop playing" could represent "a subtle caress of relief" because to find the solution and stop playing could be a finality.

continuing seemed to me an empty endeavor (21). I felt disoriented and confused, not having found the last two pieces. Then Angeles, Ignacio's mother, entered the room (22). She smiled when she saw us, and calmly sat on the floor next to Ignacio. She looked at him, looked at the puzzle, looked at me with a great smile, patted Ignacio's head, and invited him to go to his bath . . . and Ignacio started picking up the pieces (23).

How can I describe my surprise when I saw such acceptance? (24) There were no arguments or complaints: "We are nearly finished!" or "Let us finish the last two pieces!" My face must have shown it. Angeles gave an answer to my confusion: "Those two pieces have been missing for quite a while. Ignacio knows it very well," she said (25).

Angeles and Ignacio went to the bathroom. I was left open mouthed. The big smile with which he confirmed his mother's "Ignacio knows it very well" told me that he did, indeed, know it very well. There was no mockery or deceit in that smile; there was only complicity and playfulness (26). We had had such a good time! (27)

Ignacio knew . . . but had been pretending to search. He was *really* interested in finding something that he knew did not exist (28). He was playing at finding what he knew was not there. *His* game was not to fill in the empty spaces. *His* game was to feel himself accompanied while he tried (29). *The enjoyment came from the experience, not from the result, since he knew there was no possibility to complete the whole* (30).

The thing is that, even though some pieces may be missing, it is still a game, and you can continue having fun (31).

(21) "An empty endeavor" along with "disoriented and confused" feelings matched what V. was experiencing.

(22) Angeles, coincidentally, was her true name, but utilizing it helped to make an association with some higher intervention: an angel.

(23) Here the main character models for V. acceptance of an unsolved puzzle.

(24) I hoped "my surprise" reflected V.'s emotion about such acceptance.

(25) The core message of the metaphor: Pieces may be missing, the puzzle may not be soluble, but even with this knowledge one can still enjoy the process.

(26) The statement that "There was no mockery," only "complicity and playfulness" is respectful of V.'s wonderings. (27) An invitation to have fun and enjoy life without always being focused on questions that can't be answered. (28) This sentence forms a paradoxical bridge to the exercise of the dot on the paper that V. knew existed but was unable to see.

(29) Here the outcome is reframed from finding a solution to enjoying company in the process.

(30) The metaphoric message is reiterated with emphasis. (31) I wanted to finish the story by reiterating the concept of fun, hoping it would resonate in V.'s thoughts and enable him to more truly enjoy his life.

I was still talking when Vicente, who had been silent and looking to me with unfocused eyes, made to get up, as if to indicate that the session was over. Before getting completely to his feet, he said, "I have no idea why you are telling me all this." There was no reproof in the remark—in fact, the opposite. His voice was deliberate, pleasant, and secure, somewhat more adult, I thought. He continued, "But it has 'reached' me. It is the first time that I feel that I have communicated with someone, that I am not alone." He changed his tone and added, in a reflective manner, "When I think of how many therapies I have done—and my therapist is fond of me, I know—but I would love to be able to tell him that what I need is this kind of communication, to feel that he is with me." As if talking to himself, he said, "Nobody told me that one can play even if one does not have all the pieces!"

A REFLECTION

If I had to justify why I am working in therapy, I would say that it is because, from time to time, I have the privilege of participating in the simplest and most basic human experience, by facing the raw reality of what we may call an existential crisis—which, in fact, is nothing more than becoming aware that we are all protagonists in this adventure of living.

Perhaps this is *the* problem, the one in which we all partake, the one that is intrinsic to life, that we cannot solve—which, however, we manage to forget, to set aside, or at least to ban from our lives without awakening in ourselves the anguished emotion that it should be granted. There are, nevertheless, some people who have not renounced the question of why and how we are here. And Vicente was one.

Two years after the session of therapy I have described here, I ran into Vicente and his daughter quite by coincidence. We said hello, and he looked at me with complicity while he touched, to show me, the pendant his daughter was wearing. It was a figure of the Little Mermaid.

1. When initially writing this chapter I used a pseudonym for Vicente. However, later we resumed contact regarding an unrelated matter, and I gave him the draft of this chapter to read. After reading it, he asked to be identified by his real name. That I have done with great pleasure. Gracias, Vicente, Ignacio, and Angeles.

REFERENCES

Erickson, M. H., Rossi, E. L., & Rossi, S. (1976). *Hypnotic realities: The induction of clinical hypnosis and forms of indirect suggestion.* New York: Irvington.

Geary, B. J., & Zeig, J. K. (Eds.). (2001). *The handbook of Ericksonian psychotherapy.* Phoenix, AZ: Milton H. Erickson Foundation Press.

Ginger, S., & Ginger, A. (1993). *La Gestalt: Una terapia de contacto.* Mexico: El manual Moderno. (Original work, in French, published 1987)

Maturana, H. R., & Verela, F. J. (1988). *The tree of knowledge: The biological roots of human understanding.* Boston: New Science Library.

Perls, F. (1969). *Gestalt therapy verbatim.* Moab, UT: Real People Press.

Rogers, C. (1970). *Carl Rogers on encounter groups.* New York: Harper & Row.

Rossi, E. L. (2004). *A discourse with our genes.* Benevento, Italy: Editris.

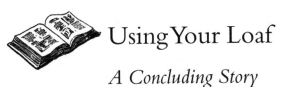

Using Your Loaf

A Concluding Story

As a therapy session draws toward its conclusion, I begin to wonder how to wrap up the session in the way that is most useful for the client. Is it helpful for me to sum up some of the points that we have covered or put emphasis upon one particular thing? Is it helpful to validate an insight or sense of empowerment that the client has discovered himself? Is it helpful to set a homework assignment like an experiential metaphor or ask the client to write a story about reaching the desired outcome?

In wrapping up a book I feel a similar challenge, and more so with this book than any of my previous books. What could I say that has not already been said in the preceding pages? How could I sum up the richness of ideas, examples, and approaches presented? And when I defined *what* might be helpful to say, *how* could I do that effectively? Of course, the idea of concluding a book on metaphors with a story was not far from my thinking. But what story would be beneficial for me to tell? The theme I ultimately chose was seeded by a couple of simple everyday experiences in my life, like taking a phone call and making a loaf of bread. Perhaps it may be helpful for me to describe that process as an illustration of how a story idea can be formulated and a metaphor developed.

My mind was pondering these challenges of how to conclude while I was baking a loaf of bread. My daughter and son-in-law had given me a bread-maker for Christmas, and I was enjoying the process of experimenting with the creation of many different types and styles of loaves. At the point that I was about to take a light rye loaf out of the oven, the phone rang. It was one of my peer reviewers, Pam Thompson, who spoke enthusiastically about the diversity of the contributions in this book. As she did, I thought to myself, *yes, that is something I would like to communicate in wrapping up.* I also wanted to invite you, as a reader, to explore and examine that variety, to see the styles of working that fit well for you and the clients you work with. Perhaps I could comment on how it might be useful to experiment with some of the approaches that do not hold immediate appeal, to see if they work in your particular therapeutic context. While it might be nice to read inspiring cases, I would also want to add that the time spent reading them only becomes meaningful if there are things you can take from them and put into practice to benefit your own clients.

Knowing what I wanted to communicate then posed me a question: "Well, how do I say these things in the most helpful and most effective way? How can I, in the words of Zeig (2006), *gift wrap* that message?"

As I hung up from speaking with Pam, put on the oven gloves and lifted my rye bread from the oven, smelling its soft and slightly sweet aroma, the seed of an idea for a story began to form. Later that day as I took a walk along the beach, the sea breeze blowing stiffly in my face, my feet sinking into soft, calf-straining sand, and waves crashing on the shore, I began to flesh out the story. A desirable outcome might be for the character to learn from the masters of his trade, and adapt that learning to his own customers and work. Resources to help him get there might be the desire to better his skills, a willingness to learn, an understanding of the processes, and an openness to adapt and experiment. The problem or challenge that might start the story off would be to improve his skills, bring joy to others, and better help them be more self-sustaining and self-nourishing—a process that was perhaps not dissimilar to what I was encountering while learning to bake bread.

Later I tested the story out on a kind friend who had already read some of the chapters. "If you were a reader of this book, would this story be a helpful or meaningful conclusion for you?" I asked. When I had written it up, I asked a similar question of my peer reviewers. This is what evolved from the process.

Once there was a young woman—though she could just as easily have been a man—who wanted to develop the craft of her calling. Ruth had enjoyed baking in her earlier years, playing, learning, and creating in the kitchen with her mother. She had enjoyed seeing the pleasure people got when she presented them with a gift of her baked goods, and she wanted to make a profession of doing something that would nourish and nurture others. Consequently, she set out on a mission to find how to make the best loaf of bread possible, the one that would be the most satisfying, enjoyable, and nourishing.

Ruth's search first took her to France, where she asked around, seeking to find the very best baker from whom she could learn. All the recommendations pointed toward Antoinette Pasquel. When they met, Antoinette happily took Ruth under her wing, teaching her both the science and the art of making the best baguettes France had to offer. People would queue up at Antoinette's doorstep early every morning. She would wrap the freshly baked bread in crisp white paper, and Ruth noticed that her customers walked away smiling happily. Knowing that this was what she wanted to do for people, too, Ruth was keen to rush home and try out the new loaves. "Wait," called Antoinette before she departed, "there is one thing you must know. Remember, you are not in this for the dough."

Ruth hurried home. She worked and worked at perfecting the art of the baguette. Smelling her fresh-baked baguettes, people began to form queues like they had at Antoinette's. Ruth similarly wrapped their bread in paper, watched them walk away happily, and felt contented. Some came back to tell her it was the best bread they had ever tasted, while others complained that it was too long or too crispy. Some said it was too small to make a decent sandwich.

Disappointed that her baguettes hadn't satisfied everyone, Ruth determined to continue on her mission. In Germany her inquiries about the best baker led her to Rolf Schneider, who was considered the master of the pumpernickel. Rolf similarly took Ruth under his wing, teaching her the science, the art, and the finesse of making heavy, dark German rye bread. Ruth saw the customers lining up early in the morning for Rolf's pumpernickel. Rolf inserted their loaves into brown paper bags, and the people left with smiles on their faces. Ruth could not wait to get home to try what she had learned. "But wait," called Rolf before she departed, "there is one thing you must know. Always remember which side your customer's bread is buttered on."

At home Ruth worked and worked to perfect the pumpernickel. Soon people were lining up at her door. She put the heavy dark loaves in brown paper bags for them and watched as they walked away happily. Over the next few days some declared her bread the best they had ever tasted, while others found it too dense, or too dark, or lacking in versatility.

Ruth was not deterred from her mission. In Italy her inquiries led her to Maria Cicero. When Ruth explained what she was seeking, Maria took her under her wing too, teaching her the science and art of making the finest focaccia. People queued up at the doorstep every morning as Maria placed the slices of focaccia in cardboard boxes and handed them to her customers, who walked away with happy expressions on their faces. "This is it," thought Ruth. "I have finally found the best bread." "Wait," called Maria as she was about to rush back home and bake her own focaccia. "There is something you should remember. Some people may not accept all that you have to offer. Sometimes half a loaf may be better than none."

Ruth worked and worked at perfecting the focaccia. People lined up at her doorstep. She put slices in little cardboard boxes, and her customers walked away with delighted expressions on their faces. Some came back over the ensuing days, saying her focaccia was definitely the best bread they had ever tasted, but others complained that they would like a lighter or plainer loaf.

Not daunted, Ruth continued on her mission to find the best bread she could offer. In Greece she learned to make pita. In India she learned the art of making naan. In fact, she traveled to several countries before arriving in Australia. There her inquiries led her to Bluey Jones. Now, Bluey didn't have your regular baker's shop on a fashionable city street. He was a shearer's cook in the outback, where he was known for his damper, an unleavened bread cooked in a cast iron camp oven over an open fire. Shearers and stock hands from all around queued up for it in the morning, and Bluey tossed the steaming hot damper on their chipped enamel plates as if he were throwing a Frisbee. Ruth watched as they walked away with happy smiles on their faces. She couldn't wait to get home to try the recipe. "Wait," called Bluey as he saw Ruth about to depart. "There is one thing you need to remember: Create your bread from your heart, and always use your loaf."

Back home Ruth worked to perfect the damper, experimenting and developing it by adding feta cheese, spinach, and other ingredients. People gathered in the morning for her bread, and she refined the process by serving it on paper plates, which people walked away holding happily. Over the next few days some sung her praises for the best bread they had ever tasted, while others complained that it was too heavy, or too salty, or didn't suit their palate.

At first Ruth was disappointed that she hadn't found the right loaf to suit everyone, but then she began to use her loaf, and thought, *The greater variety of bread or buns I have in the oven, the greater my chances of contributing to the happiness and well-being of the people I serve.* So instead of trying to fit people to the loaf, she began to match her loaves to each of her individual customers. Ruth observed what crusty loaf Mrs. Smith requested each day, what variety of naan Mr. Singh favored, what style of bread suited the sandwiches Mr. Thomas liked to make for lunch, and how Ms. Garcia could not tolerate gluten. Each loaf she packaged individually to suit both the bread and the customer, excitedly wondering what joy her customers might experience when unwrapping it.

Continually mindful of everything she had learned along the way, and particularly of Bluey's comment about remembering to use your heart and your loaf, she came upon the idea of teaching others to make their own loaves. *This,* she thought, *is where my journeys and learning have taken me: to be a little part of the process of empowering others to discover the art of sustaining and nourishing themselves.*

And that is how the story evolved.

REFERENCE

Zeig, J. K. (2006). *Confluence: The selected papers of Jeffrey K. Zeig.* Phoenix, AZ: Zeig, Tucker & Theisen.

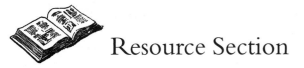

Resource Section

FURTHER READING RESOURCES

At times, as you have read the preceding chapters, you may have found yourself thinking I would like to know more about this author's work with metaphor or in other areas. Rather than requiring the reader to wade through all the references for each chapter in which some contributors have cited some of their work, and some haven't, I thought it might be helpful to have a succinct list of their books and major book chapters in this separate section. Many contributors have been very prolific communicators of their work in the published form, while for some the chapter here is their first major publication. Therefore not all contributors are in the following list. In addition, I specifically asked that they not include journal articles (of which a number of authors have published many), first, because such a list would prove to be too lengthy and, second, because articles may not be as readily available as books to most practitioners.

Battino, R. (1999). *Meaning: A play based on the life of Viktor E. Frankl.* Carmarthen, UK: Crown House.

Battino, R. (2000). *Guided imagery and other approaches to healing.* Carmarthen, UK: Crown House.

Battino, R. (2001). *Coping: A practical guide for people who have life-challenging diseases and their caregivers.* Carmarthen, UK: Crown House.

Battino, R. (2002). *Metaphoria: Metaphor and guided metaphor for psychotherapy and healing.* Williston, VT: Crown House.

Battino, R. (2006). *Expectation: The very brief therapy book.* Carmarthen, UK: Crown House.

Battino, R. (2006). *That's right, is it not? A play based on the life of Milton H. Erickson, M.D.* Phoenix, AZ: Milton H. Erickson Foundation Press.

Battino, R., & South, T. L. (2005). *Ericksonian approaches: A comprehensive manual* (2nd ed.). Carmarthen, UK: Crown House.

Burns, G. W. (1995). Psychoecotherapy: An hypnotic model. In G. Burrows & R. Stanley (Eds.), *Contemporary international hypnosis* (pp. 279–284). London: Wiley.

Burns, G. W. (1998). *Nature-guided therapy: Brief integrative strategies for health and wellbeing.* Philadelphia: Brunner/Mazel.

Burns, G. W. (2001). *101 healing stories: Using metaphors in therapy.* New York: Wiley. (Also published in Chinese, Spanish, and Indonesian)

Burns, G. W. (2001). Jay Haley: The man who made therapy an ordeal. In J. K. Zeig (Ed.), *Changing directives: The strategic therapy of Jay Haley* (pp. 154–170). Phoenix, AZ: Milton H. Erickson Foundation Press.

Burns, G. W. (2005). *101 healing stories for kids and teens: Using metaphors in therapy.* Hoboken, NJ: Wiley. (Also published in Italian, Spanish, Korean, and Chinese)

Burns, G. W. (2005). Naturally happy, naturally healthy: The role of the natural environment in well-being. In F. Huppert, B. Keverne, & N. Baylis (Eds.), *The science of well-being* (pp. 405–431). Oxford: Oxford University Press.

Burns, G. W. (2006). Building coping skills with metaphors. In M. D. Yapko (Ed.), *Hypnosis and treating depression: Applications in clinical practice* (pp. 49–69). New York: Routledge.

Burns, G. W., & Street, H. (2003). *Standing without shoes: Creating happiness, relieving depression, enhancing life.* Sydney, Australia: Prentice Hall. (Also published in Portuguese and Spanish)

Cecchin, G., Lane, G., & Ray, W. (1994). *The cybernetics of prejudices in the practice of psychotherapy.* London: Karnac Books. (Also published in Italian)

Cecchin, G., Lane, G., & Ray, W. (2003). *Irreverence: A strategy for therapists' survival.* London: Karnac Books. (Originally published 1992; also published in Spanish, Italian, and German)

Cone, J. D., & Hayes, S. C. (1980). *Environmental problems / behavioral solutions.* Monterey, CA: Brooks/Cole. (Republished in 1986 by Cambridge University Press)

Dahl, J., Wilson, K. G., Luciano, C., & Hayes, S. C. (2005). *Acceptance and commitment therapy for chronic pain.* Reno, NV: Context Press.

Erickson, B. A., & Erickson Klein, R. (1991). Milton H. Erickson's increasing shift to less directive hypnotic techniques as illustrated by work with family members. In S. Lankton, S. Gilligan, & J. Zeig (Eds.), *Views on Ericksonian brief therapy, process and action* (Ericksonian Monographs No. 8; pp. 106–116). New York: Brunner/Mazel.

Erickson, B. A., Erickson, E., & Erickson Klein, R. (1999). Erickson: A framework of therapy and living. In W. Mathews & J. Edgette (Eds.), *Current thinking and research in brief therapy: Solutions, strategies, narratives* (pp. 7–18). New York: Taylor & Francis.

Erickson Klein, R. (1988). How Milton H. Erickson encouraged individuality in his children. In J. Zeig & S. Lankton (Eds.), *Developing Ericksonian therapy* (pp. 498–501). New York: Brunner/Mazel.

Erickson Klein, R. (1990). Pain control interventions of Milton H. Erickson. In J. Zeig & S. Gilligan (Eds.), *Brief therapy: Myths, methods and metaphors* (pp. 273–291). New York: Brunner/Mazel.

Erickson Klein, R. (2004). True friendship. In S. Kane & K. Olness (Eds.), *The art of therapeutic communication: The therapeutic works of Kay F. Thompson* (pp. 509–516). Carmarthen, UK: Crown House.

Frusha, V., Ray, W., & Hale, D. (1999). Intentional use of implication: An unexplored aspect of the MRI brief therapy model. In W. Ray & S. de Shazer (Eds.), *Evolving brief therapies* (pp. 57–67). Iowa City, IA: Geist & Russell.

Hayes, S. C. (Ed.). (1989). *Rule-governed behavior: Cognition, contingencies, and instructional control.* New York: Plenum Press.

Hayes, S. C., Barlow, D. H., & Nelson-Grey, R. O. (1999). *The scientist-practitioner: Research and accountability in the age of managed care* (2nd ed.). New York: Allyn & Bacon.

Hayes, S. C., Barnes-Holmes, D., & Roche, B. (2001). (Eds.). *Relational frame theory: A post-Skinnerian account of human language and cognition.* New York: Plenum Press.

Hayes, S. C., Follette, V. M., Dawes, R. M., & Grady, K. E. (Eds.). (1995). *Scientific standards of psychological practice: Issues and recommendations.* Reno, NV: Context Press.

Hayes, S. C., Follette, V. M., & Linehan, M. M. (Eds.). (2004). *Mindfulness and acceptance: Expanding the cognitive behavioral tradition.* New York: Guilford Press.

Hayes, S. C., & Hayes, L. J. (Eds.). (1992). *Understanding verbal relations.* Reno, NV: Context Press.

Hayes, S. C., Hayes, L. J., Reese, H. W., & Sarbin, T. R. (Eds.). (1993). *Varieties of scientific contextualism.* Reno, NV: Context Press.

Hayes, S. C., Hayes, L. J., Sato, M., & Ono, K. (Eds.). (1994). *Behavior analysis of language and cognition.* Reno, NV: Context Press.

Hayes, S. C., & Heiby, E. (1998). *Prescription privileges for psychologists: A critical appraisal.* Reno, NV: Context Press.

Hayes, S. C., Jacobson, N. S., Follette, V. M., & Dougher, M. J. (Eds.). (1994). *Acceptance and change: Content and context in psychotherapy.* Reno, NV: Context Press.

Hayes, S. C., & Smith, S. (2005). *Get out of your mind and into your life: The new acceptance and commitment therapy.* Oakland, CA: New Harbinger.

Hayes, S. C., & Strosahl, K. D. (Eds.). (2004). *A practical guide to acceptance and commitment therapy.* New York: Springer-Verlag.

Hayes, S. C., Strosahl, K., & Wilson, K. G. (1999). *Acceptance and commitment therapy: An experiential approach to behavior change.* New York: Guilford Press.

Keeney, B., & Ray, W. (1990). Hilda's gallery: Orchestration of a case. In B. Keeney, *Therapeutic improvisations: A practical guide for creative clinical strategies,* (pp. 82–106). New York: Guilford. (also published in German, Spanish, Italian, & Japanese)

Keeney, B., & Ray, W. (1996). Resource focused therapy. In M. Hoyt (Ed.), *Constructive therapies: Vol. 2* (pp. 334–346). New York: Guilford Press.

Kopp, R. (1995). *Metaphor therapy: Using client-generated metaphors in psychotherapy.* New York: Brunner/Mazel/ Taylor & Francis.

Kopp, R. (2001). Metaphor therapy. In R. Corsini (Ed.), *Handbook of innovative psychotherapies* (pp. 381–391). New York: Wiley.

Lankton, C. (1985). Elements of an Ericksonian approach. In S. Lankton (Ed.), *Elements and dimensions of an Ericksonian approach* (Ericksonian Monograph No. 1; pp. 61–75). New York: Brunner/Mazel.

Lankton, C. (1988). Task assignments: Logical and otherwise. In S. Lankton & J. Zeig (Eds.), *Developing Ericksonian psychotherapy: State of the arts* (pp. 257–279). New York: Brunner/Mazel.

Lankton, C. (2000). Using hypnosis to transform sleep disruptions with active intention. *Sleep and Hypnosis, 2*(4), 163–170.

Lankton, C. (2001). Marriage contracts that work. In B. Geary & J. Zeig (Eds.), *The handbook of Ericksonian psychotherapy* (pp. 416–431). Phoenix, AZ: Milton H. Erickson Foundation Press.

Lankton, C. (2004). Therapeutic alliances in the pursuit of sexual pleasure. In D. Flemons & S. Green (Eds.), *Quickies: Brief sex therapy* (pp. 45–67). New York: Norton.

Lankton, C., & Lankton, S. R. (1989). *Tales of enchantment: Goal-oriented metaphors for adults and children in therapy.* New York: Brunner/Mazel.

Lankton, S. R., & Lankton, C. (1983). *The answer within: A clinical framework of Ericksonian hypnotherapy.* New York: Brunner/Mazel.

Lankton, S. R., & Lankton, C. (1985). Ericksonian styles of paradoxical therapy. In G. Weeks (Ed.), *Promoting change through paradoxical therapy* (pp. 134–186). Homewood, IL: Dorsey Press.

Lankton, S. R., & Lankton, C. (1986). *Enchantment and intervention in family therapy: training in Ericksonian hypnosis.* New York: Brunner/Mazel.

Lankton, S. R., & Lankton, C. (1996). Application of Ericksonian principles to larger systems. In W. Matthews & J. Edgette (Eds.), *The evolution of brief therapy: Vol. 1* (pp. 215–238). New York: Brunner/Mazel.

Lankton, S. R., & Lankton, C. (1998). Ericksonian emergent epistemologies: Embracing a new paradigm. In M. Hoyt (Ed.), *The handbook of constructive therapies* (pp. 116–136). San Francisco: Jossey-Bass.

McNeilly, R. B. (2000). *Healing the whole person: A solution-focused approach to using empowering language, emotions, and actions in therapy.* New York: Wiley.

McNeilly, R. B. (2001). Creating a context for hypnosis. In B. B. Geary & J. K. Zeig (Eds.), *The handbook of Ericksonian psychotherapy* (pp. 57–65). Phoenix, AZ: Milton H Erickson Foundation Press.

McNeilly, R. B. (in press). *Learning solutions in counseling and hypnosis: A series of DVD demonstrations.* Carmarthen, UK: Crown House.

McNeilly, R. B., & Brown, J. (1994). *Healing with words.* Melbourne, Australia: Hill of Content. (Translated into Portuguese)

Mills, J. C. (1994). *Gentle willow: A book for children about dying.* Washington, DC: Magination Press.

Mills, J. C. (1999). *Reconnecting to the magic of life: A tapestry of healing stories and practical stepping stones that inspire our natural abilities to rekindle joy and embrace change.* Phoenix, AZ: Imaginal Press. (Translated into French and Portuguese)

Mills, J. C. (2001). Dreaming pots: A natural healing approach for helping children with fears and trauma. In H. G. Kaduson & C. E. Schaefer (Eds.), *101 more play therapy techniques* (pp. 152–158). North Vale, NJ: Jason Aronson.

Mills, J. C. (2001). Ericksonian play therapy: The spirit of healing with children and adolescents. In B. B. Geary and J. K. Zeig (Eds.), *The handbook of Ericksonian psychotherapy* (pp. 506–521). Phoenix, AZ: Milton H. Erickson Foundation Press.

Mills, J. C. (2003). *Little tree: A book for children with serious medical problems* (2nd ed.). Washington, DC: Magination Press.

Mills, J. C. (2006). The bowl of light: A story-craft for healing. In L. Carey (Ed.), *Expressive and creative arts methods for trauma survivors* (pp. 207–213). London: Jessica Kingsley.

Mills, J. C., & Crowley, R. (1985). *Fred Flintstone helps protect the vegetables.* A therapeutic comic book commissioned by Childhelp USA.

Mills, J. C., & Crowley, R. (1986). *Therapeutic metaphors for children and the child within.* Philadelphia: Taylor & Francis. (This book was awarded the 1988 Clark Vincent Award for an outstanding contribution to the profession through a literary work by the California Association of Marriage and Family Therapists. Also available in French, German, Italian, and Russian)

Mills, J. C., & Crowley, R. (1988). *Cartoon magic.* Washington, DC: Magination Press.

Mills, J. C., & Crowley, R. (1988). *Sammy the elephant and Mr. Camel.* Washington, DC: Magination Press.

Nelson, R. O., & Hayes, S. C. (Eds.). (1986). *Conceptual foundations of behavioral assessment.* New York: Guilford Press.

O'Donohue, W. T., Henderson, D. A., Hayes, S. C., Fisher, J. E., & Hayes, L. J. (2001). *A history of the behavioral therapies: Founders' personal histories.* Reno, NV: Context Press.

Ray, W. (1995). The interactional therapy of Don D. Jackson. In J. Weakland & W. Ray (Eds.), *Propagations: Thirty years of influence from the mental research institute* (pp. 37–70). New York: Haworth Press.

Ray, W. (2001). "Rabid" and "rapid" psychotherapy on the jet propelled couch: Pivotal moments in the evolution of paradoxical prescription. In J. Zeig (Ed.), *Changing directives: The strategic psychotherapy of Jay Haley* (pp. 29–41). Phoenix, AZ: Zeig, Tucker & Theisen.

Ray, W. (2005). The theory and therapy of Don D. Jackson. In Keizo Hasagawa (Ed.), *The pragmatics of communication in clinical psychology: Vol. 2* (pp. 50–58). Tokyo: Kaneko Shobo. (In Japanese)

Ray, W. (Ed.). (2006). *Don D. Jackson: Selected essays at the dawn of an era: Vol 1.* Reading, MA: Zeig, Tucker & Theissen.

Ray, W., & de Shazer, S. (Eds.). (1999). *Evolving brief therapies.* Iowa City, IA: Geist & Russell.

Ray, W., & Díaz, B. (2004). "Don't get too bloody optimistic": John Weakland at Work. In S. Green & D. Flemons (Eds.), *Quickies: Brief sex therapy* (pp. 213–249). New York: Norton.

Ray, W., & Keeney, B. (1993). *Resource focused therapy.* London: Karnac Books.

Ray, W., Keeney, B., & Stormberg, J. (1999). Resource focused therapy with a "poly-substance" abusing young adult. In W. Ray & S. de Shazer (Eds.), *Evolving brief therapies* (pp. 97–131). Iowa City, IA: Geist & Russell.

Ray, W., & Schlanger, K. (1999). John Weakland: A bibliography. In W. Ray & S. de Shazer (Eds.), *Evolving brief therapies* (pp. 233–236). Iowa City, IA: Geist & Russell.

Ray, W., & Watzlawick, P. (2005). El enfoque interaccional Conceptos perdurables del Mental Research Institute (MRI). In Arturo Roizenblatt (Ed.), *Terapia Familiar y de Pareja* (pp. 191–208). Santiago, Chile: Editorial Mediterráneo.

Short, D., Erickson, B. A., & Erickson Klein, R. (2005). *Hope and resiliency: Understanding the psychotherapeutic strategies of Milton H. Erickson, MD.* Norwalk, CT: Crown House.

Weakland, J., & Ray, W. (Eds.). (1995). *Propagations: Thirty years of influence from the mental research institute.* New York: Haworth Press.

Yapko, M. D. (1988). *When living hurts: Directives for treating depression.* New York: Brunner/Mazel.

Yapko, M. D. (Ed.). (1989). *Brief therapy approaches to treating anxiety and depression.* New York: Brunner/Mazel.

Yapko, M. D. (1992). *Free yourself from depression.* Emmaus, PA: Rodale Press.

Yapko, M. D. (1992). *Hypnosis and the treatment of depressions: Strategies for change.* New York: Brunner/Mazel.

Yapko, M. D. (1994). *Suggestions of abuse: True and false memories of childhood sexual trauma.* New York: Simon & Schuster.

Yapko, M. D. (1995). *Essentials of hypnosis.* New York: Brunner/Mazel.

Yapko, M. D. (1997). *Breaking the patterns of depression.* New York: Random House/Doubleday.

Yapko, M. D. (1999). *Hand-me-down blues: How to stop depression from spreading in families.* New York: St. Martin's.

Yapko, M. D. (2001). *Treating depression with hypnosis: Integrating cognitive-behavioral and strategic approaches.* New York: Brunner/Routledge.

Yapko, M. D. (2004). *Trancework: An introduction to the practice of clinical hypnosis* (3rd ed.). New York: Brunner/Routledge.

Yapko, M. D. (Ed.). (2006). *Hypnosis and treating depression: Applications in clinical practice.* New York: Routledge.

CONTRIBUTORS' FAVORITE METAPHOR BOOKS

As I read the preceding chapters, I found myself wondering what books had influenced the contributors' thinking about metaphor, which authors or thinkers had guided their practice, and what had shaped their work to its current state, so I decided to ask them. I requested each to list his or her three favorite metaphor books and write a sentence or two about what the contributor liked about each. There were no other guidelines, which allowed contributors to choose from discourses on metaphor, practitioner texts, storybooks that have given them ideas or inspiration, books of cross-cultural tales, and so on. The following list, presented in alphabetical order with the contributors' initials after their comments, is the result of that inquiry. I hope it is a helpful guide for extending your reading in the field of metaphor or harking back to some of the original sources.

Barker, P. (1985). *Using metaphors in psychotherapy.* New York: Brunner/Mazel.
>   *Barker provides a warm and compassionate yet clinical consideration of the role of metaphor in a variety of clinical contexts, helping the reader develop both an effective framework for designing and delivering metaphors.* [MY]

Battino, R. (2002). *Metaphoria: Metaphor and guided metaphor for psychotherapy and healing.* Williston, VT: Crown House.

    This book couples an analysis of the nuts and bolts of metaphor creation with the written metaphors of a gifted storyteller. Reframing Erickson's task-oriented assignments, such as ordeals and ambiguous function assignments, as metaphors cannot help but provide the reader with a new perspective. [GS]

    Battino reviews what many of the acknowledged experts say about metaphor and then goes well beyond them by adding his own insightful stories and perspectives, providing a broad and deep array of therapeutic possibilities for employing metaphors in treatment. [MY]

Bettelheim, B. (1984). *Freud and man's soul.* New York: Vintage Books.

    In this small but important book Bettelheim offers unique insight into Freud's humanism that is literally lost in the English translation. The author vividly demonstrates the essential role of metaphor in Freud's thought and theory. [RK]

Brahm, A. (2004). *Opening the door of your heart: And other Buddhist tales of happiness.* Melbourne, Australia: Lothian Books.

    Build a wall of 1,000 bricks, and what do you notice—the well-laid 998 or the 2 you misaligned? Brahm, a Western monk, offers 108 such modern, everyday experiences as samples of spiritual tales to delightfully communicate ancient wisdom for living the happy life. A great opportunity to observe a skillful teller of wise and compassionate healing stories. [GB]

Bruchac, J. (2003). *Our stories remembered.* Golden, CO: Fulcrum.

    This book is a treasure trove of stories honoring the complexity of the Native American culture, history, and values. The stories open the inner door to wisdom through which begs each of us to look within the stories of our own culture in order to learn more about our families. [JM]

Burns, G. W. (2001). *101 healing stories: Using metaphors in therapy.* New York: Wiley.

    Having predominantly worked with cultural myths and client-generated metaphors, I found this book a lovely introduction to the use of therapist-created metaphors. The myriad of stories reflecting the wisdom of the world are a practical and immensely useful source for using metaphors in therapy. Burns's suggestions and ideas about the use of metaphors are also a helpful guidance for people beginning to apply metaphors in therapy. [AE]

    A very practical and creative resource that awakened my interest in adapting and developing stories or metaphors as an indirect, non-threatening way to engage and empower clients throughout the therapeutic process. The underlying themes in these stories from around the world impart cross-cultural values, wisdom, and understanding that help clients effect change in their lives. [CP]

    Not only are Burns's stories entertaining and engaging, but he provides a practical framework for employing metaphors and identifying the contexts where the stories might best be used. A sensible approach to an approach where sense isn't always immediately evident. [MY]

Burns, G. W. (2005). *101 healing stories for kids and teens: Using metaphors in therapy.* Hoboken, NJ: Wiley.

    Though I had long been working with and teaching metaphors, this book opened new relaxed, playful and vivid ways for children and adolescents to discover their own answers and healing stories. A must-read, must-use book for therapists, teachers, parents, or anyone working and relating with children. [TGS]

Campbell, J. (1986). *The inner reaches of outer space: Metaphor as myth and as religion.* New York: Harper & Row.

    Joe Campbell's prose is lucid and his ideas are profound. He explains how myth can only be understood as metaphor and reveals metaphoric themes common across cultures throughout human history. [RK]

Campbell, J. (1988). *The power of myth.* New York: Doubleday.

   This book is a must for understanding not just the techniques involved in creating metaphors, but more importantly the heart of myth, story, and metaphor. It is one I refer to again and again to review the cultural values embedded in each story shared. The myths are what souls are made of and I know all who read it will be enthralled. [JM]

Campbell, J. (1993). *Myths to live by.* New York: Arkana.

   Joseph Campbell's work touched and influenced me while I was exploring the use of metaphors in cross-cultural counseling. The universality of myths and their meaning spoke to me when I first discovered this book and has continued to guide my work ever since. His amazing knowledge of myths has awakened my hunger and interest in hearing stories and metaphors forever more. [AE]

Chodron, P. (1997). *When things fall apart: Heart advice for difficult times.* Boston: Shambala.

   This book is full of Buddhist wisdom, including stories that can be readily applied to difficulty in accepting thoughts, emotions, and situations. [LF]

Coelho, P. (1988). *The alchemist: A fable about following your dream.* San Francisco, CA: HarperCollins.

   This a story of a journey in which a boy learns that "fear of suffering is worse than the suffering itself." [LF]

Eifert, G. H., & Forsyth, J. P. (2005). *Acceptance and commitment therapy for anxiety disorders: A practitioner's treatment guide to using mindfulness, acceptance, and values-based behavior change strategies.* Oakland, CA: New Harbinger.

   I consult this book frequently for appropriate metaphors for clients with sleep disorders. [LF]

Estes, C. P. (1992). *Women who run with the wolves.* New York: Ballantine Books.

   This collection of myths and stories of the wild woman archetype is a deeply spiritual book, honoring what is tough, smart, and untamed in us all. This volume reiterates that the soul is still wild, and the recovery of that vitality will set us right in the world. I like the story where the wise woman collects the far-flung bones of the wild creature and sings over the reassembled pieces until the spirit can return and transformation is complete. [CH-L]

   This book is like a rich box of chocolates. You read one story at a time and digest the delicious soul healing messages. It is one that remains by my bedside and a must for all training. If you want to truly know the heart of storytelling, read this book. [JM]

Freedman, J., Epston, D., & Lobovits, D. (1997). *Playful approaches to serious problems: Narrative therapy with children and their families.* New York: Norton.

   Stories seem to me one of the most natural tools in working with children and families. This book has absorbed and encouraged me to use stories and metaphors with refugee children and their parents in somewhat different ways than the cultural-based stories and metaphors I tend to work with. I enjoyed reading the stories in the chapters and see the book as a valuable source of guidance in family work. [AE]

   What a beautiful book on how to work and communicate with children. The case vignettes and case stories guide the reader in understanding how we as therapists can utilize the words, stories, pictures, and thoughts of our clients to cocreate hope. Moreover, this book has taught me to find ways of communicating with my clients, through collaborative narrative play. A must have if you are conversing with children in your practice! [JN]

Friedman, E. (1990). *Friedman's fables.* New York: Guilford Press.

   In this delightfully engaging book, Edwin Friedman reveals inspiring use of stories to promote change in seemingly impossible situations. Flowers that wilt because they don't appreciate their own beauty, birds that refuse to fly "just because their parents want them to," scavenger fish that stop "taking crap," and 21 other tales are presented in ways relevant to physical and spiritual healing, teaching, marriage, and child rearing. [WR & JS]

Haley, J. (1973). *Uncommon therapy.* New York: Norton.

>   *Categorized according to the stages of development all individuals traverse in the life cycle, these stories of Erickson's healing encounters created a paradigm shift for me in living and practicing therapy. I never get tired of repeating these same stories and enjoy the jolt of their impact on all who hear them.* [CH-L]

Hammond, D. C. (1990). *Handbook of hypnotic suggestions and metaphors.* New York: Norton.

>   *It looks like a dictionary and sometimes gives the idea that metaphor is like a prescription, but it covers a big range of problems and is easily accessible. If you look at it as a box of painting tubes, it might be helpful for creating your own mixture of colors.* [TGS]

Hayes, S. C., Strosahl, K. D., & Wilson, K. G. (1999). *Acceptance and commitment therapy: An experiential approach to behavior change.* New York: Guilford Press.

>   *The ACT book introduced me to using metaphors with clients. In addition to providing a rationale for treatment, it includes several metaphors that can be used to illuminate the psychological processes functioning for the client. Throughout the book, the authors encourage clinicians to use and generate metaphors creatively and spontaneously with clients.* [MH]

Hurnard, H. (1993). *Hinds' feet in high places: The beloved story of Much-Afraid and her exciting journey to the high places.* Wheaton, IL: Tyndale House.

>   *Based on the Song of Solomon, this allegory is a story of Christian faith, where the main character, Much-Afraid, takes a spiritual journey through difficult places. With the help of her companions, Sorrow and Suffering, she is able to reach the high places and commune with the loving Shepherd she has been seeking. Although this story was not explicitly intended for use within clinical settings, it provides a nice tale of how the acceptance of personal trials can be an aid in the pursuit of valued life directions.* [MH]

Kane, S., & Olness, K. (Eds.). (2004). *The art of therapeutic communication: The therapeutic works of Kay F. Thompson.* Carmarthen, UK: Crown House.

>   *Kay Thompson was a masterful hypnotherapist with an elegant ability to integrate metaphor and multilevel suggestion into therapeutic communication. This tribute seeks to capture the essence of what Thompson so skillfully demonstrated through her professional work.* [REK]

>   *Jump into Thompson's altered state vehicle, shift into drive, and cruise down the mindway as she provides numerous examples of word play, metaphor language development, and actual metaphors from her vast repertoire of knowledge. This book demonstrated to me the depth of enjoyment that work play can bring to the listener and gave me the confidence to use my own unique ideas.* [GS]

Kopp, R. R. (1995). *Metaphor therapy: Using client-generated metaphors in psychotherapy.* New York: Brunner/Mazel.

>   *The paradigmatic shift in Kopp's work from therapist-generated to client-generated metaphors was like that light bulb going off in my head in terms of discovering a way of using metaphors that really made sense in a therapeutic setting. His work also inspired me to put together my way of working, which I call "guided metaphor," and which is based on the client's own life stories.* [RB]

>   *This book inspired my excitement and current bias towards noticing and exploring the client's own metaphoric language to bring about therapeutic change. The author provided me with an initial methodological framework for utilizing and transforming metaphoric imagery, and I now frequently work with client-generated metaphors in my counseling practice.* [CP]

Kopp, S. (1972). *If you meet the Buddha on the road, kill Him: The pilgrimage of psychotherapy patients.* New York: Bantam Books.

One of the first psychotherapy books I ever read. Sheldon Kopp uses tales and metaphors to teach us that we all have our own Buddhahood! This book consistently reminds me that we are our own experts in the journey of our lives. No one else is or can ever be. If we can hold on to that thought and see our clients as their own Buddhas, then and only then can we be successful and respectful in our conversations with our clients! [JN]

Kotzé, E., & Morkel, E. (2002). *Matchboxes, butterflies and angry foots*. Pretoria, South Africa: Ethics Alive.

This is a remarkable book, with remarkable stories from remarkable children. This book is a reminder of the difficulties that children face in their lives, which shows us as adults, parents, educators, and therapists that children have an amazing inner strength that no problem can extinguish. This book gives us wonderful insight into how children solve problems through telling stories and using metaphors to heal and grow. [JN]

Krakauer, J. (1997). *Into thin air*. New York: Anchor.

In 1996, 15 climbers died in the worst disaster of Everest mountaineering. This book tells of the passion and struggle to reach a goal, of facing situations outside our control, of death and survival, of guilt and selflessness, and of heroic companionship. Such real life accounts of how people deal with overwhelming adversity can metaphorically provide both inspiration and means for others facing their own challenges. [GB]

Lakoff, G., & Johnson, M. (1980). *Metaphors we live by*. Chicago: University of Chicago Press.

This book changed the way I view metaphor. The authors, a philosopher and a linguist, show how we construct our reality metaphorically and how metaphor organizes our thoughts and actions. [RK]

Lankton, S. R., & Lankton, C. (1983). *The answer within: A clinical framework of Ericksonian hypnotherapy*. New York: Brunner/Mazel.

Their systematic approach to the use of metaphor opened my eyes to the possibilities of conscious design in metaphor usage rather than "simple" storytelling. [RB]

This book was my first experience with therapeutic metaphor. In this classic, the Lanktons show how a metaphor can be built brick by brick to utilize the multiple dimensions of client experience to affect therapeutic outcomes. The multiple embedded metaphor approach expanded my worldview to new possibilities. [GS]

Oliver, M. (2000). *The leaf and the cloud*. New York: Da Capo Press.

This poem speaks of questioning and discovery, about what is observable and what is not, about what passes and what persists. Oliver communicates the beauty she finds in the world and makes it unforgettable. I feel as if I am perceiving with brand new, reawakened senses when I return to the all-is-sacred world she eloquently describes. [CH-L]

Rubaiyat of Omar Khayyam.

This piece of literature comes to us from Persia, where it was written 1600 years ago. Through varied translations it integrates numerous and beautiful metaphors into its poetry, which tells a long story filled with intriguing characters of that epoch. The combination of art and elements that we cannot possibly understand speak to me of the richness within each of us. [REK]

Remen, R. N. (1996). *Kitchen table wisdom: Stories that heal*. New York: RiverheadBooks.

Remen's work added a dimension of compassion and humanity to metaphor that took it out of the realm of "intervention" into the realm of one person connecting with another on the most basic level—two human beings journeying through this life. I still read her books with a sense of awe. [RB]

This collection of stories helped me realize that every person is a story; it's when we share our own experiences and listen to each other's stories that we begin to know who we are and where we belong. The author gave me a renewed appreciation for the stories we shared around the kitchen table when I was a child – a source of enduring wisdom and entertainment. [CP]

Reps, P., & Senzaki, N. (1998). *Zen flesh, Zen bones.* New York: Tuttle.
> *Zen stories can be overdone in therapy, but when timed correctly there are none better for clinical purposes.* [SH]
> *Another favorite, these short, pithy tales speak of the unexpected and the obvious, expanding appreciation and options in the reader's life.* [RM]

Rosen, S. (1982). *My voice will go with you: The teaching tales of Milton H. Erickson.* New York: Norton.
> *This is my very favorite metaphor book. Erickson's teaching tales are everyday, dramatic, and light-hearted—an engaging combination.* [RM]
> *Rosen wrote down many of the stories that Dad liked to tell over and over. He told the stories to students, to colleagues, and to his family. As he repeated stories, he emphasized different messages. I like this book because it is so familiar and because I find new meaning each time I listen to his voice.* [REK]
> *Rosen's well-organized compilation achieves several goals. First, it makes it easy to find metaphor ideas, second, the selection allows the reader to have fun and interest, third, it is perfect to give to clients as a reading book, and finally, it provides an understanding of Erickson's use of metaphors in psychotherapy. I have included this book in our training courses from the beginning.* [TGS]
> *A priceless collection of the teaching tales of Milton Erickson, the definitive master of healing through the use of metaphor. Presented in useful categories such as "Changing the Unconscious Mind," "Motivating Tales," "Trust the Unconscious," and "Observe: Notice Distinctions," stories and examples from Erickson invite readers to trust the abilities and experiences of clients, and their own.* [WR & JS]

Silverstein, S. (1976). *The missing piece.* New York: Harper & Row.
> *This classic, pictorial metaphor for all ages is about being stuck and needing to change. Written by one of children's favorite poets, this seemingly simple story inspired me to use simple and humorous metaphors to initiate and motivate change in people who sought my help.* [JL]

Silverstein, S. (1981). *The missing piece meets the big O.* New York: Harper & Row.
> *A sequel to the previous title, this book continues the metaphor with the message that everyone has to do his or her own work to change. It is one I share a great deal with my clients to underline any metaphorical work we may be doing together.* [JL]

Steinberg, F. E., & Whiteside, R. G. (2006). *Becoming dragon.* Auckland, New Zealand: Phac.
> *Written for therapists rather than clients, this beautiful parable inspiringly shows the way out of professional burnout with guiding characters who represent different aspects of the good therapist. However, it is much more. Study the processes by which these skillful therapist/writers conceptualize, construct, and tell their tale, and you will know all you need to know about effective therapeutic storytelling.* [GB]

Stewart, I., Barnes-Holmes, D., Hayes, S. C., & Lipkens, R. (2001). Relations among relations: Analogies, metaphors, and short stories. In S. C. Hayes, D. Barnes-Holmes, & B. Roche (Eds.), *Relational frame theory: A post-Skinnerian account of human language and cognition* (pp. 73–86). New York: Kluwer Academic/Plenum.
> *This chapter presents a basic analysis of human language and cognition that explains why the clinical use of metaphors is important and potent. By explicating to the verbal relations among events, relational frame theory explains how the functions of these events can also be translated from one thing to another, as with the use of metaphor.* [MH]

The Bible.

    The stories in the Old and New Testaments are rich sources of clinical metaphors. Many people have been exposed to these stories, and they have deep resonance. It is important to know your client, however, since any stories that come from a religious tradition can disturb some clients even when used in a secular context. [SH]

Thomson, L. (2005). *Harry the hypno-potamus: Metaphorical tales for the treatment of children.* Norwalk, CT: Crown House.

    This book is tremendously useful when you need a good story to address such problems as anxiety, enuresis, encopresis, pain management, or chronic illnesses in children. Children can easily identify with the animal characters and can utilize the strategies the animals develop with Harry and Dr. Dan's help. While fairy tales teach social solutions, these stories are practical for the myriad of medical situations that children face. [JL]

Wallas, L. (1985). *Stories for the third ear: Using hypnotic fables in psychotherapy.* New York: Norton.

    Underscoring the vital importance of basic premises of establishing rapport, understanding and utilizing the client's story, language, frame of reference, and pacing before leading, Lee Wallas clearly discusses the nature of the multiple levels of experience and understanding that are so intimately a part of human behavior. Even those readers who do not use formal hypnotic techniques will be inspired by these engaging stories for the third ear. [WR & JS]

Index